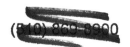
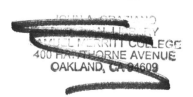

D1556263

2/9/2003

Oxford Medical Publications

The muscular dystrophies

The muscular dystrophies

Edited by

Alan E.H. Emery,

Department of Neurology,
Royal Devon & Exeter Hospital,
Exeter, U.K.

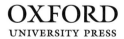

OXFORD

UNIVERSITY PRESS

Great Clarendon Street, Oxford OX2 6DP

Oxford University Press is a department of the University of Oxford.
It furthers the University's objective of excellence in research, scholarship,
and education by publishing worldwide in

Oxford New York

Athens Auckland Bangkok Bogotá Buenos Aires Cape Town
Chennai Dar es Salaam Delhi Florence Hong Kong Istanbul Karachi
Kolkata Kuala Lumpur Madrid Melbourne Mexico City Mumbai Nairobi
Paris São Paulo Shanghai Singapore Taipei Tokyo Toronto Warsaw
with associated companies in Berlin Ibadan

Oxford is a registered trade mark of Oxford University Press
in the UK and in certain other countries

Published in the United States
by Oxford University Press Inc., New York

British Library Cataloguing in Publication Data
Data available

Library of Congress Cataloging in Publication Data
Data available

ISBN 0–19–263291–4

10 9 8 7 6 5 4 3 2 1

Typeset by Newgen Imaging Systems (P) Ltd., Chennai, India
Printed in Great Britain
on acid-free paper by T. J. International Ltd, Padstow

DEDICATED TO KIICHI ARAHATA

1946–2000

Contents

Preface ix
Contributors xi

1 Muscular dystrophy – an evolving concept   *1*
   Alan E. H. Emery

2 Congenital muscular dystrophies   *10*
   Eugenio Mercuri and Francesco Muntoni

3 Fukuyama congenital muscular dystrophy   *39*
   Kayoko Saito and Makio Kobayashi

4 Duchenne muscular dystrophy or Meryon's disease   *55*
   Alan E. H. Emery

5 Becker muscular dystrophy   *72*
   Marianne de Visser and Edo M. Hoogerwaard

6 Emery – Dreifuss muscular dystrophy   *95*
   Daniela Toniolo

7 The limb-girdle muscular dystrophies   *109*
   Katharine M. D. Bushby

8 Facioscapulohumeral muscular dystrophy   *137*
   Meena Upadhyaya and David N. Cooper

9 Distal muscular dystrophy   *173*
   Bjarne Udd and Hannu Somer

10 Oculopharyngeal muscular dystrophy: the muscular dystrophies   *189*
   Bernard Brais and Fernando M. S. Tomé

11 Dilated cardiomyopathy and related cardiac disorders in
   muscular dystrophy   *202*
   J. Andoni Urtizberea, Denis Duboc, Ketty Schwartz, and Gisèle Bonne

12 Medical management and treatment of muscular dystrophy   *223*
   Adnan Y. Manzur

13 Respiratory care in muscular dystrophy   *247*
   Anita K. Simonds

14 Gene and cell therapy for primary myopathies   *261*
Giulio Cossu and Paula R. Clemens

15 Surgical management of muscular dystrophy   *284*
Luciano Merlini and Jürgen Forst

16 Animal models of muscular dystrophy   *297*
Satoru Noguchi and Yukiko K. Hayashi

Index   310

Preface

The muscular dystrophies are an important group of inherited disorders. They are all characterized by muscle wasting and weakness but vary considerably in their clinical manifestations and severity. Based on the distribution of muscle involvement coupled with muscle protein and molecular genetic studies over 30 different types are now recognized. The aim of this text is to review the current state of out knowledge of these diseases.

Inevitably, there is some variation in the different approaches to these diseases which reflects the present state of our knowledge. For example, in the case of congenital muscular dystrophy, current emphasis is centred on defining the various clinical phenotypes and when so defined, searching for the responsible genes. In the case of facioscapulohumeral muscular dystrophy, though the responsible gene locus appears to have been located, the function of the particular gene (or genes) responsible is not yet clear. In this disorder the authors explain the various approaches being pursued to define the molecular basis for this intriguing disease. Myotonic dystrophy has been excluded from the discussions because it clearly stands alone among muscle diseases with its very distinctive and unique clinical presentation and multisystem involvement.

Following the identification in 1987 that dystrophin was the protein defective in Duchenne and Becker muscular dystrophies and which then proved to be localized to the sarcolemma, it seemed that the resultant disruption of the muscle membrane would provide a plausible explanation for the phenotype in muscular dystrophy. This idea gained additional credence as some other forms of dystrophy, such as congenital dystrophy and certain types of limb girdle dystrophy, also proved to be due to defects in other muscle-membrane associated proteins. But this idea now seems to be an oversimplification as defects in sarcomeric and even myonuclear membrane proteins have now been identified as the basic defects in certain dystrophies. But whatever the basis of these disorders their prevention as well as management and treatment remain preeminently important and these matters are addressed by several contributors.

One of the most important contributors to this volume was to have been Kiichi Arahata, who unfortunately died prematurely during its preparation. This book is dedicated to his memory. He contributed so much to the study of muscle diseases and his early death has robbed the medical and scientific community of a valued researcher.

Kiichi had a love of Japanese Haiku poetry which (in English translation) I too shared. Some months before his death he sent me this one which he had just written and which he entitled 'Spring'

In the early Spring
A sprinkle of rain has passed
Natural primroses in a group.

This seems in some ways a fitting tribute to a close and dear friend.

Exeter AEHE
Spring 2001

Contributors

Gisèle Bonne, INSERM U 523 Institut de Myologie, Bâtiment Joseph Babinski, Groupe Hospitalier Pitié-Salpêtrière, 47 boulevard de l'Hôpital, 75651 Paris Cedex 13, France

Bernard Brais, Hôpital Notre-Dame-CHUM, 1560 rue Sherbrooke Est, Montreal, Quebec H2L 4M1, Canada

Katharine M.D. Bushby, University of Newcastle upon Tyne, Department of Human Genetics, 19/20 Claremont Place, Newcastle upon Tyne NE2 4AA

Paula R. Clemens, Department of Neurology, Rm S-515 Biomedical Science Tower South, University of Pittsburgh, Pittsburgh PA 15213, USA

David Cooper, Institute of Medical Genetics, University of Wales College of Medicine, Health Park, Cardiff CF14 4XN

Giulio Cossu, Neurology Service, Pittsburgh Veterans Administration, Medical Centre & Department of Neurology, University of Pittsburgh, Pittsburgh PA, USA

Marianne de Visser, Academic Medical Centre (AMC), Department of Neurolgy H2-216, Meibergdreef 9, 1105 AZ Amsterdam, The Netherlands

Denis Duboc, Service de Cardiologie, Groupe Hospitalier Cochin-St Vincent de Paul, Bd de Port Royal, 75014 Paris, France

Alan E.H. Emery, Department of Neurology, Royal Devon and Exeter Hospital, Exeter EX2 5DW, UK

Jürgen Forst, Orthopaedic Clinic, University Erlangen-Nürngerg, Rathsbergerstr 57, D-91054 Erlangen, Germany

Yukiko Hayashi, Department of Neuromuscular Research, National Institute of Neuroscience, NCNP, 4-1-1 Ogawa-Higashi, Kodaira, Tokyo 187-8502, Japan

Edo M. Hoogerwaard, Academic Medical Centre (AMC), Department of Neurology H2-216, Meibergdreef 9, 1105 AZ Amsterdam, The Netherlands

Makio Kobayashi, Department of Pathology, Tokyo Women's Medical University, School of Medicine, Tokyo, Japan

Adnan Y. Manzur, Dubowitz Neuromuscular Centre, Department of Paediatrics, Hammersmith Hospital, Du Cane Road, London W12 0NN

Eugenio Mercuri, The Dubowitz Neuromuscular Centre, Department of Paediatrics & Neonatal Medicine, Hammersmith Hospital, Du Cane Road, London W12 0NN

Luciano Merlini, Istituto Ortopedico Rizzoli, Neuromuscular Laboratory, Via Pupilli 1, 40136 Bologna, Italy

Francesco Muntoni, The Dubowitz Neuromuscular Centre, Department of Paediatrics & Neonatal Medicine, Hammersmith Hospital, Du Cane Road, London W12 0NN

Satoru Noguchi, Department of Neuromuscular Research, National Institute of Neuroscience, NCNP, 4-1-1 Ogawa-Higashi, Kodaira, Tokyo 187-8502, Japan

Kayoko Saito, Department of Paediatrics, Tokyo Women's Medical University, School of Medicine, 8-1 Kawada-cho, Shinjuku-ku, Tokyo 162-8666, Japan

Ketty Schwartz, INSERM U 523, Institut de Myologie, Hôspital Pitié-Salpêtrière, 47 boulevard de l'Hôpital, 75651 Paris Cedex 13, France

Anita K. Simonds, Consultant in Respiratory Medicine, Royal Brompton & Harefield NHS Trust, Sydney Street, London SW3 6NP

Hannu Somer, Helsinki University Central Hospital, Department of Neurology, PO Box 340, Haartmaninkatu 4, FIN-00290 Helsinki, Finland

Fernando M.S. Tomé, INSERM U153, Institut de Myologie, Bâtiment Babinski, 47 boulevard de l'Hôpital, 75651 Paris Cedex 13, France

Daniela Toniolo, Institute of Genetics, Biochemistry & Evolution, CNR, Via Abbiategrasso 207, 27100 Pavia, Italy

Bjarne Udd, Department of Neurology, Vaasa Central Hospital, Vaasa 65130, Finland

Meena Upadhyaya, Institute of Medical Genetics, University of Wales College of Medicine, Heath Park, Cardiff CF14 4XN

J Andoni Urtizberea, INSERM U153, Institut de Myologie, Bâtiment Babinski, 47 boulevard de l' Hôpital, 75651 Paris Cedex 13, France

Chapter 1

Muscular dystrophy – an evolving concept

Alan E.H. Emery

Introduction

Muscular dystrophy is one of the fastest growing fields in medicine, at both the clinical and laboratory level. Over the last 50 years or so, many important innovations in medical science have actually been initiated in studies of muscular dystrophy (Emery and Emery 1995). For example, the first application in medicine of discriminant function statistical analysis was in the 1950s for resolving clinical and genetic heterogeneity in these diseases. A little later the first application of Bayseian statistics was in risk calculations in muscular dystrophy, a statistical method subsequently applied in genetic counselling in general as well as in many other branches of medicine and science. In the early 1980s, Duchenne muscular dystrophy (DMD) was the very first inherited disorder in which the causative gene was located by linkage to a DNA marker (a restriction fragment length polymorphism). In 1987 it was also the first inherited disorder in which the defective protein was identified by the revolutionary technique of reverse genetics or, more precisely, positional cloning. This technique has subsequently been applied with great success to other forms of dystrophy as well as to many other genetic disorders.

Knowing the protein defect in a particular dystrophy has led to the application of immunohistochemistry and Western blot analysis in diagnosis. Furthermore, knowing the molecular genetic defect in a disorder provides not only a precise diagnosis to be made in an individual case, but also opens up the possibility of prenatal diagnosis.

Protein defects

So far over 30 different forms of muscular dystrophy have been identified of which no less than half have been classified as limb girdle types of dystrophy (LGMD). In some dystrophies the genetic defect has been found to affect one of the muscle membrane-associated proteins such as dystrophin, laminin α-2 chain (merosin), various sarcoglycans, caveolin-3 and dysferlin. Here, the absence of these proteins in particular dystrophies with resultant disruption of the muscle membrane provides a plausible explanation for the phenotype. But there are several notable exceptions. For example in oculopharyngeal muscular dystrophy the defective protein is retained within the nucleus itself (triplet expanded poly-A binding protein). In some other dystrophies the defective protein is localized to the sarcoplasm and myonuclei (calpain-3 in LGMD 2A) or appears to be exclusively sarcomeric (myotilin in LGMD 1A, telethonin in LGMD 2G). Finally in Emery–Dreifuss muscular dystrophy (EDMD) the protein defects in the X-linked and autosomal dominant forms reside in the nuclear membrane (Table 1.1). Clearly, the underlying pathogenesis must be different in these various dystrophies, though in order to account for all these diseases having at least some degree of muscle weakness, they must presumably share some common final pathway (Emery 1998). However, the nature of this common final pathway is not yet clear. Perturbation of the dystrophin-glycoprotein complex (which includes dystrophin and the sarcoglycans) leads to disruption of the linkage between the extracellular matrix and the cytoskeleton (Cohn and Campbell 2000a). The idea that such perturbations would help to explain muscle weakness in those dystrophies associated with defects in proteins of this complex is attractive. But the clinical features of other dystrophies are not so easily explained. The possible role of apoptosis (Morris 2000) and neuronal nitric oxide synthase or n NOS (Sander *et al.* 2000) are currently attracting attention in attempts to understand the pathogenesis of these disorders. Recent developments in the fields of structural genomics and proteomics may well prove helpful in this regard.

Table 1.1 Disease associated proteins in various muscular dystrophies (Fukutin, the protein responsible for Fukuyama congenital dystrophy, has not yet been precisely localized)

Muscle membrane (sarcolemma & extracellular matrix)
    Dystrophin
    Laminin α 2 chain (merosin)
    α 7 Integrin
    Dysferlin
    Caveolin-3
    Sarcoglycans

Sarcomeric
    Telethonin
    Myotilin

Cytosol (muscle enzyme)
    Calpain-3

Nuclear inclusions
    Poly-A binding protein

Nuclear membrane
    Emerin
    Lamin A/C

Table 1.2 Some muscle proteins not yet associated with any specific neuromuscular disorders

Muscle membrane associated
  Rapsyn
  Sarcospan
  ε- sarcoglycan
  Dystroglycans (α and β)
  Syntrophins (α and β)
  Dystrobrevin
  Utrophin
  Biglycan

Muscle and nuclear membrane associated
  Myoferlin

Cytoplasmic
  Melusin

Studies of muscle proteins have not only revealed specific defects in various forms of muscular dystrophy, but have also led to the discovery of many other proteins which so far have not yet been associated with any specific neuromuscular disorders in humans (Table 1.2). However, studies of transgenic mice suggest that a complete absence of dystroglycan for example, may be lethal *in utero*.

Definition of dystrophy

In the classical study of Walton and Nattrass (1954), the dystrophies were defined as inherited, primary diseases of muscle characterized by progressive muscle wasting and weakness in which the muscle histology revealed muscle fibre degeneration and necrosis and later invasion by connective tissue and fat. But as more clinically distinct types of dystrophy have been recognized and their molecular genetic and protein defects identified, this simple definition is no longer tenable.

Clinical variability

Some disorders are severe and progressive while others are not. For example, DMD begins in early childhood and is relentlessly progressive, whereas some cases of Becker muscular dystrophy may not present until mid-life and be relatively slowly progressive. In fact, mutations which retain the open reading frame and are related to the central rod region of the dystrophin protein may only result in muscle cramps in old age. Furthermore, some mutations of this gene can result in a cardiomyopathy with very mild muscle weakness or with no weakness at all. Predicting the likely outcome in an individual case is becoming clearer in all dystrophies as we learn more of genotype-phenotype correlations.

Genetic heterogeneity

The complexity of the situation is exemplified in the case of the *LMNA* gene which encodes lamins A and C of the nuclear lamina, a fibrous meshwork underlying the inner nuclear membrane. At first it was thought that certain phenotypes could be related to specific functional domains of the gene (Fatkin *et al.* 1999). But this has proved to be an oversimplification. In fact, mutations in different exons of the gene result in a whole variety of clinical conditions ranging from normality to autosomal dominant or autosomal recessive EDMD, LGMD 1B, dilated cardiomyopathy and conduction defects, and even Dunnigan partial lipodystrophy (Table 1.3).

Furthermore, the *same* mutation of the *LMNA* gene within a family may result in different phenotypes. For example, families of EDMD have been described in which some individuals have the complete phenotype but others may only develop the cardiomyopathy (Bonne *et al.* 2000; Canki-Klain *et al.* 2000). And families have also been reported in which an identical mutation of the dysferlin gene is associated with LGMD 2B in some individuals but with Miyoshi type distal muscular dystrophy in other family members (Weiler *et al.* 1999). Such intra-familial variability must result from the effects of other, as yet unidentified, modifier genes segregating in these families. The role of particular SNPs (Single Nucleotide Polymorphisms) in this regard has yet to be evaluated, but it is an intriguing possibility that this could provide the molecular basis for at least some of this intra-familial variability.

Cardiac involvement

The discovery of the molecular basis of a particular type of muscular dystrophy has often then resulted in further gene studies revealing an extension of the associated phenotype. Many forms of muscular dystrophy for example have now been found to be

Table 1.3 Distribution of mutations in the *LMNA* gene producing autosomal dominant (AD) or autosomal recessive (AR) Emery–Dreifuss muscular dystrophy (EDMD), limb girdle muscular dystrophy 1B (LGMD 1B), dilated cardiomyopathy and conduction defects (DCM & CD) and Dunnigan-type partial lipodystrophy (PLD)

	Exons											
	1	2	3	4	5	6	7	8	9	10	11	12
AD EDMD	+			+	+	+	+	+	+			
AR EDMD												
Affected homozygote				+								
Symptomless heterozygote				+								
LGMD 1B			+			+			+			
DCM + CD	+		+			+				+		
PLD								+			+	

Table 1.4 Gene mutations associated with dilated cardiomyopathy (DCM) in certain dystrophies and myopathies. This list is not exhaustive because DCM has also been reported in rare, isolated cases of other inherited disorders

Gene locus	Protein defect	Disorder
1q	* Lamin A/C	AD DCM
		LGMD 1B
		AD EDMD
2q	* Desmin	AD DCM
6p	* Desmoplakin	AR DCM + keratoderma
15q	Actin	AD DCM
—	α–δ Sarcoglycans	LGMD 2 C–F
Xq28	* Emerin	XR EDMD
Xq28	'Tafazzin'	Barth syndrome
Xp21	Dystrophin	XR DCM
		DMD
		BMD

* = conduction defect also.

associated with a cardiomyopathy which in some cases is associated with a conduction defect. Roughly 30 per cent of cases of dilated cardiomyopathy are inherited and then often associated with various dystrophies and myopathies (Table 1.4). In fact in many cases the associated cardiomyopathy can be the predominant feature rather than muscle weakness. At least in certain sarcoglycanopathies, perturbations of the microvascular smooth muscle in the heart, as well as disruption of cardiac muscle membrane proteins, may play an important role in the pathogenesis of dilated cardiomyopathy (Cohn and Campbell 2000b).

Muscle histology

The single unifying feature of the dystrophies was previously considered to be their muscle histology. But here again as studies have extended beyond DMD it has become clear that there are no *specific* diagnostic features that are common to all forms of dystrophy. Some of the variations in histology are illustrated in Fig. 1.1. For example, in some of the more severe forms of dystrophy, such as DMD, the earliest findings can be little more than variation in fibre size and fibre splitting, but later in the course of the disease fibre necrosis and invasion by macrophages becomes evident and finally the tissue is replaced by connective tissue and fat. But in facioscapulohumeral dystrophy and dysferlin deficiency, invasion of the tissue by mononuclear cells ("inflammatory" changes) is often found. In fact in dysferlin deficiency the occurrence of "inflammatory" change and the associated very high SCK levels may lead to confusion with polymyositis. In oculopharyngeal muscular dystrophy rimmed vacuoles and nuclear inclusion bodies are typical and in distal muscular dystrophy rimmed vacuoles are also a frequent finding though often, as in mild cases of other dystrophies, the only finding may be some variation in fibre size.

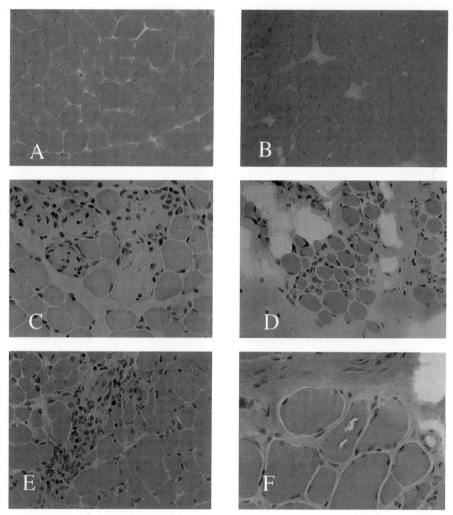

Fig. 1.1 Some of the variations in muscle histology observed in different types of dystrophy (A, normal; B, fibre splitting and internal nuclei; C, necrosis and phagocytosis; D, variations in fibre size; E, 'inflammatory' changes; F, rimmed vacuoles). (Haematoxylin & eosin stain). Reproduced by kind permission of Dr. Caroline Sewry. Please see four colour plate section between pages 20 and 21.

Muscle proteins and acquired diseases

Certain muscle proteins now known to be defective in certain dystrophies seem likely to be targets for damage caused by various micro-organisms in infectious diseases. In fact several recent reports indicate that this may well help provide molecular explanations for the clinical features of some of these diseases. For example, the enteroviral protease 2A of the Coxsackievirus B3 has been shown to specifically cleave cardiac muscle dystrophin and this would explain the cardiomyopathy resulting from such infections (Badorff *et al.* 1999; Lee *et al.* 2000). Other viruses, such as adenovirus and human immunodeficiency virus also cleave various muscle proteins (actin, desmin, myosin, tropomyosin) which could therefore account for some of the clinical effects of infections by these viruses.

Infectious agents may also produce disease through mechanisms not directly involving muscle proteins yet are known to be the basis of certain dystrophies. For example, poly(A)-binding protein II (PAB II) is responsible for polyadenylation of mRNA. In oculopharyngeal muscular dystrophy, mutant PAB II results in *lengthening* of the mRNA poly(A) tail which is subsequently sequestrated in the nucleus, forming intranuclear inclusions. Interestingly influenza A virus NS 1 protein inhibits the same protein (PAB II) which then results in the generation of pre-mRNAs having only *short* poly(A) tails (Fig. 1.2), which are also not exported from the nucleus (Chen *et al.* 1999). Clearly poly(A) tails must be of the correct length to ensure their export from the nucleus. Some other examples are given in Table 1.5. The pathogenicity of acquired infections is complex and often involves many proteins other than those listed (Donnenberg 2000). Nevertheless our understanding of the molecular basis of the dystrophies may perhaps

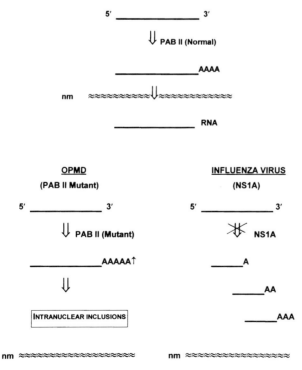

POLYADENYLATION OF mRNA

(PAB II + PAP + CPSF + CFI + C$_{St}$F)

5' ——————— 3'

⇓ PAB II (Normal)

——————AAAA

nm ≈≈≈≈≈≈≈≈⇓≈≈≈≈≈≈≈≈≈

——————— RNA

OPMD
(PAB II Mutant)

5' ——————— 3'

⇓ PAB II (Mutant)

——————AAAAA↑

⇓⇓

INTRANUCLEAR INCLUSIONS

nm ≈≈≈≈≈≈≈≈≈≈≈≈≈≈≈≈

INFLUENZA VIRUS
(NS1A)

5' ——————— 3'

✳ NS1A

———A

———AA

———AAA

nm ≈≈≈≈≈≈≈≈≈≈≈≈≈≈≈≈

Fig. 1.2 Poly(A)-binding protein II (PAB II) along with several other factors (PAP, CPSF, CFI, C$_{St}$F) is responsible for the synthesis and processing of pre-mRNA poly(A) tails. In oculopharyngeal muscular dystrophy (OPMD) mutant PAB II results in lengthening of poly(A) tails; influenza A virus NS1 protein (NS1A protein) inhibits PAB II resulting in short poly(A) tails. (nm, nuclear membrane).

Table 1.5 Involvement of certain muscle proteins in the pathogenicity of some acquired infections

Protein	Infection	Action	Result
Dystrophin (& Sarcoglycans)	Coxsackie B3	Protease 2A	DCM
PAB 2	Influenza A	NS1 (blocks host metab)	Virulence, DCM/myositis
Cardiac myosin	Haemolytic streptococcus	Antibodies	Carditis
Cardiac laminins			Valvular disease
Laminin α 2 (G domain)	Mycobacterium leprae	Receptor in peripheral nerves	Neuropathy
Laminin α 2	Parvovirus B19	?Receptor	DCM
Actin cytoskeleton	Yersinia Sp	Protein kinase	Disrupts cytoskeleton & inhibits phagocytosis
	Clostridial Sp	Various	"
	Pasteurella Haemolytica	Polymerization	Toxicity
	Candida Albicans	Attachment	Cell disruption
	Various bacteria	Uptake/binding	Virulence

contribute to our understanding of the molecular pathology underlying diseases produced by various infectious agents. It is also just possible that (subclinical) infections by such agents may in some instances contribute to clinical variability observed in certain dystrophies.

Conclusions

Early studies, which were largely concerned with DMD led to a definition of muscular dystrophy which is no longer tenable. A great variety of genetically distinct conditions are now included under this rubric which vary considerably in their clinical features, muscle histology, molecular genetic and protein defects. Unless some unifying biochemical feature is found which is shared by all the dystrophies, which seems unlikely on present evidence, then the only features common to these disorders can be summarized as follows. Firstly, inherited conditions characterized by some degree of muscle weakness which is not of neurogenic origin. Secondly, associated with specific defects in proteins normally expressed at least in skeletal muscle tissue. Finally, by exclusion, mitochondrial myopathies and other myopathies associated with well-recognized histological abnormalities such as central cores or nemaline rods. But definitions which depend on exclusion criteria may not always be easy to sustain. The best solution would therefore be to use a nomenclature based on their specific protein defects such as dystrophinopathies, sarcoglycanopathies, merosinopathies and laminopathies. However, for the sake of tradition the currently accepted term "muscular dystrophy" will be retained in the present text.

References

Badorff, C., Lee, G., Lamphear, B.J. and Martone, M.E. *et al.* (1999). Enteroviral protease 2A cleaves dystrophin: evidence of cytoskeletal disruption in an acquired cardiomyopathy. *Nature Medicine*, **5**, 320–26.

Bonne, G., Mercuri, E., Muchir, A., Urtizberea, A., Bécane, H.M., Recan, D. *et al.* (2000). Clinical and molecular genetic spectrum of autosomal dominant Emery–Dreifuss muscular dystrophy due to mutations of the lamin A/C gene. *Annals of Neurology*, **48**, 170–80.

Canki-Klain, N., Recan, D., Milicic, D., Llense, S., Leturcq, F., Deburgrave, N. *et al.* (2000). Clinical variability and molecular diagnosis in a four-generation family with X-linked Emery–Dreifuss muscular dystrophy. *Croatian Medical Journal*, **41**, 389–95.

Chen, Z., Li, Y. and Krug, R.M. (1999). Influenza A virus NS 1 protein targets poly(A)-binding protein II of the cellular 3′-end processing machinery. *EMBO Journal*, **18**, 2273–83.

Cohn, R.D. and Campbell, K.P. (2000a) Molecular basis of muscular dystrophies. *Muscle & Nerve*, **23**, 1456–71.

Cohn, R.D. and Campbell, K.P. (2000b). Pathogenetic role of the sarcoglycan-sarcospan complex in cardiomyopathies. *Acta Myologica*, **19**, 171–80.

Donnenberg, M.S. (2000). Pathogenic strategies of enteric bacteria. *Nature*, **406**, 768–74.

Emery, A.E.H. (1998). The muscular dystrophies. *British Medical Journal*, **317**, 991–95.

Emery, A.E.H. and Emery, M.L.H. (1995). *The history of a genetic disease.* Royal Society of Medicine Press, London.

Fatkin, D., MacRae, C., Sasaki, T., Wolff, M. R., Porcu, M., Frenneaux, M. *et al.* (1999). Missense mutations in the rod domain of the lamin A/C gene as causes of dilated cardiomyopathy and conduction-system disease. *New England Journal of Medicine*, **341**, 1715–24.

Lee, G-H., Badorff, C. and Knowlton, K.U. (2000). Dissociation of sarcoglycans and the dystrophin carboxyl terminus from the sarcolemma in enteroviral cardiomyopathy. *Circulation Research*, **87**, 489–95.

Morris, G.E. (2000). Nuclear proteins and cell death in inherited neuromuscular disease. *Neuromuscular Disorders*, **10**, 217–27.

Sander, M., Chavoshan, B., Harris, S.A., Iannaccone, S.T. *et al.* (2000). Functional muscle ischaemia in neuronal nitric oxide synthase-deficient skeletal muscle of children with Duchenne muscular dystrophy. *Proceedings of the National Academy of Sciences, USA*, **97**, 13818–23.

Walton, J.N. and Nattrass, F.J. (1954). On the classification, natural history and treatment of the myopathies. *Brain*, **77**, 169–231.

Weiler, T., Bashir, R., Anderson, L.V.B., Davison, K., Moss, J.A., Britton, S. *et al.* (1999). Identical mutation in patients with limb girdle muscular dystrophy type 2B or Miyoshi myopathy suggests a role for modifier gene(s). *Human Molecular Genetics*, **8**, 871–77.

Chapter 2

Congenital muscular dystrophies

Eugenio Mercuri and Francesco Muntoni

Introduction

The congenital muscular dystrophies (CMD) are a heterogeneous group of autosomal recessively inherited diseases, presenting at birth or within the first few months of life, with hypotonia, muscle weakness, contractures and characterized by dystrophic changes on the muscle biopsy. Recent epidemiological data suggest that the incidence and prevalence of CMD is 4.65×10^{-5} and 8×10^{-6} (Mostacciuolo *et al.* 1996). These figures indicate that this myopathy is among the most frequent neuromuscular diseases with autosomic recessive transmission.

The clinical diversity of CMD is suggested by the different degrees of motor developmental delay, physical disability and muscle pathology, and by the variable presence of mental retardation. Most of the efforts aimed at delineating and subdividing the various CMD forms have originated from the International Consortium on CMD, that, under the auspices of the European Neuromuscular Centre (ENMC), has convened six dedicated workshops, whose proceedings have been published in Neuromuscular Disorders (Dubowitz 1994; 1997; 1999; Dubowitz and Fardeau 1995; Muntoni and Guicheney 2001). The classification proposed in this chapter, that takes into account the recent advances in the molecular genetic studies, is largely a reflection of the data presented at these workshops.

In the last six years it has become increasingly evident that the classification of the different forms of CMD is a difficult task. In 1994 the International Consortium on CMD separated three forms of CMD with structural brain changes from a classical or 'pure' CMD without structural brain abnormalities (Dubowitz 1994). A significant advance came from a further subdivision of the 'pure' form into two groups according to the presence or deficiency of merosin: merosin-deficient and merosin-positive CMD (Dubowitz and Fardeau 1995). However, each of these groups still showed a significant clinical and pathological heterogeneity and a number of new syndromes have been described. At the last workshop on CMD the classification has been updated separating the forms of CMD which have been mapped (CMD diseases) from the ones with clearly defined clinical and pathological features which however have not yet been mapped (CMD syndromes).

Six CMD forms have been mapped up to now, and the genes responsible for three of them have been identified (see Table 2.1).

Table 2.1 CMD Diseases in which the gene loci have been identified

Name	Abbreviation	Gene symbol	OMIM	Location	Protein
Merosin deficient CMD	MDC1A	LAMA2	156225	6q2	Laminin α2
Fukuyama CMD	FCMD	FKT1	253800	9q3	Fukutin
Integrin α7 deficiency		ITGA7	600536	12q	Integrin α7
Muscle–Eye–Brain disease	MEB	?	253280	1p3	?
CMD/rigid spine syndrome	RSMD1	?	602771	1p3	?
CMD/muscle hypertrophy	MDC1B	?	604801	1q4	?
CMD/muscle hypertrophy2	MDC1C	KKRP		19q	KPRP
Ullrich disease	UCMD	COL6	254090	21q	Collagen6

Clinical and pathological evidence suggests, however, that several other CMD syndromes exist, some associated with mental retardation and others without.

A useful way to approach the diagnosis of a child with congenital muscular dystrophy is to consider a few important details. Firstly, is there a central nervous system involvement, in terms of severe mental retardation and/or structural brain defect and is there eye involvement? Secondly, is merosin normally expressed in the muscle? Finally, is there early and severe rigidity of the spine or distal joint laxity?

In this chapter we will first describe the CMD conditions usually *not* associated with mental retardation, and then consider the forms in which this is invariable and severe finding.

CMD without significant mental retardation

A proposed classification of the CMD syndromes without mental retardation is indicated below:

(i)   CMD with absent merosin, linked to the LAMA2 locus

(ii) CMD with reduced merosin

    (a) primary deficiencies, linked to the LAMA2 locus

    (b) secondary deficiencies

        (1) MDC1B, linked to chromosome 1q

        (2) form(s) unlinked to MDC1B or LAMA2

(iii) CMD with normal merosin and rigidity of the spine (RSMD1, linked to chromosome 1p)

(iv) CMD with normal merosin and distal joint laxity

(v)   Integrin α7 deficiency

(vi) Other forms

Merosin-deficient congenital muscular dystrophy (MDC1A)

In 1994 a major breakthrough in the field of CMD research came with the demonstration by a group of French investigators that merosin was deficient in the muscle biopsy of a significant proportion of patients with the form of CMD without mental retardation, also known as the 'pure form' of CMD (Tomé et al. 1994; see also Tomé 1999 for a review). Merosin (laminin 2) is a heterotrimeric basement membrane protein that acts as extracellular ligand for the α-dystroglycan. It is expressed in striated muscles, Schwann cells and placenta (Engvall 1993; Voit et al. 1994; Vuolteenaho et al. 1994). The availability of antibodies against the three laminin components, led to the demonstration that it was the laminin α2 chain deficient in these patients. Ten additional laminin variants have so far been identified, each of which is composed of a heterotrimer of an alpha, beta, and gamma chain and differentially expressed in different tissues. The predominant variants in muscle are laminin-2 (α2-β1-γ1) and laminin-4 (α2-β2-γ1). This means that both laminin-2 and -4 (this latter predominantly expressed at the myotendinous and neuromuscular junctions) are affected by mutations in the gene for the laminin α2 chain. The laminins influence cell adhesion, differentiation, growth, shape and migration. Merosin, in particular, is believed to promote myotube stability and prevent apoptosis (Vachon et al. 1995).

While most patients studied were found to have either no or trace expression of the protein in skeletal muscle, in some the residual levels were appreciable (Fig. 2.1). This led to a complication in the interpretation of the pathological changes in individual cases that will be further discussed under 'partial merosin deficiency'. In the following paragraphs we will describe the clinical features of those patients with absent laminin α2 chain expression, or with just a trace in the muscle biopsy. In keeping with other authors, we will use the terms 'merosin deficiency' as equivalent of 'laminin α2 chain deficiency'.

Merosin deficient-CMD represents approximately 40 per cent of CMD cases in France and UK (Philpot et al. 1995a; Tome et al. 1994). Lower incidence of this form occurs, however, in different populations (e.g. Italy, personal observation).

Clinical findings

Children affected by merosin-deficient CMD invariably present at birth or in the first few months of life with hypotonia, weakness (Fig. 2.2), respiratory and feeding problems (Philpot et al. 1995a). Contractures (hip flexion contractures; talipes) may also occur, but severe fetal immobility leading to arhrogryposis is uncommon. Weakness often affects upper limbs more severely than lower limbs, where antigravity movements are preserved. Prominence of the calves and facial weakness can be observed in the neonatal period. Serum CK is invariably markedly elevated, usually >10 times normal values in the early phases of the disease. Motor development is delayed and the maximal motor ability is only sitting unsupported; this is usually achieved by the age of 3 years. Children may be able to stand with some form of support or, in rare instances,

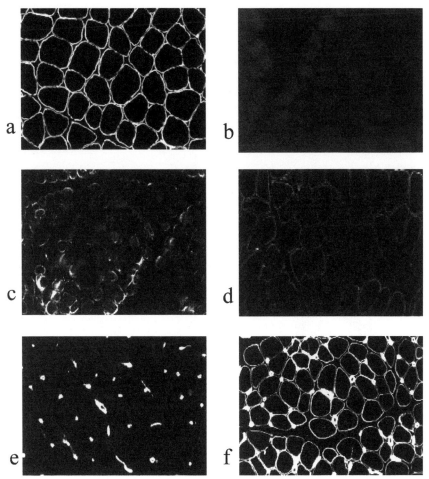

Fig. 2.1 Panel a: normal skeletal muscle immunostained with a Chemicon antibody against laminin α2 chain: note the normal uniform sarcolemmal expression of the protein. Panel b: muscle biopsy from a patient with merosin-deficient CMD, showing total absence of laminin α2 chain. Panel c: muscle biopsy from a patient showing trace expression of laminin α2 chain. Panel d: muscle biopsy of a patient showing partial reduction of laminin α2 chain expression. Panel e: normal skeletal muscle immunostained with an antibody against laminin α5 chain: only blood vessels are stained. Panel f: muscle biopsy from a patient with partial merosin deficiency: upregulation of laminin α5 at the sarcolemma. The magnification in all staining is ×180.

walk with support. Although muscle power remains static in most cases, increase inflexion deformity at the hips, knees, elbows and ankles, followed by rigidity and scoliosis of the spine, occur almost invariably, leading to increased limitation of functional abilities (Fig. 2.3). In view of the severe muscle weakness and contractures, conservative

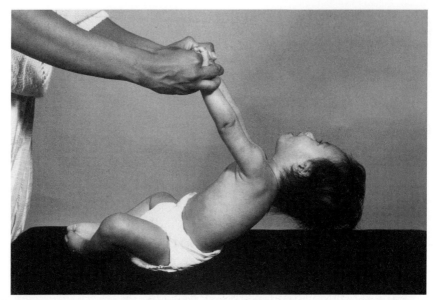

Fig. 2.2 Two months old boy affected by merosin-deficient CMD. Note the severe hypotonia and the head lag.

management is usually preferred to aggressive orthopaedic procedures. Spinal surgery can only rarely be performed in these children because of poor respiratory function.

A useful clinical sign that helps in the clinical distinction between merosin-positive and deficient cases is the limitation of eye movements that occurs only in the latter category (Philpot and Muntoni 1999). Limitation of upward gaze can be seen in the majority of merosin-deficient CMD children, usually by the end of the first decade of life.

Frequent complications in merosin-deficient CMD are respiratory failure, feeding problems and failure to thrive. Regarding the *respiratory aspects*, these children invariably have severely impaired respiratory function and frequently develop night time hypoventilation. The symptoms can be subtle and may occur over a short period of time even in early childhood. Treatment with night time non-invasive positive pressure ventilation delivered by nasal mask or facemask provides resolution of the symptoms and is likely to affect the long term prognosis of this condition (Simonds *et al.* 2000); we now perform at least yearly overnight oxygen saturation monitoring in younger children and six monthly studies in children older than eight years.

Regarding the *feeding problems*, failure to thrive occurs in more than 80 per cent of affected children; weak and uncoordinated swallowing, leading to increased risk of aspiration pneumonias, is a frequent finding in these children. Early gastrostomy

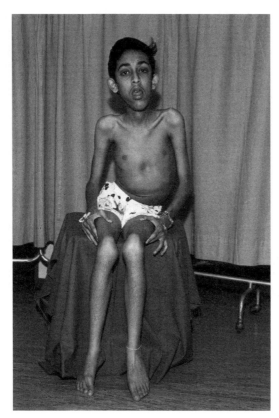

Fig. 2.3 Merosin-deficient boy aged 10 years. Note the facial weakness, the generalized thinning of the muscles and the severe scoliosis. The boy is able to sit unsupported but not to stand.

should be given serious consideration because of the progressive nature of failure to thrive together with swallowing difficulties (Philpot *et al.* 1999).

Central nervous system involvement

Brain Magnetic resonance imaging studies invariably show white matter changes in patients with merosin-deficient CMD despite there being no significant mental retardation. These changes can be demonstrated as increased signal intensity of white matter on T_2-weighted magnetic resonance images (MRI) (Philpot *et al.* 1995b; 1999b). The changes are diffuse, resembling a leucodystrophy and affect both hemispheres (Fig. 2.4a) but spare the internal capsule, corpus callosum, basal ganglia, thalami, and cerebellum (Cook *et al.* 1992; Mercuri 1995a,b; 1999; Philpot *et al.* 1995a,b). These changes can be best visualized after six months (Mercuri *et al.* 1996) and are concordant within siblings (Philpot *et al.* 1995b). More recently we were able to demonstrate abnormal white matter changes even in the newborn period (Mercuri *et al.* 2001) using a fast spin echo, resulting in an increased T_2 weighting, that results in an increased contrast and an overall better detection of the white matter changes. This observation

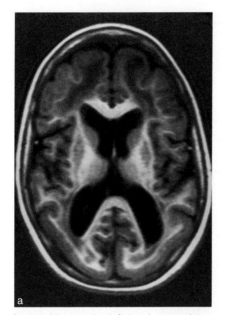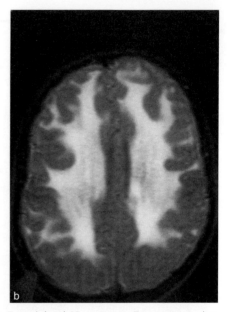

Fig. 2.4 (a) Merosin-deficient boy aged 7 years. T_2-weighted SE sequence. Transverse section showing extensive white matter lesions, seen as high signal on T_2, in both hemispheres. (b) Merosin-deficient boy aged 10 years: T_1 weighted image. Transverse section showing bilateral occipital cortical dysplasia. Note also the diffuse abnormal signal in the white matter (seen as low signal on T_1) in both hemispheres.

suggests that abnormalities are detectable in white matter before it is myelinated and that processes other than dysmyelination are involved. The basis for this increase in signal in part of the white matter is not entirely resolved; using immunohistochemical and ultramicroscopic techniques, laminin $\alpha2$ chain has been localized to the basal lamina of cerebral blood vessels, leading to the suggestion that this molecule might be important for the selective filtration of the blood–brain barrier (Villanova *et al.* 1997). While recent pathological studies in an infant with merosin-deficient CMD failed to detect any significant white matter abnormality (Taratuto *et al.* 1999), Echenne reported an increased white matter spongiosis and oedema in an older patient with merosin-deficient CMD (Echenne *et al.* 1984; personal communication).

Structural brain changes, including occipital agyria (Brett *et al.* 1998; Pini *et al.* 1996; Sunada *et al.* 1995; Taratuto *et al.* 1999) (Fig. 2.4b), and cerebellar hypoplasia (Philpot *et al.* 1999b) can be demonstrated in a proportion of children with merosin-deficient CMD. The former is a striking form of pachygyria that is present in approximately 5 per cent of cases, and associated with mental retardation and epilepsy. Cerebellar hypoplasia was present in 20 per cent of our cases (Philpot *et al.* 1999b) but has been rarely reported by others. It was, however, present in the case whose brain pathology was reported by Taratuto (1999).

Cognitive function is usually normal in children with "pure" CMD irrespective of the merosin status (Mercuri *et al.* 1999); noticeable exceptions are represented by patients with the occipital pachygyria. In a recent detailed neurocognitive study we were also able to demonstrate lower scores on the performance scales in patients with cerebellar hypoplasia. Visual function is normal (Mercuri *et al.* 1998).

Electrophysiologic studies have confirmed functional central nervous system (CNS) changes in merosin-deficient CMD. Visual and somatosensory evoked responses are usually abnormal in merosin-deficient cases but normal in all the merosin-positive cases (Mercuri *et al.* 1995a). Brainstem evoked potentials, in contrast, are always normal and this is in agreement with the sparing of the brainstem on brain MRI.

Epilepsy is a frequent complication of merosin-deficient CMD, and includes cases with partial deficiency (see below); it affects approximately 30 per cent of cases (Voit 1998). A peculiar form of epilepsy (periodic spasms) has been reported in patients with occipital agyria (Pini *et al.* 1996) but is not an invariable finding (Brett *et al.* 1998; personal observation).

Peripheral nervous system involvement

As a result of the lack of merosin in the Schwann cells, children with merosin-deficient CMD have a *demyelinating neuropathy*, which can be demonstrated by reduced peripheral motor nerve conduction velocity. In contrast, sensory nerve function appears unaffected (Shorer *et al.* 1995); this parallels the observation of a motor but not sensory neuropathy in the d*y*/d*y* animal model of merosin-deficient CMD. A detailed description of the d*y*/d*y* mouse model is presented in Chapter 16.

Cardiac involvement

We have recently shown that a proportion of merosin-deficient cases have a mild to moderate hypokinesia, while cardiac function is normal in merosin-positive CMD (Spyrou *et al.* 1998).

Muscle pathology

The muscle biopsy shows a classical dystrophic picture with a wide variation in fibre size and an increase in endomysial connective tissue and adipose tissue (Sewry *et al.* 1996; 1997a; Tomé *et al.* 1994). Immunofluorescent techniques can readily demonstrate the reduction or absence of laminin α2 chain. In most cases, this laminin chain is totally absent or only present in traces (Fig. 2.1). The cases characterized by partial reduction will be discussed below. The preservation of the basal lamina has to be proven in each case with the parallel study of other relevant merosin chains (γ1 and β1) (Sewry *et al.* 1995). Furthermore, the overexpression of laminin α5 in the non-regenerating muscle fibres is a useful secondary marker of merosin deficiency (Fig. 2.1). The expression of lamina α2 can also be demonstrated in the skin, at the dermo–epidermal junction. The expression of this protein can, therefore, be studied in the skin when muscle is not available (Sewry *et al.* 1997a). The results are of easy interpretation in patients with total absence of the protein; cases with partial deficiency need more careful interpretation.

Molecular genetics

The laminin α2 chain gene has been mapped to chromosome 6q22–23 (the LAMA 2 gene) (Vuolteenaho *et al.* 1994). By homozygosity mapping and linkage analysis, Hillaire *et al.* (1994) demonstrated that the merosin-deficient CMD locus is on chromosome 6q2 within the region of the LAMA 2 gene. This is composed of 64 exons, with a transcript of 9.4 kb. Several mutations have now been found, most of which are nucleotide substitutions, small deletions or insertions, resulting in nonsense or splice site changes (Guicheney *et al.* 1997; 1998; Mendell *et al.* 1998; Nissinen *et al.* 1996; Pegoraro *et al.* 1996; 1998). One large deletion (Pegoraro *et al.* 1998) and a *de novo* nucleotide substitution (Naom *et al.* 2000) have been reported. The large size of the gene hampers identification of mutations, and even using the protein truncation test not all mutations could be identified (Pegoraro *et al.* 1998). Linkage analysis, combined with immunocytochemistry, therefore continues to be of importance in establishing the primary involvement of the LAMA2 gene, and in prenatal diagnosis (Naom *et al.* 1997a). The expression of merosin in the trophoblast (Voit *et al.* 1994) allows us to directly study its presence by chorionic villus sampling (CVS) (Muntoni *et al.* 1995; Naom *et al.* 1997b).

Congenital muscular dystrophy with normal intelligence and reduced merosin

These patients can be broadly divided in two groups; those linked to the LAMA2 chain gene and those unlinked. They are both characterized by a reduction of merosin documented using immunohistochemistry (Fig. 2.1) or western blot analysis. The detection of laminin α2 chain in cases with partial expression may depend on which, and how many, antibodies are used. As it is the case for dystrophinopathies, it is now apparent that it is important to assess all cases of CMD with more than one antibody to the laminin α2 chain. This chain is processed into two fragments on immunoblots, of 80 and 300 kDa, but the antibodies available only recognize one or other of the fragments. Differential immunolabelling of sections is seen using antibodies to each fragment in cases of partial deficiency, and a reduction is often easier to observe with antibodies to the 300 kDa fragment (Sewry and Muntoni 1999; Sewry *et al.* 1995; 1996). The majority of cases that show no protein expression with antibodies to the globular 80 kDa fragment also show an absence with all antibodies. One exception, however, has been observed, as a result of a mutation in the globular region (Dubowitz 1999). While merosin is abnormal in most of these patients, these changes are at times subtle, and visible only once laminin α2 has been studied using a panel of antibodies. The laminin α5 upregulation can provide additional helpful information, as this is almost invariably seen (in non-regenerating fibres) when laminin α2 chain is decreased. A recent case of a primary partial deficiency without up-regulation of LAMA5 has, however, been reported (Pegoraro *et al.* 2000). Laminin β2 expression may also provide additional information as it is often reduced in cases with (partial or total) merosin deficiency (Cohn *et al.* 1997).

Regarding the two groups of patients characterized by partial merosin deficiency: In the primary cases, the phenotype is often milder compared to patients with absent merosin (Fig. 2.5). Affected individuals usually achieve independent ambulation, and in some cases onset of symptoms may be delayed to the second decade of life (Allamand *et al.* 1997; Cohn *et al.* 1998; Herrmann *et al.* 1996; Mora *et al.* 1996; Naom *et al.* 1997a; Sewry *et al.* 1997b; Tan *et al.* 1997). A few cases with partial deficiency and a severe phenotype, indistinguishable from that observed in classical merosin-deficient CMD, have also been described (Cohn *et al.* 1998; Morandi *et al.* 1999, personal observation). These cases typically have only mild or moderate deficiency with the 80 kDa antibodies but a severe depletion, or absent staining with the 300 kDa antibodies. Cases of partial deficiency and severe phenotype often have mutations (missense mutations or other mutations that are compatible with a residual expression of the protein) in highly functional domains of the protein, such as the G (globular) domain, that interacts with α dystroglycan (Mercuri *et al.* in preparation).

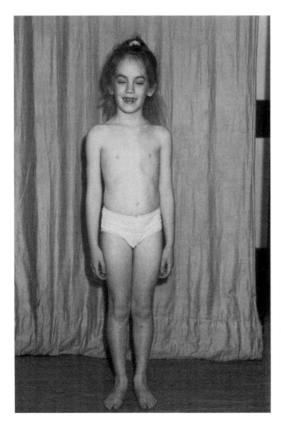

Fig. 2.5 Seven-year-old girl with partial merosin deficiency. Note that the phenotype is much milder than that observed in patients with absent merosin (Fig. 2.3).

Diagnostic clues for the primary forms are the mild electrophysiological demyelinating peripheral neuropathy and the white matter changes on brain MRI that are indistinguishable from those observed in patients with absence of the protein. Neuronal migration disorder (occipital pachygyria and, in one instance, cerebellar polymicrogyria) has been described also in patients with partial laminin α2 chain deficiency (Pegoraro *et al.* 2000).

From a diagnostic and counselling point of view it is, therefore, important to acknowledge that partial protein expression can be associated with a severe outcome. In the milder cases, onset of symptoms is often delayed and the phenotype more closely resembles limb-girdle muscular dystrophy. Presentation as late as the second decade of life with proximal weakness, elevated serum CK and a dystrophic muscle biopsy has been reported. Epilepsy (partial seizures) is at least as common in partial deficiency compared to classical merosin-deficient CMD (Cohn *et al.* 1998).

A homozygous in frame deletion in the LAMA2 chain gene (Allamand *et al.* 1997) and compound heterozygosity between a null allele and various splice site mutations have now been reported in several cases with partial deficiency and a mild phenotype (Allamand *et al.* 1997; Naom *et al.* 1998; 2000).

Regarding the secondary cases (with normal intelligence), these include a recently described form mapped to chromosome 1q42 (MDC1B); and several other pedigrees unlinked to either the LAMA2, MDC1B, or other CMD loci.

Congenital muscular dystrophy 1B (MDC1B): muscle hypertrophy and secondary merosin deficiency, linked to chromosome 1q42

This is a form initially described in one family from the United Arab Emirates and one family from Germany, and is characterized by delayed motor milestones but acquisition of independent ambulation (Brockington *et al.* 2000; Muntoni *et al.* 1998). Muscle weakness was predominantly proximal but with a significant axial component and mild facial weakness and head lag. The only clear disease progression was limited to the development of early respiratory failure in one of the two families; generalized muscle hypertrophy, combined with wasting of the neck muscle, was also observed. Serum CK was grossly elevated, and the muscle biopsy showed a partial deficiency of merosin (see below). Both children in the German family developed at least one episode of spontaneous myoglobinuria.

Genetic studies have localized the locus responsible for this form of CMD to chromosome 1q42 in both families (Brockington *et al.* 2000).

Biochemical studies: antibodies to laminin α2 showed reduced labelling on several fibres. Other proteins of the extracellular matrix, including integrins α7 and β1D, were also reduced on the same fibres; α dystroglycan showed a severe deficiency in both families.

Congenital muscular dystrophy 1C (MDC1C): muscle hypertrophy and secondary merosin deficiency, linked to chromosome 19q.

This represents a clinically heterogeneous group of conditions for which the primary defect has been recently mapped to chromosome 19q (Brockington *et al.*, submitted). Although rare, these forms might be confused both clinically and pathologically with merosin deficient CMD.

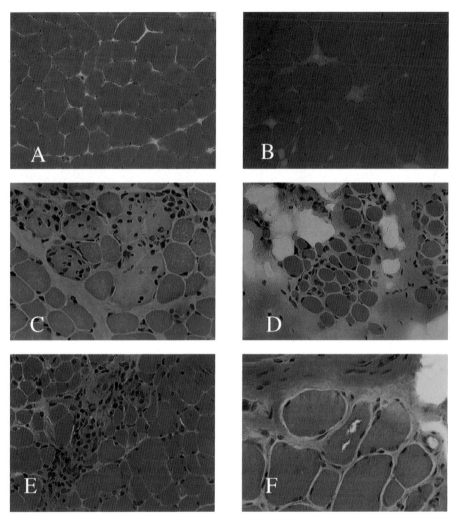

Fig. 1.1 Some of the variations in muscle histology observed in different types of dystrophy (A, normal; B, fibre splitting and internal nuclei; C, necrosis and phagocytosis; D, variations in fibre size; E, 'inflammatory' changes; F, rimmed vacuoles). (Haematoxylin & eosin stain). Reproduced by kind permission of Dr. Carolyn Sewry.

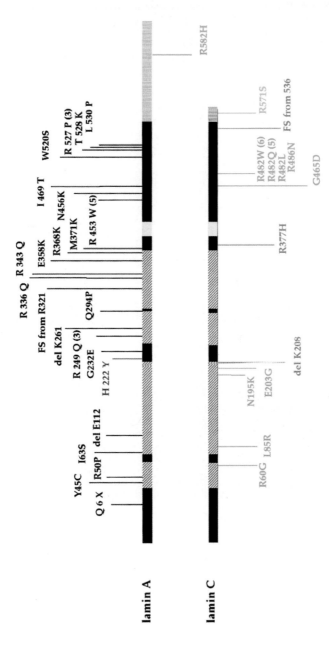

Fig. 6.2 Distribution along the lamins of the mutations in LMNA gene. The molecular organization of lamins A and C is schematically represented. Dashed boxes are the coil coiled domains. In yellow is the chromatin binding domain. Striped are the two alternative N terminal regions. Above, in black, are the mutations in AD-EMD; in red the mutation in AR-EMD. Below are the mutations in the other three disorders, in light blue, mutations in DCM-CD; in orange, mutations in LGMD1B; in green, mutations in OFPLD.

The spectrum of the phenotype includes cases with a severe phenotype and inability to walk unsupported but also children with milder course. At the moment it is not clear if these represent variants of the same disorder or different genetic entities.

Regarding patients with the severe phenotype, we recently described a Scottish family with reduced laminin α2 chain on both muscle and skin biopsy and a severe clinical phenotype characterized by poor functional achievements, prominent feeding problems, markedly elevated serum CK but with normal brain MRI (Mercuri *et al.* 2000). Both children were unable to stand unsupported and the distribution and severity of weakness was similar to the 6q merosin-deficient CMD. Noticeable differences between these two siblings and the 6q merosin-deficient CMD were the normal peripheral nerve electrophysiology and the absence of white matter changes on brain MRI. These features distinguish this form also from Fukuyama congenital muscular dystrophy, Muscle–Eye–Brain disease or other forms of CMD with secondary partial merosin deficiency, abnormal brain MRI and mental retardation (see below).

The muscle biopsy showed a significant depletion of several proteins of the extracellular matrix, including laminin α2, β1 and γ1 chains. Laminin α2 and β1 chains were

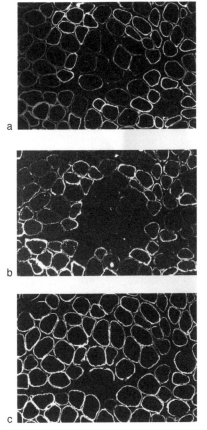

Fig. 2.6 Panel a: skeletal muscle from a patient with partial merosin deficiency immunostained with antibodies against laminin α2 chain. Panel b: serial sections from the same patient shown in panel a, stained with anti-α dystoglycan antibodies: note the more severe depletion of α dystroglycan compared to laminin α2 chain. Panel c: serial section of the same patient showing preserved expression of β-dystroglycan. The magnification in all staining is ×180.

also reduced in skin. An almost total absence of α-dystroglycan has been recently demonstrated in this case (Voit and Brown, personal observation) (Fig. 2.6).

A group of patients with similar features, characterized by striking calf muscle hypertrophy macroglossia, and early respiratory failure have recently been reported by Estournet at an ENMC meeting (Muntoni and Guicheney 2001). All these patients had early flexion deformity of the fingers, a feature shared by the Scottish children described by Mercuri *et al.* Serum CK were grossly elevated.

Milder cases of ambulant children with similar features to the ones described above (muscle hypertrophy and secondary merosin deficiency) and unlinked to the all known loci have been recently described by Voit (Muntoni and Guicheney 2001). Genetic studies will eventually clarify if these represent allelic or genetically distinct CMD forms.

CMD with rigidity of the spine and normal merosin: RSMD1, linked to 1p

A locus for congenital muscular dystrophy in association with rigidity of the spine has recently been mapped to chromosome 1p35–p36 (Moghadaszadeh *et al.* 1998). The original paper described five patients from three families from Morocco, Turkey and Iran. Since then several other cases have been reported (Flanigan *et al.* 2000; Moghadaszadeh *et al.* 1999). The consistent clinical features are early rigidity of the spine and restrictive respiratory syndrome. These children generally have mild hypotonia and weakness in the first few months of life with some improvement in muscle power by the end of the first year and achieve independent walking by 18 months of age. Overtime muscle power remains relatively stable or only shows a mild decrease and mainly concerns the axial muscles and to a lesser extent the proximal muscles. There is however a progressive atrophy of the muscles which can be observed on MRI, showing a selective pattern of involvement of the thigh muscles in the early stages of the disease followed by a widespread diffusion of the muscle abnormalities (Flanigan *et al.* 2000). Rigid spine and Achilles tendon contractures are a constant feature after 5–6 years and scoliosis is also frequently observed. Respiratory failure is an invariable and early feature, requiring nocturnal ventilatory support in the second decade of life, when patients are still ambulant. Serum CK are normal or minimally elevated.

Muscle biopsy generally shows a dystrophic process varying in severity, and in one of the cases reported by Flanigan *et al.* (2000), only minimal changes could be observed. The variability of these findings might be explained by the age of the patients at the time of the biopsy or by the muscle sampled, as in the initial phases of the disease, a selective muscle involvement can be present. Merosin is normally expressed. The locus is on chromosome 1p35–36, but the gene has not been identified yet.

CMD with distal joint laxity and normal merosin (Ullrich disease)

In 1930 Ullrich described two boys with early onset weakness and contractures of the proximal joints but striking laxity of wrists and ankles. Since Ullrich's original description several other cases have been reported (Nonaka *et al.* 1981). These children usually show contractures and hypotonia since birth and some of them acquire the ability to walk independently. The course of the disease is static of slowly progressive and loss of ambulation may occur. All patients developed rigidity of the spine, often associated with scoliosis, failure to thrive and early and severe respiratory involvement. Several patients in our personal series went into respiratory failure in the first or second decade or life. Serum CK are normal and merosin is also normally experssed. A recent study has reported collagen VI deficiency on muscle and skin in 2 patients with Ullrich disease (Higuchi *et al.* 2001). Soon after that, recessive mutations in collagen VI were found in 4 patients who also showed a near total absence of collagen VI in fibroblasts and muscle on immunofluorescence (Camacho *et al.* 2001). Our data on 15 patients with similar phenotype show that not all the patients with this phenotype link to collagen VI loci, suggesting further genetic heterogeneity.

Integrin α7 deficiency

Mutations have recently been described in the gene for the integrin α7 on chromosome 12q13 in three Japanese patients (Hayashi *et al.* 1998). Motor milestones were delayed in all three and one was in addition globally retarded. Weakness was mild and predominantly proximal and CK was mildly raised. A muscle biopsy showed fatty replacement and variation in fibre size and was described as a myopathy. However, features of degeneration and regeneration were present in one of the patients. Brain MRI was normal. Although integrin α7 is a ligand for laminin α2, the expression of the latter is normal in this condition. This contrasts with the secondary reduction of integrin α7/β1D complex when laminin α2 is deficient. No further cases have been reported since.

Other forms

CMD with epidermolysis bullosa—Kletter *et al.* (1989) described three children from an inbred pedigree with CMD and epidermolysis bullosa simplex. The patients had infantile hypotonia and progressive weakness and the muscle biopsy revealed changes consistent with a muscular dystrophy. The epidermolysis bullosa and the weakness were severe and the eldest child could not walk at the age of 4.5. Since this original description, mutations in the plectin gene (PLEC1) gene at 8q24 have been described in several patients with epidermolysis bullosa, but their muscle weakness does not appear before the second or third decade of life (Pulkkinen *et al.* 1996). As mutations in the PLEC1 gene have not been reported yet in the infants with the severe phenotype, it is not clear if this gene is responsible also for the congenital form of muscular dystrophy.

"Pure" merosin positive CMD is a highly heterogeneous group of conditions; few large families have been described, including one Palestinian family affected by a CMD form characterized by generalized muscle weakness and hypotonia at birth and a relatively benign clinical course with normal or moderately increased CK, normal intelligence, normal brain imaging and peripheral nerve electrophysiology (Mahjneh *et al.* 1999).

CMD with severe mental retardation

Several well defined forms of CMD are associated with severe mental retardation and structural brain changes and include CMD-Fukuyama CMD (FCMD), muscle– eye–brain disease (MEB), and Walker–Warburg syndrome (WWS). An increasing number of other conditions with severe mental retardation have more recently been reported by various authors and are invariably associated with structural brain defects and eye involvement A list of these conditions is indicated below.

CMD syndrome with mental retardation

(i)   Fukuyama CMD

(ii)   Muscle–Eye–Brain Disease

(iii)   Walker–Warburg syndrome

(iv)   CMD with cerebellar hypoplasia

(v)   Microcephaly-muscle hypertrophy-cerebellar hypoplasia

(vi)   CMD with cerebellar cysts

(vii)   Microcephaly-normal structural brain

(viii) Microcephaly-pachigyria-peripheral neuropathy

(ix)   CMD + cataracts

(x)   CMD with adducted thumbs

The overlap between some of these conditions is significant (e.g. between the various subtypes characterized by cerebellar involvement, such as forms iv–viii)) and genetic studies will eventually confirm whether these represent variant of the same disorder or not. However, differences in the expression of merosin, CNS and peripheral nerve involvement suggest that these might well be separate diseases; some of them will be briefly described below.

Fukuyama congenital muscular dystrophy

Fukuyama congenital muscular dystrophy (FCMD, OMIM 253800) is an autosomal recessive disorder characterized by muscular dystrophy with severe mental retardation (Fukuyama et al. 1960). It is the second most common form of childhood muscular dystrophy in Japan after Duchenne muscular dystrophy (DMD), with an incidence of 7–12/100,000 (Fukuyama et al. 1981). The initial impression that this syndrome is exceedingly rare outside Japan has been recently confirmed from the recent molecular genetic investigations following the identification of the responsible gene.

Clinical features   The clinical features of the disease were reviewed extensively by Fukuyama et al. (1981) and Fukuyama et al. (1997). Onset was early and severe, with hypotonia and poor sucking during the neonatal period. Severe artrogryphosis is not usual. Muscle weakness is typically generalized and involves the facial muscles with pseudohypertrophy of the cheeks, giving a typical appearance. Enlargement of the calves and forearms are also common. Motor milestones are markedly delayed; a minority of patients are unable to achieve the sitting position or even head control; most, however, achieved the ability to sit unaided and to crawl on the knees, with the maximal motor ability acquired between the ages of 2 and 8 years (Fukuyama *et al.* 1981). Rare patients achieve independent ambulation; with time, however, weakness and contractures progress, with loss of functional abilities. By the age of 10 years, most of these children had become immobile, and the majority die by their late teens (Fukuyama *et al.* 1981).

Intellectual retardation can vary but is usually severe; Fukuyama recognized three subtype of the disorder based on intellectual function; the first characterized by severe mental retardation and absent speech; the second by moderate mental retardation and acquistion of a limited vocabulary, usually less than 20 words; the third category by mild mental retardation where the children generally learn to speak in short phrases (Fukuyama *et al.* 1997). The patients with better mental function tended to be those with the least motor disability.

Epilepsy is common. In a series of 83 cases, 44 per cent had no seizures, 37 per cent febrile seizures, and 20 per cent persistent epilepsy unassociated with fever (Fukuyama *et al.* 1997).

Central nervous system involvement   Early CNS imaging with CT showed that some patients had distinct white matter hypodensity (Fukuyama *et al.* 1981; Mukoyama *et al.* 1979; Yoshioka *et al.* 1980; 1991). Ventricular dilation was sometimes present, probably secondary to brain atrophy, but progressive hydrocephalus was rare and cephalocoeles, were not seen. This remains a diagnostic feature of WWS (Fukuyama *et al.* 1981; Yoshioka *et al.* 1980). More recent MRI studies showed areas of polymicrogyria, macrogyria, and agyria (Fukuyama *et al.* 1981; Yoshioka *et al.* 1991). This has been confirmed at autopsy, which reveals a disorganized cortex with loss of the usual cortical layers and proliferation of gliovascular bundles or septa, separating the cortex into clumps of cells with neurons lying at irregular angles to one another (Fukuyama *et al.* 1981; Kamoshita *et al.* 1976; Takada *et al.* 1984). There is also often focal fusion of the cerebral hemispheres due to an intense fibroglial proliferation of the leptomeninges. A reduction of neurones in the brainstem has also been recently reported (Itoh *et al.* 1996).

Sequential MRI studies have demonstrated that the abnormal signal in the white matter is most likely to be due to delayed myelination rather than dysmyelination, as it improves with age.

Eye involvement   Eye abnormalities are not consistently seen in every patient and are usually not severe, but they do occur in approximately 60–70 per cent of these patients. Myopia is the most frequent abnormality (Honda and Yoshioka 1978). More severe ocular changes, such as optic nerve atrophy, cataract, and retinal detachment, have been reported, but are rare (Chijiiwa *et al.* 1983; Fukuyama *et al.* 1981; Honda and Yoshioka 1978; Yoshioka *et al.* 1990).

Muscle pathology   All cases of FCMD have a high CK, even in the early stages of the disease that tends to decline with age (Dubowitz 1994; Fukuyama *et al.* 1981). The muscle histology shows a consistently dystrophic picture. Muscle immunocytochemistry has revealed a reduction of dystrophin-associated glycoproteins (Matsumura *et al.* 1993). In addition, merosin expression in the muscle is also reduced (Hayashi *et al.* 1993); more recently, a severe depletion of α-dystroglycan was reported by Hayashi and Arahata, further indicating a severe basal lamina defect in this condition (Muntoni and Guichney 2001).

Molecular genetics   Fukuyama CMD is inherited as an autosomal recessive trait. The gene for FCMD has been localized to chromosome 9q31–33 (Toda *et al.* 1993) and the gene product named fukutin (Kobayashi *et al.* 1998). The mechanism of mutation in the FCMD results from an ancient retrotransposon insertion located in the 3′ untranslated region of the gene encoding a novel 461-amino acid protein. The fukutin protein contains an amino-terminal signal sequence, which together with results from transfection experiments suggested that fukutin is initially localized in the Golgi and than secreted into the extracellular matrix. Efforts to generate antibodies against fukutin and therefore to provide localization and functional data on this protein have so far not been achieved.

Muscle–eye–brain disease

Clinical features   Muscle–eye–brain disease (MEB, OMIM: 236670) was first described by Santavuori *et al.* (1977, 1978). With the exception of few cases, the vast majority of reported patients come from Finland (Santavuori *et al.* 1989).

In 1989, Santavuori *et al.* reviewed the clinical features of 19 patients with MEB. Severe hypotonia, sucking difficulties, and failure to thrive are already evident by two months, and in only in some cases, by six months. The children often share similar faces, with a large head, prominent forehead, flat midface and short nose and philtrum. They have generalized weakness, involving the limbs and trunk and their motor development is extremely delayed and only a small minority eventually achieve ambulation. Over time, the involvement of the CNS becomes more evident, with the lower limbs becoming spastic with increased reflexes (Santavuori *et al.* 1989). The CK levels can be normal during the first year of life with highest values recorded between the ages of 5 and 15 years (Dubowitz 1994; Santavuori *et al.* 1989).

Mental retardation is a constant feature and it is generally severe, with only few cases achieving limited speech. Epilepsy is also very common (Santavuori *et al.* 1989).

Overall, the disease is progressive, with patients gradually losing their few acquired skills with time. The disease progression is however not as severe as FCMD or Walker–Warburg syndrome, and survival into early adulthood is common (85 per cent) with descriptions of cases surviving into their 4th or 5th decade (Dubowitz 1994; Muntoni and Guicheney 2001; Santavuori *et al.* 1989).

Central nervous system involvement   In all patients, MRI shows that the grossly abnormal gyral formation, often associated with pachygyria over the frontal, temporal, and parietal regions and polymicrogyria over the occipital region. Enlarged ventricles, brainstem hypoplasia and cerebellar hypoplasia are also present in most cases. Patchy white matter changes can occasionally be observed but, if present, they are localized to the periventricular white matter and are less severe than those observed in WWS (Dubowitz and Fardeau 1995; Muntoni and Guicheney 2001). Neuropathological studies have shown coarse gyri with nodular appearance of surface and agyric areas. Microscopically the cortex appeared disorganized without horizontal lamination.

Eye involvement   Ocular involvement is constantly present in MEB (Raitta *et al.* 1978; Santavuori *et al.* 1977; 1978; 1989). Severe myopia and retinal hypoplasia are the most common findings but other abnormalities such as congenital and infantile glaucoma, nystagmus, and cataract are also frequently found (Dubowitz 1994; Muntoni and Guicheney 2001; Santavuori *et al.* 1989).

Muscle pathology   The muscle biopsy has a dystrophic picture, with variation in fibre size and necrotic and regenerative fibres in the infantile period and progressive increase in connective tissue and adipose tissue at a later stage (Santavuori *et al.* 1989).

Merosin is reduced, while laminin β2 chain is overexpressed in Western blot studies (Auranen *et al.* 2000; Haltia *et al.* 1997). These findings may reflect a yet unidentified primary disturbance in the basement membrane composition in MEB.

Molecular genetics   The MEB has been recently mapped to chromosome 1p32–34 (Cormand *et al.* 1999) by linkage in Finnish MEB families. The MEB locus was refined to a less than 1-cM interval using linkage disequilibrium and haplotype analysis. Several candidate genes have been excluded from the critical region and the defected gene underlying MEB remains to be identified (Muntoni and Guicheney *et al.* 2001).

Walker–Warburg syndrome

Walker–Warburg syndrome is a rare autosomal recessive disorder reported in patients from many different nationalities and races, presenting with eye abnormalities, brain malformations and muscular dystrophy (Dobyns *et al.* 1989).

Walker originally described a severe developmental disorder with an abnormal cerebral gyral pattern, hydrocephalus, and retinal dysplasia (Walker 1942) and only relatively recently has it become evident that muscular dystrophy is also a feature of this condition (Dambska *et al.* 1982; Towfighi *et al.* 1984). In 1989 Dobyns reviewed the literature and expanded the phenotype of WWS to include CMD (Dobyns *et al.* 1989).

Clinical features   Walker–Warburg syndrome has the most severe phenotype of the muscle–eye–brain syndromes (Dobyns 1993). Decreased fetal movements and polyhydramnios are generally reported. Resuscitation is commonly required at birth and a significant majority of the infants affected by WWS are stillborn or die in the perinatal period. The median survival for all liveborn infants is 18 weeks, although about 5–10 per cent can survive more than five years (Dobyns *et al.* 1989). The survivors can be slightly less affected and although they might acquire the ability to sit and roll, they all have profound mental and motor retardation. Seizures are common and can be difficult to control.

Central nervous system involvement   MRI generally shows severe gyral changes, with agyria and additional areas of macrogyria and polymicrogyria. The corpus callosum and septum pellucidum are absent or hypoplastic. On pathology the cortex is abnormally thick and shows the typical cobblestone lissencephaly. The leptomeninges can obliterate the interhemispheric fissure and subarachnoid space (Dobyns *et al.* 1985; 1989; Towfighi *et al.* 1984). Microscopically, the cortex is severely disrupted with no recognizable neuronal layers. The white matter is extensively involved with diffuse changes throughout the cortex (Dobyns *et al.* 1985; 1989; Towfighi *et al.* 1984), in contrast to MEB and FCMD which are both associated with less severe involvement of the white matter.

Ventricular dilation, with or without progressive hydrocephalus, is also extremely common frequently requiring the insertion of a shunt.

The cerebellum is hypoplastic, particularly the posterior vermis, and the gyral pattern of the cerebellar cortex is abnormal. Other brain malformation, such as Dandy-Walker, meningocoeles and encephalocoeles have also been described (Dobyns *et al.* 1989).

Eye involvement   Patients with WWS show a wide spectrum of eye abnormalities. Retinal abnrmalities, of various degree, are present in all patients (Dobyns *et al.* 1989). Severe abnormalities include microphthalmia, colobomatous malformation, and retinal detachment secondary to retinal dysplasia. Milder changes include abnormal retinal vascularization, absent macular, and optic disc hypoplasia. Anterior chamber malformation can also be found in some patients, common abnormalities including corneal clouding, narrowing of the iridocorneal angle, with or without glaucoma and cataract (Dobyns *et al.* 1989; Dubowitz and Fardeau 1995).

Muscle pathology   The CK level is usually elevated (Dobyns *et al.* 1989; Dubowitz 1994; Muntoni and Guicheney 2001), but newborn infants can have normal or only mildly elevated levels. Muscle biopsy is dystrophic, but there have been reports of apparently normal muscle biopsies in infants during the first months of life (Dobyns *et al.* 1989; Dubowitz 1994) and it has been suggested that the biopsy becomes more dystrophic with time (Dobyns *et al.* 1989; Towfighi *et al.* 1984).

Merosin is usually normally expressed in the muscle biopsy of WWS patients (Voit *et al.* 1995). In one single case a slight reduction of laminins $\alpha 2$ and $\beta 2$ at the age of one year has been recently reported (Villanova *et al.* 1998).

Molecular genetics   The locus responsible for WWS has not been identified yet. The identification of the locus for MEB disease has allowed to screen all the cases with overlap in phenotypes with WWS demonstrating that they are genetically distinct entities (Dubowitz 1999; Muntoni and Guicheney 2001). A Turkish patient with WWS who carried a *de-novo* translocation of chromosomes 5q35 : 6q21 has been recently reported. Linkage analysis in 11 consanguineous WWS families performed by van Broekhoven however, excluded either of these two breakpoints from containing a common gene responsible for WWS (Muntoni and Guicheney 2001). The identification of the WWS locus will eventually answer the question whether or not WWS is genetically homogeneous.

CMD with cerebellar hypoplasia

A patient reported by Knubley and Bertorini (1988) was noted in the neonatal period to have a mild tremor and to be hypotonic. Motor milestones was delayed, and speech was mildly delayed and slurred. Ataxia and jerky eye movements were noted. Her CPK was markedly raised and a biopsy confirmed a dystrophy. A CT and NMR confirmed cerebellar atrophy, though intelligence was normal. Similar cases were reported more recently by Echenne *et al.* (1998). He described four patients, two of whom were sibs, with congenital muscular dystrophy, mild intellectual impairment, and moderate to severe cerebellar atrophy. Onset was in the neonatal period or the first few months of life. Creatine kinase was markedly elevated. Merosin immunostaining of skeletal muscle showed no abnormality while the brain MRI failed to show white matter abnormalities or neuronal migration disorder, effectively ruling out the diagnosis of FCMD or MEB (Echenne *et al.* 1998).

Microcephaly-muscle hypertrophy-cerebellar hypoplasia

Villanova *et al.* (2000) have recently reported five patients from four Italian families with severe mental retardation and structural brain changes. All patients had hypotonia, weakness and joint contractures since birth and showed a severe global retardation. They never acquired the ability to walk (or to sit in two cases) and also had severe cognitive impairment with absent speech. On examination all patients showed an enlargement of the calf and quadriceps muscles and microcephaly. Structural ocular abnormalities were not present but two patients had severe myopia. Brain MRI showed an abnormal posterior cranial fossa with enlargement of the cisterna magna, variable hypoplasia of the vermis of cerebellum and periventricular white matter changes. The muscle biopsy showed a dystrophic pattern in all with significant reduction of laminin 2 and upregulation of laminin 5; more recently we demonstrated a severe depletion of α-dystroglycan in these cases (personal observation). Linkage analysis excluded the known loci for CMD.

CMD with cerebellar cysts

A consanguineous Turkish family with this phenotype was recently reported (Talim *et al.* 2000). Characteristic features were early-onset hypotonia, generalized muscle wasting, with weakness involving especially the neck muscles, joint contractures and high CK. The patient was unable to walk and her IQ was 59. Muscle biopsy showed dystrophic changes with partial deficiency of the laminin α2 chain. Brain MRI revealed multiple small cysts in the cerebellum, without cerebral cortical dysplasia or white matter changes. The loci responsible for FCMD, LAMA2 and MEB were all excluded by linkage analysis.

Microcephaly-normal structural brain

Another form of CMD with mental retardation but normal structural brain was reported in two siblings by Topaloglu *et al.* (1998). These siblings had severe mental retardation and weakness, and were unable to walk. Merosin was partially reduced in the muscle biopsy and the brain MRI was normal in both sibs, including the white matter. All the relevant CMD loci (FCMD; LAMA2; MEB) were excluded.

Microcephaly-pachigyria-peripheral neuropathy

Two separate families have been described with this unusual phenotype. In the first one four affected siblings were characterized by congenital hypotonia, severe mental retardation, microcephaly, delayed psychomotor development, generalized muscular wasting and weakness with mild facial involvement, calf pseudohypertrophy and joint contractures. Peripheral nerve studies were consistent with a demyelinating peripheral neuropathy, while brain MRI disclosed pontocerebellar hypoplasia, bilateral opercular abnormalities and focal cortical dysplasia as well as minute periventricular white matter changes. Opthalmological examination was normal and haplotype analysis excluded the FCMD, LAMA2 and MEB disease loci. Merosin expression was normal in the dystrophic muscle biopsy using antibodies against both the 80 and 320 kDa fragments (Ruggieri *et al.* 2001, in press). An almost identical family had been reported in the past (Belpaire-Dethiou *et al.* 1999).

CMD and cataracts

Topaloglu reported three cases in two families with merosin-positive congenital muscular dystrophy, mild mental retardation, bilateral cataracts and normal cranial MRI (Topaloglu *et al.* 1997).

A second family was reported by Reed *et al.* (1999) with cataracts first observed at six months, microcephaly and mild retardation. Brain MRI was normal. CPK was moderately elevated. Merosin was normally expressed in both families.

Three more families with similar features were reported at a recent CMD workshop by Bushby and Merlini (Muntoni and Guicheney 2001). MEB and other CMD loci were excluded in all.

CMD with adducted thumb

This is a rare syndrome characterized by adducted thumbs, weakness and ophthalmoplegia. Kunze *et al.* (1983) reported a female infant who died at the age of three months.

She had bulbar weakness and difficulty in swallowing, ophthalmoplegia, hypotonia, and areflexia. There were multiple joint contractures with camptodactyly and adducted thumbs. More recently, an almost identical family was decribed by Voit at a recent CMD workshop, who reported two siblings with mild mental retardation, and cerebellar hypoplasia with ptosis, ophthalmoplegia, moderate elevation of serum CK and a dystrophic muscle biopsy with normal expression of merosin (Muntoni and Guicheney 2001).

Conclusion

The congenital muscular dystrophies represent a common group of disorders, in which clinical and genetic heterogeneity has only started to be appreciated in the last few years. Since the first two major breakthroughs in 1994, with the discovery of the Fukuyama gene and of merosin deficiency, there have been considerable advances in the classification of these disorders. In addition to the forms that have been mapped, a number of syndromes have been described on the basis of the clinico-pathological findings, and a list of these is provided in Table 2.2. Regarding the pathogenesis of CMD, both laminin α2 and integrin α7 are abundant extracellular matrix proteins. The primary or secondary deficiency of these proteins in a number of CMD forms together with the recent observation of a profound depletion of α-dystroglycan in several forms, provides further evidence for a role of the extracellular matrix. However, preservation of these proteins in several other syndromes (such as RSMD1), suggests that other pathogenetic mechanisms are likely to exist, which will be fully understood only after the genes responsible for these forms have been isolated and characterized.

Acknowledgements

The authors would like to thank all the CMD families that attend the Hammersmith Hospital and Dr. Caroline A. Sewry and Dr. Sue Brown for the immunohistochemical pictures. A significant part of the work mentioned in this chapter was presented by various members of the ENMC–CMD Consortium; we are particularly in debt to Victor Dubowitz, Thomas Voit, Pascale Guicheney, Luciano Merlini and Haluk Topaloglu. The generous support of the Muscular Dystrophy Campaign of Great Britain and Northern Ireland is gratefully acknowledged, together with the EU grant "Myocluster".

Further reading

We recommend the reader interested in a detailed historical review to read the recent manuscript from Tome (1999). An excellent book mainly focused on Fukuyama muscular dystrophy and other CMD syndromes with mental retardation is the one edited by Fukuyama, Osawa and Saito in (1997). The ENMC–CMD Workshop reports will also provide further details on the individual syndromes discussed in this chapter. Details on most of the syndromes reported in this chapter can also be found in the London Neurogenetic database edited by Michael Baraister and Robin Winter, Oxford

Table 2.2 CMD syndromes in which the responsible gene loci have not been identified

Name	Features	Severity	Merosin status
1. Without mental retardation			
Secondary merosin deficiency	Muscle hypertrophy Markedly elevated CK	Variable (severe to moderate)	Reduced
With distal Joint laxity (Ullrich type with normal collagen VI)	Distal joint laxity CK normal	Mild to moderate	Normal
With epidermolysis bullosa	Junctional epidermolysis Bullosa; elevated CK Plectin gene involved in mild and late onset cases	Variable (mostly mild)	Normal
2. With mental retardation			
Walker-Warburg syndrome	Cobblestone lissencephaly Eye dysgenesis; CK $\neq\neq$	Fatal in infancy	Normal
Microcephaly / calf hypertrophy	Cerebellar hypoplasia; megacisterna magna; CK: $\neq\neq$	Inability to walk	Reduced
Microcephaly	Severe mental retardation Normal brain MRI	Inability to walk	Normal
With cerebellar hypoplasia	Isolated cerebellar hypoplasia CK normal or $\neq$	Variable	Normal
Microcephaly, pachigyria, peripheral neuropathy	Pontocerebellar hypoplasia occipital pachigyria	Inability to walk	Reduced
Cerebellar cysts	Cerebellar cysts; CK: $\neq\neq$	Inability to walk	Reduced
With cataracts	Cataracts in the first year of life CK normal, $\neq$ or $\neq\neq$	Ability to walk	Normal
CMD with adducted thumbs	Mental retardation Opthalmoplegia	Ability to walk	Normal

University Press. A recent biochemical review of diseases associated with extracellular matrix defects can be found in Sewry and Muntoni (1999).

References

Allamand, V., Sunada, Y., Salih, M.A., Straub, V., Ozo, C.O., Al Turaiki, M. *et al.* (1997). Mild congenital muscular dystrophy in two patients with an internally deleted laminin alpha2-chain. *Human Molecular Genetics*, **6**, 747–52.

Auranen, M., Rapola, J., Pihko, H., Haltia, M., Leivo, I., Soinila, S. *et al.* (2000). Muscle membrane-skeleton protein changes and histopathological characterization of muscle–eye–brain disease. *Neuromuscular Disorders*, **10**, 16–23.

Belpaire-Dethiou, M.C., Saito, K., Fukuyama, Y., Kondo Iida, E., Toda, T., Duprez, T. *et al.* (1999). Congenital muscular dystrophy with central and peripheral nervous system involvement in a Belgian patient. *Neuromuscular Disorders*, **9**, 251–6.

Brett, F.M., Costigan, D., Farrell, M.A., Heaphy, P., Thornton, J. and King, M.D. (1998). Merosin-deficient congenital muscular dystrophy and cortical dysplasia. *European Journal of Paediatric Neurology*, **2**(2), 77–82.

Brockington, M., Sewry, C.A., Herrmann, R., Naom, I., Dearlove, A., Rhodes *et al.* (2000). Assignment of a form of congenital muscular dystrophy with secondary merosin deficiency to chromosome 1q42. *American Journal of Human Genetics*, **66**(2), 428–35.

Camacho-Vanegas O., Bertini E., Zhang R.Z., Petrini S., Minosse C., Sabatelli P., *et al.* (2000). Ullrich scleroatonic muscular dystrophy is caused by recessive mutations in collagen type VI. *PNAS*, **98**, 7516–21.

Chijiiwa, T., Nishimura, M., Inomata, H. *et al.* (1983). Ocular manifestations of congenital muscular dystrophy (Fukuyama type). *Annals of Ophthalmology*, **15**, 921–8.

Cohn, R.D., Herrmann, R., Wewer, U.M. and Voit, T. (1997). Changes of laminin beta2 chain expression in congenital muscular dystrophy. *Neuromuscular Disorders*, **7**(6–7), 373–8.

Cohn, R.D., Herrmann, R., Sorokin, L., Wewer, U.M. and Voit, T. (1998). Laminin alpha2 chain-deficient congenital muscular dystrophy: variable epitope expression in severe and mild cases. *Neurology*, **51**(1), 94–100.

Cook, J.D., Gascon, G.G., Haider, A. *et al.* (1992). Congenital muscular dystrophy with abnormal radiographic myelin pattern. *Journal of Child Neurology*, suppl. **7**, S51–S63.

Cormand, B., Avela, K., Pihko, H. *et al.* (1999). Assignment of the muscle–eye–brain disease gene to 1p32–p34 by linkage analysis and homozygosity mapping. *American Journal of Human Genetics*, **64**, 126–35.

Dambska, M., Wisniewski, K., Sher, J. and Solish, G. (1982). Cerebro-oculo-muscular syndrome: a variant of Fukuyama congenital cerebromuscular dystrophy. *Clinical Neuropathology*, **1**, 93–8

Dobyns, W.B., Kirkpatrick, J.B., Hittner, H.M. *et al.* (1985). Syndromes with lissencephaly II: Walker–Warburg and cerebro-oculo-muscular syndromes and a new syndrome with type II lissencephaly. *American Journal of Human Genetics*, **22**, 157–95.

Dobyns, W.B., Pagon, R.A., Armstron, D. *et al.* (1989). Diagnostic criteria for Walker–Warburg syndrome. *American Journal of Human Genetics*, **32**, 195–210

Dobyns, W.B. (1993). Classification of the cerebro-oculo-muscular syndrome(s). *Brain & Development* **15**, 242–4.

Dubowitz, V. (1994). 22nd ENMC sponsored workshop on congenital muscular dystrophy held in baarn, the Netherlands, 14–16 may 1993. *Neuromuscular Disorders*, **4**(1), 75–81.

Dubowitz, V. and Fardeau, M. (1995). Proceedings of the 27th ENMC Sponsored Workshop on Congenital Muscular Dystrophy. *Neuromuscular Disorders*, **5**, 253–8.

Dubowitz, V. (1997). 50th ENMC International workshop: congenital muscular dystrophy. 28 February 1997 to 2 March 1997, Naarden, The Netherlands. *Neuromuscular Disorders*, **7**, 539–47.

Dubowitz, V. (1999). 68th ENMC international workshop (5th international workshop): On congenital muscular dystrophy, 9–11 April 1999, Naarden, The Netherlands. *Neuromuscular Disorders*, **9**, 446–54.

Echenne, B., Pages, M. and Marty-Double, C. (1984). Congenital muscular dystrophy with cerebral white matter spongiosis. *Brain Development*, **6**, 491–5.

Echenne, B., Rivier, F., Tardieu, M. *et al.* (1998). Congenital muscular dystrophy and cerebellar atrophy. *Neurology*, **50**, 1477–80.

Engvall, E. (1993). Laminin variants: why, where and when? *Kidney International*, **43**, 2–6.

Flanigan, K.M., Kerr, L., Bromberg, M.B., Leonard, C., Tsuruda, J., Zhang, P. *et al.* (2000). Congenital muscular dystrophy with rigid spine syndrome: a clinical, pathological, radiological, and genetic study. *Annals of Neurology*, **47**(2), 152–61.

Fukuyama, Y., Kawazura, M. and Haruna, H. (1960). A peculiar form of congenital progressive muscular dystrophy. *Pediatria University Tokyo*, **4**, 5–8.

Fukuyama, Y., Osawa, M. and Suzuki, H. (1981). Congenital progressive muscular dystrophy of the Fukuyama type—clinical, genetic and pathological considerations. *Brain & Development*, **3**, 1–29.

Fukuyama, Y., Osawa M. and Saito, K. (eds) (1997). *Congenital muscular dystrophies*, Elsevier, Tokyo.

Guicheney, P., Vignier, N., Zhang, X., He, Y., Cruaud, C., Frey, V. *et al.* (1998). PCR based mutation screening of the laminin alpha2 chain gene (LAMA2): application to prenatal diagnosis and search for founder effects in congenital muscular dystrophy. *Journal of Medical Genetics*, **35**(3), 211–7.

Guicheney, P., Vignier, N., Helbling-Leclerc, A., Nissinen, M., Zhang, X., Cruaud, C. *et al.* (1997). Genetics of laminin alpha2 chain (or merosin) deficient congenital muscular dystrophy: from identification of mutations to prenatal diagnosis. *Neuromuscular Disorders*, **7**(3), 180–6.

Haltia, M., Leivo, I., Somer, H., Pihko, H., Paetau, A., Kivela, T. *et al.* (1997). Muscle–eye–brain disease: a neuropathological study. *Annals of Neurology*, **41**, 173–80.

Hayashi, Y.K., Engvall, E., Arikawa-Hirasawa, E. *et al.* (1993). Abnormal expression of laminin subunits in muscular dystrophies. *Journal of Neurological Sciences*, **119**, 53–64.

Hayashi, Y.K., Chou, F.L., Engvall, E., Ogawa, M., Matsuda, C., Hirabayashi, S. *et al.* (1998). Mutations in the integrin alpha7 gene cause congenital myopathy. *Nature Genetics*, **19**, 94–7.

Herrmann, R., Straub, V., Meyer, K., Kahn, T., Wagner, M. and Voit, T. (1996). Congenital muscular dystrophy with laminin alpha2 chain deficiency: identification of a new intermediate phenotype and correlation of clinical findings to muscle immunohistochemistry. *European Journal of Pediatrics*, **155**(11), 968–76.

Higuchi I., Suehara M., Iwaki H., Nakagawa M., Arimura K., Osame M. (2001). Collagen VI deficiency in Ullrich's disease. *Annals Neurology*, **49**, 544.

Hillaire, D., Leclerc, A., Faure, S., Topaloglu, H., Chiannilkulchai, N., Guicheney, P. *et al.* (1994). Localization of merosin-negative congenital muscular dystrophy to chromosome 6q2 by homozygosity mapping. *Human Molecular Genetics*, **3**(9), 1657–61.

Honda, Y. and Yoshioka, M. (1978). Ophthalmological findings of muscular dystrophies: a survey of 53 cases. *J Pediatr Ophthalmol Strabismus*, **15**, 236–8.

Itoh, M., Houdou, S., Kawahara, H. and Ohama, E. (1996) Morphological study of the brainstem in Fukuyama type congenital muscular dystrophy. *Pediatric Neurology*, **15**, 327–31.

Kamoshita, S., Konishi, Y., Segawa, M. and Fukuyama, Y. (1976) Congenital muscular dystrophy as a disease of the central nervous system. *Archives of Neurology*, **33**, 513–6.

Kletter, G., Evans, O.B., Lee, J.A. *et al.* (1989). Congenital muscular dystrophy and epidermolysis bullosa simplex. *Journal of Pediatrics*, **114**, 104–7.

Knubley, W.A. and Bertorini, T. (1988). Congenital muscular dystrophy with cerebellar atrophy. *Developmental Medicine Child Neurology*, **30**, 378–90.

Kobayashi, K., Nakahori, Y., Miyake, M. *et al.* (1998). An ancient retrotransposal insertion causes Fukuyama-type congenital muscular dystrophy. *Nature*, **394**, 388–92.

Kunze, J., Park, W., Hansen K.H. and Hanefeld F. (1983). Adducted thumb syndrome. Report of a new case and a diagnostic approach. *European Journal of Pediatrics*, **141**: 122–6.

Mahjneh, I., Bushby, K., Anderson, L., Muntoni, F., Tolvanen-Mahjneh, H., Bashir, R. *et al.* (1999). Merosin-positive congenital muscular dystrophy: a large inbred family. *Neuropediatrics*, **30**(1), 22–8.

Matsumura, K., Nonaka, I. and Campbell, K.P. (1993). Abnormal expressions of dystrophin-associated proteins in Fukuyama-type congenital muscular dystrophy. *Lancet*, **341**, 521–2.

Mendell, J.T., Panicker, S.G., Tsao, C.Y., Feng, B., Sahenk, Z., Marzluf, G.A. *et al.* (1998). Novel compound heterozygous laminina2-chain gene (LAMA2) mutations in congenital muscular dystrophy. Mutations in brief no. 159. *Human Mutations*, **12**(2), 135.

Mercuri, E., Berardinelli, A., Philpot, J. and Dubowitz, V. (1995a). Somatosensory and visual evoked potentials in congenital muscular dystrophy: correlation with MRI changes and muscle merosin status. *Neuropediatrics*, **26**, 3–7.

Mercuri, E., Dubowitz, L., Muntoni, F., Berardinelli, A., Pennock, J., Sewry, C. *et al.* (1995b). Minor neurological and perceptuo-motor deficits in children with congenital muscular dystrophy: correlation with brain MRI changes. *Neuropediatrics*, **26**, 156–62.

Mercuri, E., Pennock, J., Goodwin, F., Cowan, F., Sewry, C., Dubowitz, V. *et al.* (1996). Sequential study of central and peripheral nervous system involvement in merosin-deficient CMD. *Neuromuscular Disorders*, **6**, 425–9.

Mercuri, E., Anker, S., Philpot, J., Sewry, C., Dubowitz, V. and Muntoni, F. (1998). Visual function in children with merosin-deficient and merosin-positive congenital muscular dystrophy. *Pediatric Neurology*, **18**(5), 399–401.

Mercuri, E., Gruter-Andrew, J., Philpot, J., Sewry, C., Counsell, S., Henderson, S. *et al.* (1999). Cognitive abilities in children with congenital muscular dystrophy: correlation with brain MRI and merosin status. *Neuromuscular Disorders*, **9**(6–7), 383–7.

Mercuri, E., Sewry, C.A., Brown, S.C., Brockington, M., Jungbluth, H., DeVile, C. *et al.* (2000). Congenital muscular dystrophy with secondary merosin deficiency and normal brain MRI: a novel entity? *Neuropediatrics*, **31**(4), 186–9.

Mercuri, E., Rutherford, M., DeVile, C., Counsell, S., Sewry, C., Brown, S. *et al.* (2001). Early white matter changes on brain Magnetic Resonance Imaging in a newborn affected by merosin-deficient Congenital Muscular Dystrophy. *Neuromuscular Disorders*, **11**, 297–9.

Moghadaszadeh, B., Desguerre, I., Topaloglu, H., Muntoni, F., Pavek, S., Sewry, C. *et al.* (1998). Identification of a new locus for a peculiar form of congenital muscular dystrophy with early rigidity of the spine, on chromosome 1p35–36. *American Journal of Human Genetics*, **62**(6), 1439–45.

Moghadaszadeh, B., Topaloglu, H., Merlini, L., Muntoni, F., Estournet, B., Sewry, C. *et al.* (1999). Genetic heterogeneity of congenital muscular dystrophy with rigid spine syndrome, *Neuromuscular Disorders*, **9**(6–7), 376–82.

Mora, M., Moroni, I., Uziel, G., Di Blasi, C., Barresi, R., Farina, L. *et al.* (1996). Mild clinical phenotype in a 12-year-old boy with partial merosin deficiency and central and peripheral nervous system abnormalities. *Neuromuscular Disorders*, **6**(5), 377–81.

Morandi, L., Di Blasi, C., Farina, L., Sorokin, L., Uziel, G., Azan, G. *et al.* (1999). Clinical correlations in 16 patients with total or partial laminin alpha2 deficiency characterized using antibodies against 2 fragments of the protein. *Archives of Neurology*, **56**(2), 209–15.

Mostacciuolo, M.L., Miorin, M., Martinello, F., Angelini, C., Perini, P. and Trevisan, C.P. (1996). Genetic epidemiology of congenital muscular dystrophy in a sample from north-east Italy. *Human Genetics*, **97**(3), 277–9.

Mukoyama, M., Sobue, I. and Kumagai, T. (1979). The brain pathology in Fukuyama type congenital muscular dystrophy-CT and autopsy findings. *Japanese Journal of Medicine*, **18**, 218–22.

Muntoni, F., Sewry, C., Wilson, L., Angelini, C., Trevisan, C.P., Brambati, B. *et al.* (1995). Prenatal diagnosis in congenital muscular dystrophy [letter]. *Lancet*, **345**(8949), 591.

Muntoni, F., Taylor, J., Sewry, C.A., Naom, I. and Dubowitz, V. (1998). An early onset muscular dystrophy with diaphragmatic involvement, early respiratory failure and secondary alpha2 laminin deficiency unlinked to the LAMA2 locus on 6q22. *European Journal of Paediatric Neurology*, **2**(1), 19–26.

Muntoni, F. and Sewry, C.A. (1998b). Congenital muscular dystrophy: from rags to riches. *Neurology*, **51**, 14–6.

Muntoni, F. and Guicheney, P. 85th ENMC international workshop (6th international CMD workshop): On congenital muscular dystrophy, 9–11 April 1999, Naarden, The Netherlands. *Neuromuscular Disorders* (in press).

Naom, I.S., D'Alessandro, M., Topaloglu, H., Sewry, C., Ferlini, A., Helbling-Leclerc, A. *et al.* (1997a). Refinement of the laminin alpha2 chain locus to human chromosome 6q2 in severe and mild merosin-deficient congenital muscular dystrophy. *Journal of Medical Genetics*, **34**(2), 99–104.

Naom, I., D'Alessandro, M., Sewry, C., Ferlini, A., Topaloglu, H., Helbling-Leclerc *et al.* (1997b). The role of immunocytochemistry and linkage analysis in the prenatal diagnosis of merosin-deficient congenital muscular dystrophy, *Human Genetics*, **99**(4), 535–40.

Naom, I., D'Alessandro, M., Sewry, C.A., Philpot, J., Manzur, A.Y., Dubowitz, V. *et al.* (1998). Laminin alpha2-chain gene mutations in two siblings presenting with limb-girdle muscular dystrophy, *Neuromuscular Disorders*, **8**(7), 495–501.

Naom, I., D'Alessandro, M., Sewry, C.A., Jardine, P., Ferlini, A., Moss, T. *et al.* (2000). Mutations in the laminin alpha2-chain gene in two children with early-onset muscular dystrophy. *Brain*, **123**(1), 31–41.

Nissinen, M., Helbling-Leclerc, A., Zhang, X., Evangelista, T., Topaloglu, H., Cruaud, C. *et al.* (1996). Substitution of a conserved cysteine-996 in a cysteine-rich motif of the laminin alpha2-chain in congenital muscular dystrophy with partial deficiency of the protein. *American Journal of Human Genetics*, **58**(6), 1177–84.

Nonaka, I., Une, Y., Ishihara, T., Miyoshino, S., Nakashima, T. and Sugita, H. (1981). A clinical and histological study of Ullrich's disease (congenital atonic-sclerotic muscular dystrophy). *Neuropediatrics*, **12**, 197–208.

Pegoraro, E., Mancias, P., Swerdlow, S.H., Raikow, R.B., Garcia, C., Marks, H. *et al.* (1996). Congenital muscular dystrophy with primary laminin alpha2 (merosin) deficiency presenting as inflammatory myopathy. *Annals of Neurology*, **40**(5), 782–91.

Pegoraro, E., Marks, H., Garcia, C.A. Crawford, T., Mancias, P., Connolly, A.M. *et al.* (1998 Laminin alpha2 muscular dystrophy: genotype/phenotype studies of 22 patients. *Neurology*, **51**(1), 101–10.

Pegoraro, E., Fanin, P.M., Trevisan, C.P., Angelini, C. and Hoffman, E.P. (2000). A novel laminin alpha2 isoform in severe laminin alpha2 deficient congenital muscular dystrophy. *Neurology*, **55**(8), 1128–34.

Philpot, J., Sewry, C., Pennock, J. and Dubowitz, V. (1995a). Clinical phenotype in congenital muscular dystrophy: correlation with expression of merosin in skeletal muscle. *Neuromuscular Disorders*, **5**, 301–5.

Philpot, J., Topaloglu, H., Pennock, J. and Dubowitz, V. (1995b). Familial concordance of brain magnetic resonance imaging changes in congenital muscular dystrophy. *Neuromuscular Disorders*, **5**, 227–31.

Philpot, J., Cowan, F., Pennock, J., Sewry, C., Dubowitz, V., Bydder, G. *et al.* (1999b). Merosin-deficient congenital muscular dystrophy: the spectrum of brain involvement on magnetic resonance imaging. *Neuromuscular Disorders*, **9**(2), 81–5.

Philpot, J. and Muntoni, F. (1999a). Limitation of eye movement in merosin-deficient congenital muscular dystrophy [letter]. *Lancet*, **353**(9149), 297–8.

Philpot, J., Bagnall, A., King, C., Dubowitz, V. and Muntoni, F. (1999a). Feeding problems in merosin-deficient congenital muscular dystrophy. *Archives of Disease in Childhood*, **80**(6); 542–7.

Pini, A., Merlini, L., Tome, F.M., Chevallay, M. and Gobbi, G. (1996). Merosin-negative congenital muscular dystrophy, occipital epilepsy with periodic spasms and focal cortical dysplasia. Report of three Italian cases in two families. *Brain Development*, **18**(4), 316–22.

Pulkkinen, L., Smith, F.J., Shimizu, H., Murata, S., Yaoita, H., Hachisuka, H. *et al.* (1996) Homozygous deletion mutations in the plectin gene (PLEC1) in patients with epidermolysis bullosa simplex associated with late-onset muscular dystrophy. *Human Molecular Genetics*, **5**, 1539–46.

Raitta, C., Lamminen, M., Santavuori, P. and Leisti, J. (1978). Ophthalmological findings in a new syndrome with muscle, eye, and brain involvement. *Acta Ophthamologica*, **56**, 465–72.

Reed, U.C., Tsanaclis, A.M., Vainzof, M., Marie, S.K., Carvalho, M.S. and Roizenblatt, J. (1999). Merosin-positive congenital muscular dystrophy in two siblings with cataract and slight mental retardation. *Brain & Development*, **21**, 274–8.

Ruggieri, V., Lubieniecki, F., Diaz, D., Ferragut, E., Saito, K., Fukuyama, Y. *et al.* Merosin positive congenital muscular dystrophy with mental retardation, microcephaly and brain abnormalities not linked to Fukutin gene. Report of 3 siblings. *Neuromuscular Disorders* (in press).

Santavuori, P., Leisti, J., Kruus, S. and Raitta, C. (1977). Muscle, eye and brain disease: a new syndrome. *Documenta Ophthalmologica*, **17**, 393–6.

Santavuori, P., Leisti, J. and Kruus, S. (1978). Muscle, eye and brain disease: a new syndrome. *Neuropädiatrie*, **8**, 553–8.

Santavuori, P., Somer, H., Sainio, K. *et al.* (1989). Muscle-eye-brain disease (MEB). *Brain & Development*, **11**, 147–53.

Sewry, C.A., Philpot, J., Mahony, D., Wilson, L.A., Muntoni, F. and Dubowitz, V. (1995). Expression of laminin subunits in congenital muscular dystrophy. *Neuromuscular Disorders*, **5**(4), 307–16.

Sewry, C.A., Naom, I., D'Alessandro, M., Ferlini, A., Philpot, J., Mercuri, E. *et al.* (1996). The protein defect in congenital muscular dystrophy. *Biochemistry Society Transactions*, **24**(2), 281S.

Sewry, C.A., D'Alessandro, M., Wilson, L.A., Sorokin, L.M., Naom, I., Bruno, S. *et al.* (1997a). Expression of laminin chains in skin in merosin-deficient congenital muscular dystrophy. *Neuropediatrics*, **28**(4), 217–22.

Sewry, C.A., Naom, I., D'Alessandro, M., Sorokin, L., Bruno, S., Wilson, L.A. *et al.* (1997b). Variable clinical phenotype in merosin-deficient congenital muscular dystrophy associated with differential immunolabelling of two fragments of the laminin alpha2 chain. *Neuromuscular Disorders*, **7**(3), 169–75.

Sewry, C.A. and Muntoni, F. (1999). Invited review: Inherited disorders of the extracellular matrix. *Current Opinion in Neurology*, **12**, 519–26.

Shorer, Z., Philpot, J., Muntoni, F., Sewry, C. and Dubowitz, V. (1995). Demyelinating peripheral neuropathy in merosin-deficient congenital muscular dystrophy. *Journal of Child Neurology*, **10**(6), 472–5.

Simonds, A.K., Ward, S., Heather, S., Bush, A. and Muntoni, F. (2000). Outcome of paediatric domiciliary mask ventilation in neuromuscular and skeletal disease. *European Respiratory Journal*, **16**, 476–81.

Spyrou, N., Philpot, J., Foale, R., Camici, P.G. and Muntoni, F. (1998). Evidence of left ventricular dysfunction in children with merosin-deficient congenital muscular dystrophy. *American Heart Journal*, **136**(3), 474–6.

Sunada, Y., Edgar, T.S., Lotz, B.P., Rust, R.S. and Campbell, K.P. (1995). Merosin-negative congenital muscular dystrophy associated with extensive brain abnormalities. *Neurology*, **45**(11), 2084–9.

Takada, K., Nakamura, H. and Tanaka, J. (1984). Cortical dysplasia in congenital muscular dystrophy with central nervous system involvement (Fukuyama type). *Journal of Neuropathology Experimental Neurology*, **43**, 395–407.

Talim, B., Ferreiro, A., Cormand, B., Vignier, N., Oto, A, Gogus, S. *et al.* (2000). Merosin-deficient congenital muscular dystrophy with mental retardation and cerebellar cysts unlinked to the LAMA2, FCMD and MEB loci. *Neuromuscular Disorders*, **10**, 548–52.

Tan, E., Topaloglu, H., Sewry, C., Zorlu, Y., Naom, I., Erdem, S. *et al.* (1997). Late onset muscular dystrophy with cerebral white matter changes due to partial merosin deficiency. *Neuromuscular Disorders*, **7**(2), 85–9.

Taratuto, A.L., Lubieniecki, F., Diaz, D., Schultz, M., Ruggieri, V., Saccoliti, M. and Dubrovsky, A. (1999). Merosin-deficient congenital muscular dystrophy associated with abnormal cerebral cortical gyration: an autopsy study. *Neuromuscular Disorders*, **9**(2), 86–94.

Toda, T., Segawa, M., Nomura, Y. *et al.* (1993). Localization of a gene for Fukuyama type congenital muscular dystrophy to chromosome 9q31–33. *Nature Genetics*, **5**, 283–6.

Tome, F.M., Evangelista, T., Leclerc, A., Sunada, Y., Manole, E., Estournet, B. *et al.* (1994). Congenital muscular dystrophy with merosin deficiency. *C.R. Acad. Sci. III*, **317**(4), 351–7.

Tome, F.M. (1999). The Peter Emil Becker Award lecture 1998. The saga of congenital muscular dystrophy. *Neuropediatrics*, **30**(2), 55–65.

Topaloglu, H., Yetuk, M., Talim, B., Akcoren, Z. and Caglar, M. (1997). Merosin-positive congenital muscular dystrophy with mental retardation and cataracts: a new entity in two families. *European Journal of Paediatric Neurology*, **1**, 127–31.

Topaloglu, H., Talim, B., Vignier, N. *et al.* (1998). Merosin-deficient congenital muscular dystrophy with severe mental retardation and normal cranial MRI: a report of two siblings. *Neuromuscular Disorders*, **8**, 169–74.

Towfighi, J., Sassani, J.W., Suzuki, K. and Ladda, R.L. (1984). Cerebro-ocular dysplasia-muscular dystrophy (COD-MD) syndrome. *Acta Neuropathologica (Berl)*, **65**, 110–23.

Vachon, P.H. and Beaulieu, J.F. (1995). Extracellular heterotrimeric laminin promotes differentiation in human enterocytes. *American Journal of Physiology*, **268**, G857–67.

Villanova, M., Sabatelli, P., He, Y., Malandrini, A., Petrini, S., Maraldi, N.M. *et al.* (1998). Immunofluorescence study of a muscle biopsy from a 1-year-old patient with Walker-Warburg syndrome. *Acta Neuropatholica (Berl)*, **96**, 651–4.

Villanova, M., Sewry, C., Malandrini, A., Toti, P., Muntoni, F., Merlini, L. *et al.* (1997). Immunolocalization of several laminin chains in the normal human central and peripheral nervous system. *J Submicr Cytol Pathol.*, **29**(3), 409–13.

Villanova, M., Mercuri, E., Bertini, E., Sabatelli, P., Morandi, L., Mora, M. *et al.* (2000). Congenital muscular dystrophy associated with calf hypertrophy, microcephaly and severe mental retardation: A new CMD syndrome. *Neuromuscular Disorders*, **1**(10): 541–7.

Voit, T. (1998). Congenital muscular dystrophies: 1997 update. *Brain & Development*, **20**(2), 65–74.

Voit, T., Fardeau, M. and Tome, F.M. (1994). Prenatal detection of merosin expression in human placenta [letter]. *Neuropediatrics*, **25**(6), 332–3.

Voit, T., Sewry, C.A., Meyer, K., Herman, R., Straub, V., Muntoni, F. *et al.* (1995). Preserved merosin M-chain (or laminin-α2) expression in skeletal muscle distinguishes Walker–Warburg syndrome from Fukuyama muscular dystrophy and merosin-deficient congenital muscular dystrophy. *Neuropediatrics*, **26**, 148–55.

Vuolteenaho, R., Nissinen, M., Sainio, K., Byers, M., Eddy, R. and Hirvonen, H. (1994). Human laminin M chain (merosin): complete primary structure, chromosomal assignment, and expression of the M and A chain in human fetal tissues. *Journal of Cellular Biology*, **124**(3), 381–94.

Walker, A.E. (1942). Lissencephaly. *Archive of Neurology and Psychiatry*, **48**, 13–29.

Yoshioka, M., Okuno, T., Nakano, Y. and Honda, Y. (1980). Computed tomography in congenital muscular dystrophy (Fukuyama type). *Prog Computed Tomography*, **2**, 341–8.

Yoshioka, M., Kuroki, S. and Kondo, T. (1990). Ocular manifestations in Fukuyama type congenital muscular dystrophy. *Brain & Development*, **12**, 423–6.

Yoshioka, M., Saiwai, S., Kuroki, S. and Nigami, H. (1991). MR imaging of the brain in Fukuyama-type congenital muscular dystrophy. *American Journal of Neuroradiology*, **12**, 63–5.

Chapter 3

Fukuyama congenital muscular dystrophy

Kayoko Saito and Makio Kobayashi

History

The first report on 15 cases of Fukuyama congenital muscular dystrophy (FCMD) was published in 1960 entitled 'A peculiar form of congenital progressive muscular dystrophy' by Fukuyama *et al.* (1960). The majority of such patients reported at that time had been treated at other institutions under an incorrect diagnosis of cerebral palsy or multiple neurological handicaps. Fukuyama *et al.* explored a different diagnosis on the basis of the following: there was no sign of spasticity or increased muscle tone; deep tendon reflexes were absent or reduced; and, muscle resistance against passive movement was always reduced. The patients were submitted for electromyography, muscle biopsy with histochemical staining and analysis of serum creatine kinase (CK) activities, a method developed only in the late 1950s. From this, Fukuyama *et al.* (1960) clearly demonstrated that the skeletal muscle of these patients showed progressive muscular dystrophy.

Fukuyama congenital muscular dystrophy was accepted as an entity by many Japanese investigators following this first report (Fukuyama *et al.* 1981; Kamoshita *et al.* 1975; Nonaka and Chou 1979), but not internationally as the prevalence of FCMD outside of Japan is extremely low. FCMD was first registered under the OMIM number 253800 in the 7th edition of McKusick 'Mendelian Inheritance in Man' in 1986. Subsequently, it was included formally as an independent subtype of muscular dystrophy in the 10th revision of the Neurological Adaptation of the International Classification of Diseases (ICD-10) published by the World Health Organization (WHO) in 1991 (G71.084). The World Federation of Neurology Research Committees on Neuromuscular Diseases also supported a similar subdivision of CMD in 1991 (G71-74, I) (Walton 1991). In this sense, an official recognition as an independent disease was given to FCMD shortly before. In the ICD-10, CMD is divided into two categories: CMD with central nervous system (CNS) abnormalities (Fukuyama), CMD without CNS abnormalities. Walker–Warburg syndrome (WWS) (Dobyns *et al.* 1985; 1989) and Muscle–Eye–Brain disease (MEBD) (Raitta *et al.* 1978; Santavuori and Leisti 1977) are also categorized as CMD with CNS, the characteristics of which are summarized in Table 3.1.

Table 3.1 Classification of CMD with CNS abnormalities

Subtype	Mental retardation	Muscle dystrophy	PNS abnormality	CNS anomalies			Eye anomalies	Gene locus
				WM	GM	CV		
FCMD	+	+ +	–	+	+ +	±	±	9q31
MEBD	+ +	+	–	+	+ + (Giant VEP)	+ +	+ +	1p32–p34
WWS	+ +	+	–	+ +	+ +	+ +	+ +	?

FCMD, Fukuyama congenital muscular dystrophy; MEBD, Muscle–Eye–Brain disease;
WWS, Walker–Warburg syndrome; PNS, peripheral nervous system;
CNS, central nervous system; WM, white matter; GM, gray matter; CV, cerebellar vermis;
VEP, visual evoked potential.

Recently, Toda *et al.* (1993) localized the FCMD gene to chromosome 9q31–q33 by genetic linkage analyses using 6 polymorphic microsatellite markers. The analysis involved 21 Japanese families, of which 13 were consanguineous parental marriages. A hint as to the gene location was provided by a FCMD patient from a consanguineous family, which was also affected with group A xeroderma pigmentosum (XP), the gene for which is localized to chromosome 9q34.1. As no other siblings were affected with either FCMD or XP, Toda *et al.* (1993) attributed the co-existence of FCMD and group A XP to homozygosity by descent in this individual. The most probable location of the FCMD gene was proposed to lie within a 7.7 CM interval between loci D9S58 and D9S59. Subsequently, the FCMD gene was localized within a region of ~5 CM between D9S127 and D9S2111 (CA246) (Toda *et al.* 1994), based on homozygosity mapping in patients born to consanguineous parents and recombination mapping analysis in other families. Linkage disequilibrium was also demonstrated between FCMD alleles and D9S306 (mfd220), which is located within a few hundred kilobases (kb) of the FCMD candidate gene region. Furthermore, new microsatellites flanking the gene were developed (Miyake *et al.* 1997; Toda *et al.* 1994; 1996). Haplotype analysis using markers closest to the gene showed that most FCMD-bearing chromosomes are derived from a single ancestral founder (Kobayashi *et al.* 1998a). The FCMD gene was cloned and the gene product was named 'fukutin' (Kobayashi *et al.* 1998b). A 3-kb retrotransposonal insertion was implicated as the founding mutation of the FCMD gene. These advances in genetic analysis have facilitated the accurate and consistent diagnosis of FCMD (Kondo-Iida *et al.* 1997a,b; 1999; Saito *et al.* 1998; 2000).

Clinical features

The clinical characteristics of FCMD according to the original description (Fukuyama *et al.* 1960) are as follows:

1. Early onset, usually before nine months

2. Hypotonia and weakness in early infancy

3. Later development of muscle wasting and joint contractures

4. Muscle involvement is diffuse and extensive, but most prominent proximally

5. Myopathic facies in nearly all cases, pseudohypertrophy present in half of cases

6. Mental and speech retardation in nearly all cases, febrile or afebrile convulsions in half of cases

7. EMG, CK and muscle biopsy findings characteristic of muscular dystrophy

8. Course is either slowly progressive or stationary

9. Autosomal recessive inheritance

FCMD is now classified into the following three clinical types, according to the patients' maximum motor abilities. (1) *The typical type* is assigned to patients who are able to sit unassisted or to slide on the buttocks (level 2–4) (Okawa and Ueda 1997) (Fig. 3.1a–e); (2) *The mild type* is assigned to patients who can stand or walk with or without support (level 5–8); and (3) *The severe type* is classified as patients who can sit only with support or with no head control (level 0–1). This classification was supported by haplotype analysis, which is described later.

The symptoms of FCMD are characterized basically by dystrophic changes in the skeletal muscle and CNS migration disturbances, including cerebral and cerebellar cortical dysplasia. The clinical features are recognized as psychomotor retardation with hypotonia and weakness. Figure 3.2 shows the motor ability level in 120 patients with FCMD, including all three types and an indication of haplotype analysis. Sixty-six (55 per cent) out of 120 were typical type, 31 (25 per cent) were mild type and 23 (20 per cent) were severe type.

Disease onset is not clear. Initial symptoms may include weak fetal movements in pregnancy, poor sucking, a mildly weak cry and floppiness. Symmetrical and generalized muscle weakness and hypotonia are noticed in early infancy. Poor weight gain has been noted in some patients, as has some limitation of hip abduction. In the typical case of FCMD, sitting without help or sliding along the floor on the buttocks is regarded as the peak motor function. Limitation of hip extension and abduction, as well as knee extension is also observed. Hyperextensibility of the joint is evident in the shoulders, wrists, elbows and trunk. Physical examination may reveal double folding (Fig. 3.1b), loose shoulder (Fig. 3.1c) and heel to ear sign. 'Puffy' cheeks, and pseudohypertrophy of the calves and forearms is evident in late infancy. Muscle consistency is classified as hard and as having a somewhat fibrous texture. Deep tendon reflexes are diminished or are absent after early infancy. Facial muscle involvement (myopathic facies) is obvious from 6 to 12 months of age (Osawa *et al.* 1997). The degree of limitation of joint movement and a myopathic face increase in severity with age. Open mouth, prognathism and macroglossia become discernible in childhood.

The characteristic CNS symptoms of FCMD include mental developmental delay (IQ range is usually 30–60) and speech delay. Figure 3.3 shows a correlation between

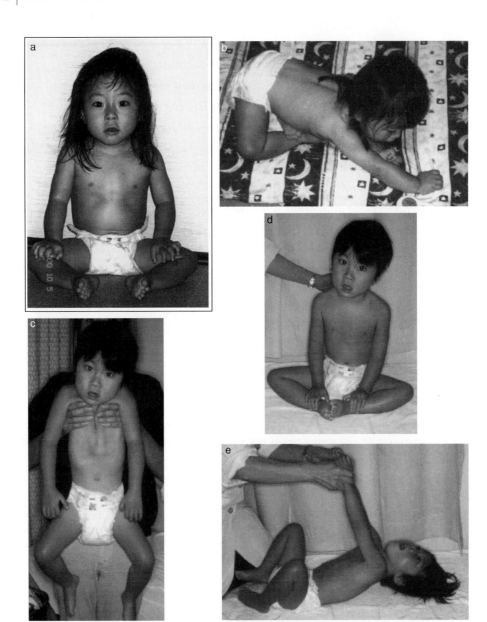

Fig. 3.1 Clinical features of the typical type of FCMD. (a) A 3 years and 3 months old girl could maintain a sitting posture in a cross-legged position. She could move around and slide on her buttocks (level 4). No remarkable muscle atrophy was present at this age except in the chest on examination. The cheeks are rounded. The tendency to keep the mouth open is noted. (b) The same patient as in (a). She showed double folding. (c) A 3 years and 5 months old boy was lifted up and showed loose shoulder. Muscle atrophy is noted in the shoulder and chest. Skin in the patellar area appears shiny. Joint contracture in the knee joint is noted. (d) The same patient as in (c). He maintained his sitting posture in a cross-legged position. The cheeks are rounded. The tendency to keep the mouth open is noted. Pseudohypertrophy of the calf muscles was evident. (e) The same patient as in (c) and (d). Head lag and elbow extension was evident with traction.

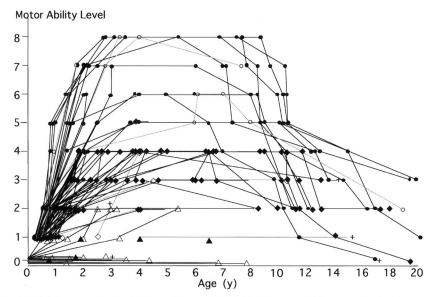

Motor Ability Level

Age (y)

Fig. 3.2 A follow-up study of 120 patients with FCMD. (a)●; ○ mild type,◆; ◇ typical type, ▲; △ severe type. Closed markers indicate the patients with homozygosity of the founding mutation in the FCMD gene; open markers indicate the patients who were heterozygote for the founding mutation in the FCMD gene. +; Deceased

The ordinate indicates motor ability level, as follows: Level 0, no neck control; 1, neck control; 2, unsupported squatting; 3, turning around; 4, moving around the floor by shuffling in a squatting posture; 5, standing by clutching; 6, gait by clutching or by hand-holding; 7, independent gait; 8, independent stair climbing.

intellectual ability and motor ability in FCMD patients. Mild type patients have an IQ of more than 35, whereas the IQ in severe type of FCMD was less than 30. Children with FCMD behave well and therefore tend to be the favourites in a nursery, kindergarten or a primary school. Even in a severe case, an FCMD patient shows eye contact, recognition of the mother and vocalization for demands. Figure 3.4 shows that social development of FCMD patients is not severely affected in comparison to physical and mental factors. An autistic tendency is not observed in FCMD patients. The typical FCMD cases can speak dozens of words.

The prevalence of seizures in FCMD patients is over 50 per cent (Osawa *et al.* 1997), with the median age of seizure onset being one year. In nearly 80 per cent of children with seizures, the seizure disorders manifest between the ages of 1 and 3 years or after age 6 years.

Ocular abnormalities observed with FCMD include disturbance of visual acuity, retinal abnormality and anterior chamber abnormality (Osawa *et al.* 1997; Tsutsumi *et al.* 1989). The opthalmologic manifestations observed in FCMD are shown in Table 3.2. Disturbance of visual acuity, including myopia and hypermetropia, was observed in all

Table 3.2 Ophthalmological manifestations of FCMD compared with Walker–Warburg syndrome (WWS)

Ophthalmological manifestations	FCMD			WWS
	mild type	typical type	severe type	Dobyns, 1997
	n=6	n=15	n=7	
Disturbance of visual acuity	4	5	6	
Severe myopia	0	0	1	3/5
Mild myopia	3	3	4	
Hypermetropia	1	2	1	
Retinal abnormality	1	4	6	32/32
Microphthalmia	0	0	1	15/36
Retinal dysplasia	1	3	5	10/23
Retinal hypoplasia (or abnormal ERG)	1	2	6	11/23
Optic nerve hypoplasia	0	1	2	20/21
Colobomas	0	0	0	3/8
Anterior chamber abnormality	1	0	3	29/38
Glaucoma	0	0	0	13/26
Angle abnormality	0	0	0	16/26
Cornea-iris-lens abnormalities	0	0	1	16/30
Cataract	0	0	3	16/28
Pupil abnormalities	0	0	0	14/24
Hyaloid abnormalities	1	0	2	12/15

three types, whereas the incidence of retinal abnormality and anterior chamber abnormality increases with the severity of the disease. One patient with severe type FCMD, who was diagnosed by DNA analysis, showed severe ocular anomalies, including microphthalmia, retinal detachment, retinal hypoplasia and cataracts, which are regarded as hallmarks of WWS or MEBD.

Fukuyama congenital muscular dystrophy children have serum creatine kinase (CK) levels 10–60 times higher than the normal range. After 6 years of age, serum CK decreases with age. A bed-ridden patient showed normal CK values.

Magnetic resonance imaging analysis of the brain revealed gyral abnormalities of a milder degree in mild cases, mild ventricular dilatation, delayed myelination but no brain stem hypoplasia (Fig. 3.5a,b). In severe cases, progressive hydrocephalus requiring a shunt operation can be observed. MRI or CT scan showed a severe degree of gyral abnormality, ventricular dilatation and brain stem hypoplasia (Fig. 3.5c) as characteristic features in severe cases (Kato *et al.* 1998). Aida *et al.* (1994) demonstrated cerebellar polymicrogyria and the presence of cerebellar cysts related to the polymicrogyria in 23 of 25 patients with CMD. These changes on MRI are distinctive enough to confer the radiological diagnosis of this disorder.

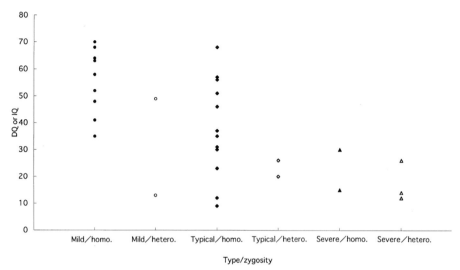

Fig. 3.3 Intellectual ability indicated by DQ or IQ in each type and showing the zygosity of the ancestral founder haplotype in FCMD. We classified the FCMD as mild (●, ○), typical (◆, ◇) and severe (▲, △) type according to the patients' maximum motor abilities.

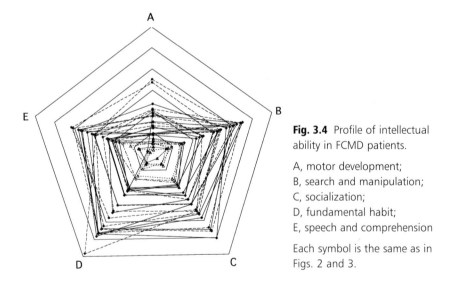

Fig. 3.4 Profile of intellectual ability in FCMD patients.

A, motor development;
B, search and manipulation;
C, socialization;
D, fundamental habit;
E, speech and comprehension

Each symbol is the same as in Figs. 2 and 3.

Pathology

Skeletal muscle pathology

Characteristic findings of FCMD muscle pathology are increased endo-, peri- and epimysial connective and fatty tissues, loss of basic muscle architecture and decreased muscle fibre numbers. Dystrophic changes are milder in early infancy than in older

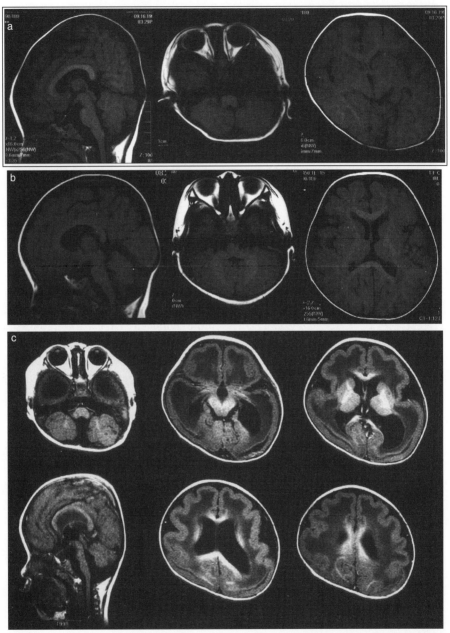

Fig. 3.5 A T1-weighted MRI of the brain. (a) 1y0m-old boy with typical FCMD. The scan showed pachygyria, including a thickened cortex and wide Sylvian fissures, giving the surface of the brain a smooth appearance. Wide gyri were observed in frontal and temporal regions. The pons, cerebellum and brain stem were not thin. (b) 0y9m-old girl with a mild type of FCMD. Gyral abnormalities were milder than those of Fig. 5a. Multiple small cysts were noted in the cerebellar hemispheres. (c) 1y2m-old boy with a severe type of FCMD. Marked pachygyria and agyria were noted in frontal, temporal and occipital regions. Heterotopia, which is observed as double cortex was identified. Cerebellar vermis, pons and brain stem hypoplasia were observed.

patients. We studied the fetal muscles of an FCMD patient who was diagnosed at 14, 17, 18 and 20 weeks gestation by haplotype analysis, and no dystrophic changes, degenerating or necrosing fibres were observed. Takada *et al.* (1987) found no evidence of dystrophic changes in the fetal muscles at 23 weeks gestation. Arahata group showed that skeletal muscle in FCMD patients exhibited a higher percentage of fibres that were immunostained abnormally for both dystrophin and spectrin (Arikawa *et al.* 1991), and for β-dystroglycan (Arahata *et al.* 1993). A dramatic reduction in laminin α2 was observed in FCMD as demonstrated by immunostaining, compared to control levels (Hayashi *et al.* 1993; 1997). These results suggest instability of the membrane cytoskeleton in the tissue of FCMD patients.

Brain Pathology (Nakano *et al.* 1996; Saito Y *et al.* 2000; Takada *et al.* 1987; Yamamoto *et al.* 1996; 1997a,b,c)
Morphological features in the CNS have been described for FCMD, and the neuropathological differences between FCMD and WWS have been discussed (Kimura *et al.* 1993; Takada *et al.* 1987). The main neuropathology is type II lissencephaly, recently termed cobblestone lissencephaly, as well as cerebellar malformations. Infant cases can show extensive areas with a lissencephalic appearance over the surface of the cerebral hemispheres, a feature which is even more prominent in the temporal lobes. In other areas, the micropolygyric pattern is frequently noted over the cortical surface of the parieto-occipital lobes (Fig. 3.6a). In the juvenile and adult cases, the agyric areas are more focal and restricted to the occipital lobes. Lissencephalic or agyric areas of malformed cortex may alternate with polymicrogyric regions, based on fusion of gyri (Fig. 3.6b) and excessive migration of glio-mesenchymal tissue extending into the subarachnoid space.

Noticeable cortical dysplasia, resembling a verrucous nodule, has even been noted on the medial aspect of the occipital and temporal lobes in a fetal case of 17 weeks gestational age. It is assumed that abnormal glio-mesenchymal interactions may contribute to the excessive neuronal migration through the breached glia limitans and finally result in the cortical dysplasia (Saito *et al.* 1998). Thus, the overmigration of CNS parenchyma into subarachnoid spaces is considered an essential pathological process resulting in cortical dysplasia.

In the cerebellum in FCMD, the cortex is also malformed even in the prenatal stage. We recently observed a patient who had a malformed or flat ventral surface of the medulla due to secondary hypoplasia accounting for the small basis of the pons, and the grooves of the spinal cord.

Eye pathology (Hino *et al.* 2001)
Pathological lesions noted in the eyes of FCMD cases are complex, most frequently evident as unilateral microphthalmia. Aside from retinal detachment, retinal pathology comprises either lack/loss of photoreceptors and retinal atrophy, or severe reduction/absence of ganglion cells in the inner retina with or without reduced retinal vasculature and dysplastic rosettes. Focal loss of outer retinal neurons may follow

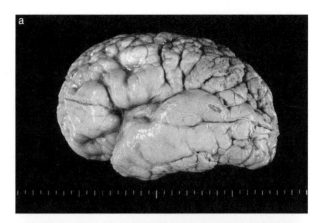

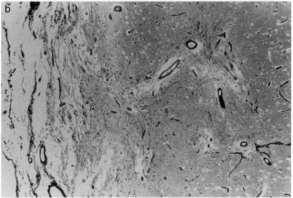

Fig. 3.6 Pathology of the cerebrum from 2y10m-old boy with severe type of FCMD. (a) Macroscopic appearance of the cerebrum of a 2y10 m-old boy with the severe type of FCMD. The cortical surface had a cobblestone appearance in the frontal lobe, a micropolygyric pattern in the parieto-occipital lobes and pachygyria or agyria in the temporal lobe. (b) Microscopically, polymicrogyric regions were noted, based on fusion of gyri and excessive migration of gliomesenchymal tissue extending into the subarachnoid space.

retrograde transneuronal degeneration in fetal life. Even in a fetal case, local folding and fusion of the retina may be observed. It is conceivable that Müller cells are implicated in the retinal pathology of FCMD.

Genetics

According to the original description, parental consanguinity was present in six out of 15 families. Judging from the high incidence of consanguineous parental marriage and sib recurrence and the absence of gender preference and vertical transmission, an autosomal recessive heredity was proposed as the most likely mode of inheritance of this disease. Detailed pedigree analyses supported this theory (Fukuyama and Ohsawa 1984; Osawa 1978) and demonstrated that the segregation ratio in sibships of 153 FCMD families did not deviate significantly from 0.25. Thus, FCMD is recognized as an autosomal recessive genetic disorder. FCMD is second in prevalence only to Duchenne type (DMD) among all subtypes of childhood progressive muscular dystrophy (PMD) in

Japan, although it is seldom reported outside of Japan. In the cohort of 337 cases of PMD followed at our paediatric neuromuscular clinic over 23 years (1971–1994), DMD and CMD accounted for 50.2 per cent (169 cases) and 35.3 per cent (117 cases) of cases, respectively (Fukuyama 1997). Based on data obtained from a recent nation-wide multi-institutional study, the annual incidence of FCMD in Japan is in the range of 1.92×10^{-5} to 3.68×10^{-5} live births (Osawa *et al.* 1997).

The founding mutation is believed to have originated in the Japanese population 100 generations (2000–2500 years) ago (Kobayashi *et al.* 1998a). Due to the apparently high consanguinity at that time, FCMD carriers with a single FCMD mutation have spread throughout Japan over time. At present, the carrier frequency is estimated at approximately one per cent of the Japanese population (Fukuyama and Ohsawa 1984; Osawa 1978).

Molecular basis and pathogenesis

Molecular genetic analyses have been conducted recently to elucidate the pathogenesis of FCMD. Since the mapping of the gene to chromosome 9q31–q33 in 1993 (Toda *et al.* 1993), new microsatellites flanking the gene have been developed (Miyake *et al.* 1997; Toda *et al.* 1994; 1996). Haplotype analysis using markers closest to the gene has shown that most of the FCMD gene-bearing chromosomes are derived from a single ancestral founder (Kobayashi *et al.* 1998a). A 3062 base pairs (bp) retrotransposonal insertion was detected as the founding mutation of the FCMD gene.

To establish a genotype–phenotype correlation, Saito *et al.* (2000) used microsatellite markers closest to the FCMD gene for haplotype analysis of 56 Japanese families, including 35 families whose children were diagnosed as FCMD with a typical pheno-type, 12 families with a mild phenotype, and nine families with a severe phenotype. Of the 12 probands with the mild phenotype, eight could walk and the other four could stand with support; 10 cases were homozygous for the ancestral founder haplotype, whereas the other two were heterozygous for the haplotype. Of the nine severe cases who lacked head control or the ability to sit without support, three had progressive hydrocephalus, two required a shunt operation, and seven showed ophthalmologic abnormalities. Haplotype analysis showed that eight of the nine cases of the severe phenotype were heterozygous for the ancestral founder haplotype and one case was homozygous for the haplotype. It was confirmed that at least one chromosome in each of the 56 FCMD patients had the ancestral founder haplotype. The frequency of heterozygosity for this haplotype was significantly higher in severe cases than in typical or mild cases ($p < 0.005$). Severe FCMD patients appeared to be compound heterozy-gotes for the founding mutation and another mutation. Kondo-Iida *et al.* (1999) undertook a systematic analysis of the FCMD gene in 107 unrelated patients and iden-tified four novel non-founding mutations in 5 of them: one missense, one nonsense, one L1 insertion, and one 1-bp insertion. As previously mentioned, we found one mis-sense mutation in a severe type of FCMD with microphthalmia. The frequency of severe phenotypes, including Walker–Warburg syndrome-like manifestations such as hydrocephalus and microphthalmia, was significantly higher among probands who were compound heterozygotes carrying a point mutation on one allele and a founding mutation on the other, than among probands who were homozygous for the 3-kb retrotransposon insertion. Remarkably, Kondo-Iida *et al.* detected no FCMD patients with non-founding (point) mutations in both alleles of the gene, suggesting that such cases might be embryonic lethal. This could explain why few FCMD cases are reported in non-Japanese populations. The results provided strong evidence that loss of function of fukutin is the major cause of FCMD, and provide some hint as to the mechanism responsible for the broad spectrum of clinical features seen in this disease.

Kobayashi *et al.* (1998) could not demonstrate fukutin in skeletal muscle using polyclonal or monoclonal antibodies. In transfected COS-7 cells, fukutin co-localized with a Golgi marker as well as showing a granular cytoplasmic distribution, suggesting that fukutin passes through the Golgi before being packaged into secretory vesicles. Unlike other muscular dystrophy-associated proteins, no staining for fukutin was seen at the plasma membrane. Kobayashi *et al.* (1998) suggested that fukutin is located in the extracellular matrix, where it interacts with and reinforces a large complex encompassing the outside and inside of muscle membranes. Alternatively, if fukutin is secreted, it may cause muscular dystrophy by an as yet unknown mechanism.

The discovery of the FCMD gene represents an important step towards greater understanding not only of the pathogenesis of muscular dystrophies but also of normal brain development. A major manifestation of FCMD is micropolygyria (type II lissencephaly), in which neuronal lamination of normal 6-layered cortex is lacking because of a defect in the migration of neurons. Other genes implicated in cortical dysgenesis disorders that appear to function in the migration and assembly of neurons during cortical histogenesis include DCX (Gleeson *et al.* 1998), LIS1 (Caspi *et al.* 2000), and RELN (Hong *et al.* 2000).

Walker–Warburg Syndrome is an extreme form of CMD with the most severe brain malformations, eye involvement and poorest prognosis. It is characterized by type II lissencephaly with progressive hydrocephalus, agyria and ocular abnormalities (Dobyns *et al.* 1985; 1989). MEBD is another rare disorder characterized by severe mental retardation, hypotonia and visual failure (Raitta *et al.* 1978; Santavuori and Leisti 1977). Clinical severity is milder in FCMD than in WWS and MEBD, particularly with respect to brain and ophthalmologic involvement (Dobyns *et al.* 1985; Fukuyama 1997). The list of clinicopathological features common to FCMD, WWS and MEBD begs the question as to whether these diseases could be allelic. However, though the chromosomal location of the WWS locus remains unknown, the MEBD locus has recently been mapped to 1p32–34 (Cormand *et al.* 1999). We reported a case diagnosed as having a mild type of WWS, who was the only child of a Japanese mother and an American father of Scandinavian descent (Saito *et al.* 1997). The patient showed neither the presence of the ancestral founder haplotype nor FCMD gene mutation on both chromosomes.

Prenatal diagnosis

We first reported prenatal diagnosis in two FCMD families using microsatellite markers in the candidate region (Kondo *et al.* 1996). Subsequently, we conducted genetic analyses for prenatal diagnosis in eight FCMD families with at least one child afflicted with FCMD, carefully considering the ethical issues in each case (Saito *et al.* 1997). Fetal materials were obtained by mid-trimester amniotic fluid sampling or from the chorionic villi. The fetuses of five families were diagnosed as being non-affected, and all proved to be healthy after birth. Those in the other three families were affected and the parents opted for abortion. The 17-, 18- and 20-week-old fetuses that were diagnosed prenatally as having FCMD were examined neuropathologically. Multiple small granular protrusions over the cerebral surface were composed of aberrant neuroglial clusters. Microscopically, the neurites, granular cells and glia migrated out through the discontinuous pial-glial barrier into the extra-cortical glial layer. Such findings are indicative of the initial stage of cortical dysplasia (Nakano *et al.* 1996; Yamamoto *et al.* 1996; 1997a). The pathological changes were less severe at earlier gestational ages.

The prenatal prediction of FCMD was shown to be correct in the families who elected to terminate the pregnancies. We anticipate a growing demand for this service. We are moving ahead slowly, in consideration of the many ethical issues inherent in prenatal diagnosis. We would like to emphasize that most of the families tested would most likely have opted for abortion without the assurance, provided by prenatal diagnosis, that their babies would be healthy. Some of these families represent a special case where having three afflicted children would be an enormous burden. Ultimately, the decision to choose prenatal diagnosis and, if chosen, what to do with the information, must be made by the parents. Our job, as physicians, is to support these families both medically and educationally.

Acknowledgements

The authors thank the family members who permitted to use photographs of their children. We also thank Prof. Yukio Fukuyama, Prof. Makiko Osawa, Drs. Haruko Suzuki, Keiko Shishikura, Yoshito Hirayama, Sawako Sumida, Kiyoko Ikeya, Eri Kondo-Iida for giving us comments and Dr. Angus Thomson for reading the manuscript. This work was supported by a research grant for Nervous and Mental Disorders (11B-1) from the Ministry of Health and Welfare of Japan, and also by a Grant-in-Aid for Scientific Research (12470173) from the Ministry of Education, Science, and Culture, Japan.

References

Aida, N., Yagishita, A., Takada, K. *et al.* (1994). Cerebellar MR in Fukuyama congenital muscular dystrophy: polymicrogyria with cystic lesions. *American Journal of Neuroradiology*, **15**, 1755–9.

Arahata, K., Hayashi, Y.K., and Ozawa, E. (1993). Dystrophin-associated glycoprotein and dystrophin co-localisation at sarcolemma in Fukuyama congenital muscular dystrophy. *Lancet*, **342**, 623–4.

Arikawa, E., Ishihara, T., Nonaka, I., Sugita, H., and Arahata, K. (1991). Immunocytochemical analysis of dystrophin in congenital muscular dystrophy. *Journal of Neurological Science*, **105**, 79–87.

Caspi, M., Atlas, R., Kantor, A., Sapir, T., and Reiner, O. (2000). Interaction between LIS1 and doublecortin, two lissencephaly gene products. *Human Molecular Genetics*, **9**, 2205–13.

Cormand, B., Avela, K., Pihko, H. *et al.* (1999). Assignment of the Muscle–Eye–Brain disease gene to 1p32-p34 by linkage analysis and homozygosity mapping. *American Journal of Medical Genetics*, **22**, 157–9.

Dobyns, W.B., Kirkpatrick, J.B., Hittner, H.M., Roberts, R.M., and Kretzer, F.L. (1985). Syndrome with lissencephaly. II: Walker–Warburg and cerebro-oculo-muscular syndromes and a new syndrome with type II lissencephaly. *American Journal of Medical Genetics*, **22**, 157–95.

Dobyns, W.B., Pagon, R.A., Armstrong, D. *et al.* (1989). Diagnostic criteria for Walker–Warburg syndrome. *American Journal of Medical Genetics*, **32**, 195–210.

Fukuyama, Y., Kawazura, M., and Haruna, H. (1960). A peculiar form of congenital progressive muscular dystrophy. Report of fifteen cases. *Pediatr Univ Tokyo*, **4**, 5–8.

Fukuyama, Y., Osawa, M., and Suzuki, H. (1981). Congenital progressive muscular dystrophy of Fukuyama type: Clinical, genetic and pathological considerations. *Brain & Development*, **3**, 1–29.

Fukuyama, Y. and Ohsawa, M. (1984). A genetic study of the Fukuyama type congenital muscular dystrophy. *Brain & Development*, **6**, 373–90.

Fukuyama, Y. (1997). Nosological establishment of congenital muscular dystrophies in the history of medicine. In *Congenital muscular dystrophies* (ed. Y. Fukuyama, M. Osawa and K. Saito) pp. 1–20. Amsterdam, Lausanne, New York, Oxford, Shannon, Tokyo: Elsevier.

Gleeson, J.G., Allen, K.M., Fox, J.W., Lamperti, E.D., Berkovic, S., Scheffer, I. *et al.* (1998). Doublecortin, a brain-specific gene mutated in human X-linked lissencephaly and double cortex syndrome, encodes a putative signaling protein. *Cell*, **92**, 63–72.

Hayashi, Y.K., Engvall, E., Arikawa-Hirasawa, E. *et al.* (1993). Abnormal localization of laminin subunits in muscular dystrophies *Journal of Neurological Science*, **119**, 53–64.

Hayashi, Y.K., Nonaka, I., and Arahata, K. (1997). Laminin a2 (or M) chain abnormality in congenital muscular dystrophy. In *Congenital muscular dystrophies* (ed. Y. Fukuyama, M. Osawa and K. Saito) pp. 259–65. Amsterdam, Lausanne, New York, Oxford, Shannon, Tokyo: Elsevier.

Hino, N., Kobayashi, M., Shibata, N., Yamamoto, T., Saito, K., Osawa, M. (2001). Clinicopathological study on eyes from cases of Fukuyama type congenital muscular dystrophy. *Brain & Development*, **23**, 97–107.

Hong, S.E., Shugart, Y.Y., Huang, D.T., Al Shahwan, S., Grant, P.E., Hourihane, J.O. *et al.* (2000). Autosomal recessive lissencephaly with cerebellar hypoplasia is associated with human RELN mutations. *Nature Genetics*, **26**, 93–96.

Kamoshita, S., Konishi, Y., Segawa, M., and Fukuyama, Y. (1975). Congenital muscular dystrophy as a disease of the central nervous system *Artch Neurol*, **33**, 513–6.

Kato, I., Osawa, M., Murasugi, H., Sumida, S., and Saito, K. (1998). Neuroimaging morphological study of brainstem and cerebellum in cases of Fukuyama type congenital muscular dystrophy (in Japanese). *Journal of Tokyo Women's Medical College*, **68**, 772–85.

Kimura, S., Sasaki, Y., Kobayashi, T. *et al.* (1993). Fukuyama-type congenital muscular dystrophy and the Walker–Warburg syndrome. *Brain & Development*, **15**, 182–91.

Kobayashi, K., Nakahori, Y., Mizuno, K. *et al.* (1998a). Founder-haplotype analysis in Fukuyama-type congential muscular dystrophy (FCMD). *Human Genetics*, **103**, 323–7.

Kobayashi, K., Nakahori, Y., Miyake, M. *et al.* (1998b). An ancient retrotransposal insertion causes Fukuyama-type congenital muscular dystrophy. *Nature*, **394**, 388–92.

Kondo, E., Saito, K., Toda, T., Osawa, M., Yamamoto, T., Kobayashi, M., and Fukuyama, Y. (1996). Prenatal diagnosis of Fukuyama type congenital muscular dystrophy by polymorphism analysis. *American Journal of Medical Genetics*, **66**, 169–74.

Kondo-Iida, E., Saito, K., Osawa, M., Ishihara, T., Toda, T., and Fukuyama, Y. (1997a). Polymorphism analysis of Fukuyama type congenital muscular dystrophy (FCMD) siblings with different phenotypes. *Brain & Development*, **19**, 181–6.

Kondo-Iida, E., Saito, K., Tanaka, H. *et al.* (1997b). Molecular genetic evidence of clinical heterogeneity in Fukuyama-type congenital muscular dystrophy. *Human Genetics*, **99**, 427–32.

Kondo-Iida, E., Kobayashi, K., Watanabe, M., Sasaki, J., Kumagai, T., Koide, H. *et al.* (1999). Novel mutations and genotype-phenotype relationships in 107 families with Fukuyama-type congenital muscular dystrophy (FCMD). *Human Molecular Genetics*, **8**, 2303–9.

Miyake, M., Nakahori, Y., Matsushita, I. *et al.* (1997). YAC and cosmid contigs encompassing the Fukuyama-type congenital muscular dystrophy (FCMD) candidate region on 9q31. *Genomics*, **40**, 284–93.

Nakano, I., Funahori, Y., Takada, K., and Toda, T. (1996). Are breaches in the glia limitans the primary cause of the micropolygyria in Fukuyama-type congenital muscular dystrophy (FCMD)? Pathological study of the cerebral cortex of a FCMD fetus. *Acta Neuropathologica* (Berlin), **91**, 313–21.

Nonaka, I. and Chou, S.M. (1979). Congenital muscular dystrophy. In *Handbook of clinical neurology* (ed. P.J. Vinken and G.W. Bruyn) Vol. 41. pp. 27–50. North Holland Amsterdam.

Okawa, Y. and Ueda, S. (1997). Rehabilitation of children with Fukuyama congenital muscular dystrophy. In *Congenital muscular dystrophies* (ed. Y. Fukuyama, M. Osawa and K. Saito) pp. 159–70. Amsterdam, Lausanne, New York, Oxford, Shannon, Tokyo: Elsevier.

Osawa, M. (1978). A genetical and epidemiological study on congenital progressive muscular dystrophy (Fukuyama type) (in Japanese). *Journal of Tokyo Women's Medical College*, **48**, 204–41.

Osawa, M., Sumida, S., Suzuki, N. *et al.* (1997). Fukuyama type congenital muscular dystrophy. In *Congenital muscular dystrophies* (ed. Y. Fukuyama, M. Osawa and K. Saito) pp. 31–68. Amsterdam, Lausanne, New York, Oxford, Shannon, Tokyo: Elsevier.

Raitta, C., Lamminen, M., Santavuori, P., and Leisti, J. (1978). Ophthalmological findings in a new syndrome with muscle, eye and brain involvement. *Acta Ophthalmologica* **56**, 465–72.

Saito, K., Suzuki, H., Shishikura, K. *et al.* (1997). A milder form of Walker–Warburg syndrome. In *Congenital muscular dystrophies* (ed. Y. Fukuyama, M. Osawa and K. Saito) pp. 345–354. Amsterdam, Lausanne, New York, Oxford, Shannon, Tokyo: Elsevier.

Saito, K., Kondo-Iida, E., Kawakita, Y. *et al.* (1998). Prenatal diagnosis of Fukuyama type congenital muscular dystrophy in eight Japanese families by haplotype analysis using new markers closest to the gene. *American Journal of Medical Genetics*, **77**, 310–6.

Saito, K., Osawa, M., Wang, Zhi-Ping. *et al.* (2000). Haplotype-phenotype correlation in Fukuyama congenital muscular dystrophy. *American Journal of Medical Genetics*, **92**, 184–90.

Saito, Y., Mizuguchi, M., Oka, A., and Takashima, S. (2000). Fukutin protein is expressed in neurons of the normal developing human brain but is reduced in Fukuyama-type congenital muscular dystrophy brain. *Annals of Neurology*, **47**, 756–764.

Santavuori, P. and Leisti, J. (1977). Muscle, eye and brain disease: a new syndrome. *Neuropaediatrie*, **8**(suppl.), 553–8.

Takada, K., Nakamura, H., and Tanaka, J. (1984). Cortical dysplasia in congenital muscular dystrophy with central nervous system involvement (Fukuyama type). *J Neuropathol Exp Neurol*, **43**, 395–407.

Takada, K., Nakamura, H., Suzumori, K., Ishikawa, T., and Sugiyama, N. (1987). Cortical dysplasia in a 23-week fetus with Fukuyama congenital muscular dystrophy (FCMD). *Acta Neuropathologica (Berlin)*, **74**, 300–6.

Toda, T., Segawa, M., Nomura, Y. *et al.* (1993). Localization of a gene for Fukuyama type congenital muscular dystrophy to chromosome 9q31–33. *Nature Genetics*, **5**, 283–6.

Toda, T., Kegawa, S., Okui, K. *et al.* (1994). Refined mapping of a gene responsible for Fukuyama type congenital muscular dystrophy: evidence for strong linkage disequilibrium. *American Journal of Human Genetics*, **55**, 946–50.

Toda, T., Miyake, M., Kobayashi, K. *et al.* (1996). Linkage-disequilibrium mapping narrows the Fukuyama-type congenital muscular dystrophy (FCMD) candidate region to 100 kb. *American Journal of Human Genetics*, **59**, 1313–20.

Tsutsumi, A., Uchida, Y., Osawa, M., and Fukuyama, Y. (1989). Ocular findings in Fukuyama type congenital muscular dystrophy. *Brain & Development*, **11**, 413–9.

Walton, J. (1991). Revised classification of neuromuscular diseases. *Neuro-Muscular Diseases News Bulletin*, March: 9–10.

Yamamoto, T., Komori, T., Shibata, N. *et al.* (1996). Fukuyama congenital muscular dystrophy: cortical dysplasia of the cerebrum in a 20 week fetus. *Neuropathology*, **16**, 184–9.

Yamamota, T., Toyoda, C., Kobayashi, M., Kondo, E., Saito, K., and Osawa, M. (1997a). Pial-glial barrier abnormalities in fetuses with Fukuyama congenital muscular dystrophy. *Brain & Development*, **19**, 35–42.

Yamamoto, T., Shibata, N., Kanazawa, M. *et al.* (1997b). Early ultrastructural changes in the central nervous system in Fukuyama congenital muscular dystrophy. *Ultrastructural Pathology*, **21**, 355–60.

Yamamota, T., Shibata, N., Kanazawa, M. *et al.* (1997c). Localization of laminin subunits in the central nervous system in Fukuyama congenital muscular dystrophy: an immunohistochemical investigation. *Acta Neuropathologica*, **94**, 173–9.

Chapter 4

Duchenne muscular dystrophy or Meryon's disease

Alan E.H. Emery

Introduction

This disease is eponymously associated with the name Duchenne because this French physician described the condition in detail in the 1860s (Duchenne 1861; 1868). His contributions were concerned with the clinical description of the condition and the muscle histology findings. However, several years previously an English physician, Edward Meryon, not only described the clinical features of the disease in some detail but also emphasized three very important points (Meryon 1851; 1852). Firstly, he emphasized that the disease affected males and was *familial* (none of Duchenne's cases were familial). Secondly, he carefully examined for the first time the spinal cord at post-mortem of a boy who had died from the disease and concluded that the cord appeared normal in all respects including the nerve tracts and 'ganglionic cells'. Duchenne did not examine the spinal cord of an affected boy until many years later and therefore could not be certain that the disease was primarily a disease of muscle and not neurogenic in origin. Finally, and most importantly, Meryon's careful muscle microscopical study led him to conclude:

> '... the striped elementary primitive fibres were found to be completely destroyed, the sarcous element being diffused, and in many places converted into oil globules and granular matter, whilst the sarcolemma or tunic of the elementary fibre was broken down and destroyed.'
>
> (Meryon 1852, p. 76)

This was a singularly important point, not made by Duchenne, since we now know that the primary defect does in fact reside in the sarcolemma.

For these various reasons it could be argued that the disease might rightfully be referred to as Duchenne muscular dystrophy or Meryon's disease (Fig. 4.1).

Clinical features

As will be discussed later, Duchenne muscular dystrophy (DMD) is due to a deficiency of the sarcolemmal associated protein dystrophin. In an affected fetus even by the second trimester of pregnancy dystrophin is absent (Bieber *et al.* 1989). Yet, clinical evidence of the disease does not appear until early childhood.

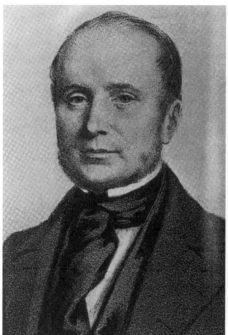 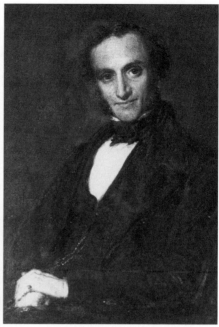

Fig. 4.1 (*Left*) Duchenna de Boulogne (1806–1875). (Reproduced from *The Founders of Neurology*, edited by Webb Haymaker, 1953. Courtesy of Charles C. Thomas, Publishers, Springfield, Illinois). (*Right*) Edward Meryon (1807–1880). (By John Linnell, private collection).

Onset

Occasionally mothers volunteer that their sons seem 'floppy' at birth, or there is some delay in motor development in early childhood. A delay in learning to walk is not uncommon. In over 50 per cent of cases walking is delayed until 18 months and roughly a quarter do not learn to walk until at least two years of age (Emery 1993). However vague the apparent onset, one thing is clear very rarely do affected boys learn to run properly. They tend to fall over more easily than normal children. Other early complaints include a waddling gait, walking on the toes and difficulty climbing stairs. In most cases the calf muscles appear enlarged, the so-called 'pseudohypertrophy' (Fig. 4.2). Any of these signs and symptoms should alert those concerned to the possibility of DMD and the need for a serum creatine kinase (SCK) test. In a significant proportion of cases there is still an unacceptable delay in making the diagnosis with the result that a mother may have a second affected child without knowing she was at risk (Bushby *et al.* 1999, Essex and Roper, 2001).

Distribution of muscle weakness

Muscle involvement is always bilateral and symmetrical. In the early stages of the disease, in general, the lower limbs are affected more than the upper limbs, and the proximal muscles more than the distal muscles. Certain muscles are predominantly affected. These include the latissimus dorsi, sternocostal head of the pectoralis major, brachio-radialis, biceps, triceps, iliopsoas, glutei, and quadriceps muscles. The involvement is highly selective: the quadriceps are more affected than the ham-strings, triceps more than biceps, wrist extensors more than flexors, neck flexors more than extensors, dorsi-flexors of the feet more than the plantar flexors. Even within a single muscle there is differential involvement. For example, the sterno-costal head of the pectoralis major muscle is more affected than the clavicular head, but in contrast the clavicular head of the sternomastoid muscle is more affected than the sternal head. This differential mus-cle involvement has been elaborated upon by Bonsett (1969). Later, slight facial weak-ness often develops and the intercostal muscles also become affected, but sphincter control, chewing, and swallowing are never affected.

Weakness of the knee and hip extensors results in Gower's manoeuvre whereby the boy climbs up his thighs pushing down on them with his hands in order to extend the hips and trunk. It is most clearly demonstrated when asked to get up from sitting on the floor. As the disease progresses it becomes actually impossible to stand up from such a sitting position. Weakness of the pectoral girdle musculature is demonstrated early on by grasping the boy around the chest from behind and attempting to lift him up when there is then a tendency to 'slip through' the examiner's arms.

Progression

Weakness is progressive but often shows periods of apparent arrest. Lumbar lordosis becomes progressively more exaggerated. Ultimately, a wheelchair becomes necessary, in most cases by the age of 12. The age at becoming confined to a wheelchair roughly correlates with age at death. The earlier a boy becomes confined to a wheelchair the poorer the prognosis (Emery 1993).

Once confined to a wheelchair contractures of the elbows, knees and hips develop. Talipes equinovarus deformity becomes marked. However, the most serious develop-ment in the later stages is thoracic deformity which restricts adequate pulmonary inflow on the compressed side. This is also aggravated by weakness of the intercostal and diaphragmatic muscles. At this point surgical correction may have to be considered (Chapter 15). The heart also becomes affected (Chapter 11). Pneumonia compounded by cardiac involvement is the commonest cause of death. Until recently, most cases of DMD died in their late teens or early twenties. However, with more attention to respi-ratory care and the use of various forms of assisted ventilation, including even tra-cheostomy (Chapter 13), many now survive into their late 20s and beyond.

Involvement of other tissues

Though skeletal muscle is clearly the tissue most obviously affected in DMD, other tis-sues and organs are also affected in the disease.

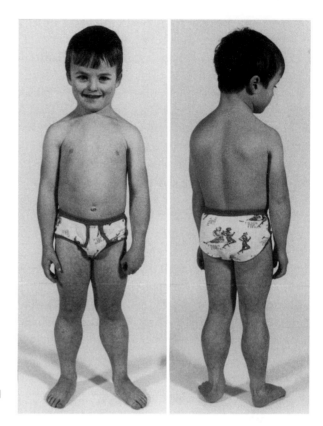

Fig. 4.2 A 4-year-old boy with Duchenne muscular dystrophy. Note the enlarged calves (From Emery 1993).

Smooth muscle

Circumstantial evidence that smooth muscle is involved is suggested by the occasional occurrence of bladder paralysis, paralytic ileus, gastric dilatation and delay in gastric emptying. At least in certain sarcoglycanopathies there is now evidence of involvement of the microvascular smooth muscle in the heart (Cohn and Campbell 2000a).

Cardiac muscle

There is clear evidence, both clinically and pathologically, of cardiac involvement in DMD. Various ECG abnormalities occur, the most obvious being high R waves in the first precordial lead (Emery 1972) which has been attributed to diffuse interstitial fibrosis in the postero-lateral part of the left ventricle (Perloff *et al.* 1967; 1984). Ultimately a dilated cardiomyopathy develops (Chapter 11) and echocardiography may reveal evidence of this before there are any related symptoms.

Central nervous system

A review of the many published data on IQ studies in DMD (Emery 1993) concluded that the overall mean IQ is about one standard deviation below the normal mean.

Around 20 per cent have an IQ less than 70. Verbal IQ is more depressed than performance IQ. These effects have been shown not to be progressive or related to the progression of the disease or to lack of educational opportunity but a genuine pleiotrophic effect of the disease gene. Epilepsy is not a manifestation of the disease. Hearing is not obviously affected but recently a locus for non-syndromic sensorineural hearing loss has been located to Xp21 (Pfister *et al.* 1998). Visual acuity is unaffected but electroretinography has revealed significant defects in many cases, perhaps related to involvement of the retinal isoforms of dystrophin (see later).

Confirmation of the diagnosis

A precise diagnosis of DMD is essential not only because of the serious prognostic implication but also for genetic counselling within an affected family. The important confirmatory tests include a SCK level, electromyography and a muscle biopsy for histology and dystrophin studies.

Serum creatine kinase

This can be carried out on a heel prick (the basis of neonatal screening for DMD) or a venous blood sample. Normally the SCK level is up to around 200 IU but in affected boys the level at the beginning is grossly elevated to 50–100 times normal. Significantly raised levels occur in some other forms of dystrophy (most notably LGMD 2B—dysferlinopathy) and in polymyositis but rarely to the levels found in preclinical and early cases of DMD. As the disease progresses SCK levels gradually decline and may approach normal levels in the late stages of the disease.

Electromyography

This is an important investigation for differentiating myogenic from neurogenic disorders. However, because of its invasive and rather unpleasant nature, it is now much less used in the diagnosis of DMD in young children. It is still widely used in the investigation of many other neuromuscular disorders in later life.

Muscle biopsy

This is nowadays performed with a needle biopsy rather than an open biopsy. The specimen obtained is examined histologically and immunohistochemically for dystrophin. In the very early stages of DMD, muscle histology may reveal little more than an increased variation in fibre size and an increase in the number of prominent rounded fibres which stain more densely with eosin—so-called eosinophilic fibres. These fibres contain increased intracellular calcium as revealed by histochemical staining with Alizarin red S (Fig. 4.3). However, by the time muscle weakness is clearly evident, muscle histology reveals clear evidence of dystrophic changes with fibre necrosis, invasion by mononuclear cells, phagocytosis, and later replacement by fat and connective tissue.

Using appropriately labelled anti-dystrophin monoclonal antibodies, in contrast to normal muscle where dystrophin is clearly localized at the periphery of all muscle fibres, in DMD there is almost a complete absence of dystrophin apart from occasional positive (revertant) fibres. In Becker muscular dystrophy (BMD), where more severe cases can clinically resemble DMD, dystrophin staining is reduced with variation between and within muscle fibres (Sewry 2000). In BMD, Western blot will demonstrate a reduction in the abundance and/or size of dystrophin.

Mutation analysis

The identification of the specific gene mutation in a case of DMD is essential for determining the carrier status of any female relatives and to aid prenatal diagnosis should this be requested at some future date. Gene studies can be performed on a blood sample. Several laboratory techniques are available for defining the nature of a dystrophin mutation and are discussed later.

Neonatal screening

DMD is among the most frequent of unifactorial disorders in Western Europe and is the most frequent X-linked condition in childhood with an incidence of 1 in 3500 newborns (Emery 1991). Since the SCK level in affected boys is grossly elevated even at birth, a number of centres throughout the world at various times have set up pilot schemes of neonatal screening based on SCK levels in a heel prick blood sample (van Ommen and Scheuerbrandt 1993). There are several reasons for justifying such schemes but the most compelling is the mother's realization that she is at risk *before* she contemplates another pregnancy. Arguably however, the idea will gain more acceptance and support when an effective treatment is found because presumably the earlier it is started the more likely its effectiveness will be.

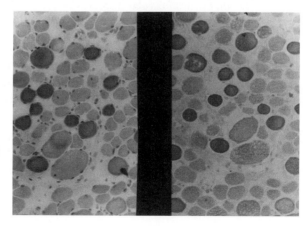

Fig. 4.3 Serial sections of gastrocnemius muscle in a preclinical (2-year-old) case of Duchenne muscular dystrophy, stained with (*left*) haematoxylin and eosin, and (*right*) alizarin red S. Note the numerous eosinophilic/calcium-positive fibres, but no evidence of muscle fibre necrosis (From Emery 1993).

Genetics

By the 1950s DMD had been proved to be X-linked. This was based on the analysis of numerous affected families and convincingly by the report of a girl with Turner's syndrome and a single X-chromosome who also had DMD. Subsequently discriminant function analysis coupled with segregation analysis confirmed DMD to be X-linked and differentiated it from dominant facioscapulohumeral dystrophy and recessive limb girdle dystrophy (Morton and Chung 1959). However it was not until some twenty years later that in 1982 the gene was localized to Xp21 (Murray *et al.* 1982). This was the very first inherited disorder in which the causative gene was located by linkage to a DNA marker (in this case a restriction fragment length polymorphism). And five years later it was the first inherited disorder in which the defective protein was identified by the revolutionary technique of reverse genetics or, more precisely, positional cloning (Kunkel *et al.* 1985; Ray *et al.* 1985). The protein was subsequently named, somewhat inappropriately, 'dystrophin', and was shown to be localized to the sarcolemma and to be deficient in DMD (Sugita *et al.* 1988; Zubrzycka-Gaarn *et al.* 1988). The chromosomal location of the genes and the identification of their protein products in other forms of dystrophy have since been achieved using similar techniques though not all these proteins have turned out to be localized to the muscle membrane (Chapter 1).

Dystrophin gene

The dystrophin gene is one of the largest in the human genome. It is 2.5 Mb in length with an mRNA of 14 kb. It consists of 79 exons with introns making up at least 98 per cent of the gene, which implies that little more than one per cent is directly involved in coding for dystrophin.

Over the years many laboratory techniques have been developed for detecting disease-associated mutations in the dystrophin gene. In roughly 70 per cent of cases gross rearrangements (mainly deletions) occur within the gene which can be detected by Southern blot and pulsed-field gel electrophoresis. These tend to be clustered around two 'hot spot' regions (proximal and central regions of the gene). The majority of these deletions can be detected by examining subsets of exons within the gene. This is possible using the so-called 'multiplex method', whereby regions of the gene which are deletion-susceptible are simultaneously analysed by amplifying these regions using the polymerase chain reaction (PCR). The technique originally developed by Chamberlain (Chamberlain *et al.* 1992) has since been modified and extended to make detection of most deletions now possible.

Regarding the 30 per cent of cases due to various point mutations, their detection presents more of a problem. Techniques now being used for this purpose include SSCP (single-strand conformation polymorphism) analysis (Sitnik *et al.* 1997), and the PTT (protein truncation test). When the latter detects a truncated band on electrophoresis, the PCR product is then sequenced in order to identify the specific mutation which has resulted in the truncated dystrophin (Roest *et al.* 1993). A variety of other laboratory techniques for identifying point mutations, which are often complex and time-consuming, are now also available in specialized centres (Bakker & van Ommen, 1998).

Dystrophin protein

This is a very large protein with a molecular weight of 427 kDa and consisting of 3685 amino acids. It is rod-shaped and composed of four domains (Koenig *et al.* 1988):

- N-terminal domain with homology to α-actinin and composed of 240 amino acids
- Central rod domain of a succession of 25 triple helical repeats similar to spectrin, and composed of roughly 3000 amino acids
- Cysteine-rich domain composed of 280 amino acids
- C-terminal domain composed of 420 amino acids

It is a costameric protein which forms a lattice which encircles the muscle fibre. It is not directly inserted into the membrane itself but via its association with various sarcoglycans forming the dystrophin–glycoprotein complex (Fig. 4.4).

This complex is clearly important for maintaining the integrity of the muscle membrane. Disruption of the complex (in DMD and certain limb girdle dystrophies) leads to disruption of the linkage between the extracellular matrix and the cytoskeleton (Cohn and Campbell 2000b).

Dystrophin is not a single protein but exists in a number of isoforms. There are three full-length transcripts (Dp 427) with associated promoters referred to as Purkinje (P), Muscle (M), and Brain (B). Each consists of a unique first exon spliced to a shared set of some 80 exons. Their differential expression in various tissues is shown in Fig. 4.5. The Brain isoform is predominantly expressed in cortical neurones and parts of the hippocampus but also to some extent in muscle. The Purkinje isoform is predominantly expressed in Purkinje cells of the cerebellum. Most relevant to the pathogenesis of DMD is perhaps the Muscle isoform. This is predominantly expressed in skeletal and cardiac muscle and to a lesser extent in the brain.

Besides these full-length isoforms there are also at least five shorter transcripts generated by internal promoters. They are each designated according to the size (in kiloDaltons) of the resultant protein and are expressed mainly in the brain or retina:

Dp 260 (retina, brain, muscle), Dp 140 (brain and spinal cord),
Dp 116 (brain and peripheral nerves), Dp 71 (various tissues) and Dp 40.

The relationship of these various isoforms to the clinical phenotype in DMD is currently an active field of research and has been the subject of a detailed review (Brown and Lucy 1997).

Pathogenesis of weakness

Though the molecular and biochemical bases of DMD are now known in some detail, a number of important questions regarding the pathogenesis of muscle

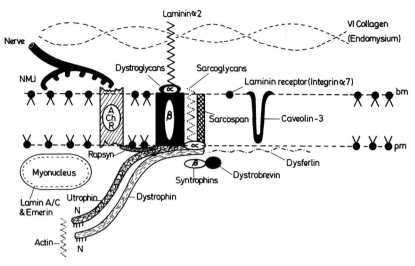

Fig. 4.4 Schematic representation of the various proteins involved directly or indirectly in different forms of muscular dystrophy. The precise relationships of these various proteins is not yet entirely clear (bm, basement membrane [basal lamina]; pm, plasma membrane [plasmalemma]; NMJ, neuromuscular junction; AChR, acetyl choline receptor). (After Emery 2000a).

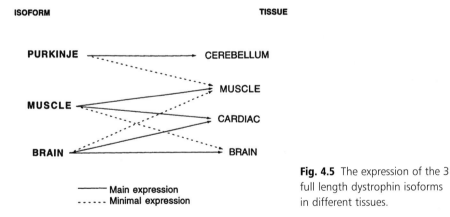

Fig. 4.5 The expression of the 3 full length dystrophin isoforms in different tissues.

weakness still remain unanswered. Some of these have been discussed previously (Emery 1994).

The deficiency of muscle dystrophin and the resultant disruption of the dystrophin–glycoprotein complex provides an attractive explanation for the development of muscle weakness in DMD, but this is clearly an over-simplification. One of the most fundamental questions which remains unanswered is why certain muscle groups become severely affected early on (e.g., quadriceps) but others only much later (e.g., soleus) and some never become affected at all (e.g., extra-ocular). Could this be related to fibre size? As fibre size increases so the surface-to-volume ratio decreases leading to higher levels of membrane stress during contraction (Petrof *et al.* 1993). And despite muscle dystrophin being deficient even in the fetus muscle weakness does not become evident until later in childhood and is thereafter progressive. Furthermore why should the postero-lateral part of the left ventricle be predominantly affected in the heart since dystrophin is deficient throughout the tissue? Could this be related to the *longitudinal* distribution of cardiac muscle fibres in this part of the heart (Cziner and Levin 1993). Answers to some of these questions may come from *in vitro* studies designed to address the role of dystrophin in shearing-type muscular injury (Kääriäinen *et al.* 2000; Loufrani *et al.* 2001). And there is a real possibility that, quite apart from the role played by essentially structural proteins in the development of muscle weakness, the reduced production of muscle membrane-associated neuronal nitric oxide (NO) synthase may well be equally important (Crosbie 2001; Sander *et al.* 2000).

Genotype–phenotype correlations

Monaco *et al.* (1988) proposed that mutations of the dystrophin gene which maintain the translational reading frame (in-frame mutations) might be expected to result in an abnormal but partially functional dystrophin. This would be the case in the milder Becker type of dystrophy (Chapter 5). On the other hand-mutations which shifted the reading frame (frame-shift mutations) would be expected to result in virtually no functional dystrophin, as in DMD. This so-called 'reading frame' hypothesis has been found to hold up in over 90 per cent of cases and is of diagnostic as well as prognostic significance. Exceptions to the rule can be explained by exon skipping in the case of out-of-frame mutations associated with a milder disease. Deletions in exons 3–7 produce a great variety of phenotypes (Muntoni *et al.* 1994). Possibly, in some of these cases there is a greater chance of a new start codon being encountered further along the gene. There is, however, no simple relationship between the *extent* of a deletion and the resultant phenotype. A very small 'out of frame' deletion can be associated with severe DMD, and a very extensive 'in frame' deletion within the central region can result in mild disease. In fact deletions in the central region are often associated with mild weakness or even be asymptomatic and associated only with a raised SCK level. For this reason the use of this region in 'mini gene' constructs for gene therapy is currently being considered (Chapter 14).

Though the majority of muscle fibres in DMD do not stain for dystrophin, occasional dystrophin-positive, so-called 'revertant fibres' do occur (Fig. 4.6). They usually occur singly but may be arranged in clusters. They are likely to result from a second site in-frame mutation which restores the reading frame (Klein *et al.* 1992).

Attempts to relate mutations at specific sites in the dystrophin gene to the occurrence of mental handicap suggest that deletions involving Dp 140 and around exon 51 (the translation start point for Dp 140) may well be relevant (Bardoni *et al.* 1999; 2000). But

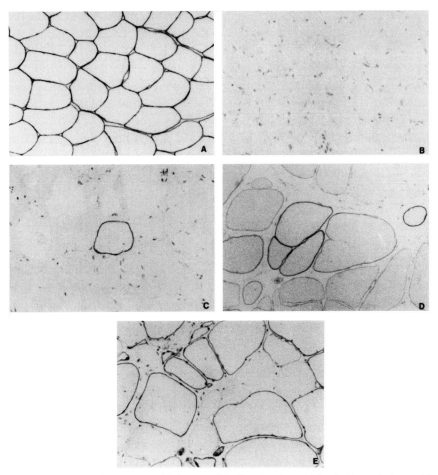

Fig. 4.6 Skeletal muscle sections with immunolabelling for dystrophin. A, Normal: dystrophin located at the sarcolemma on all fibres. B, DMD with frame-shift deletion: no dystrophin is present, (counterstained with haematoxylin and eosin). C, DMD with frame-shift deletion: single positive fibre ('revertant'). D, BMD with in-frame deletion: no dystrophin labelling shows marked variation both between and within fibres. E, Manifesting carrier of DMD: dystrophin labeling shows variation between fibres. Magnification ×250; indirect immunoperoxidase labeling with a monoclonal antibody (Dy8/6C5) which recognizes an epitope at the extreme C-terminus of dystrophin. (Reproduced by kind permission of Dr. Louise Anderson and Dr. Margaret Johnson).

it is not yet entirely clear in what way dystrophin, and in particular Dp 140, affects brain function (Gorecki and Barnard 1997). Dp 71 is the major dystrophin isoform expressed in adult brain tissue but its function is as yet poorly understood (Austin *et al.* 2000).

In the case of X-linked dilated cardiomyopathy, two main regions of the dystrophin gene appear to be involved: the 5′ end and the central region around exons 48–49, the more severe cases being associated with mutations involving the 5′ end. In the latter case, dystrophin is reduced or absent in cardiac muscle but normal in skeletal muscle. The reason for these differences in transcription levels in different tissues, it has been argued, may reflect differences in splicing or exon skipping (Ferlini *et al.* 1999). There is even a suggestion that in DMD, those with deletions of exons 48–49 die more frequently from a cardiomyopathy compared to others with mutations elsewhere in the gene (Nigro *et al.* 1994).

Recent profiling of muscle cDNA arrays has revealed that the expression of many genes, some as yet unidentified, are changed in DMD. This will require explanation and may well contribute to a better understanding of the pathogenesis of DMD in future (Chen *et al.* 2000; Tkatchenko *et al.* 2001).

Manifesting carrier

It has been known for sometime that female carriers of DMD may occasionally exhibit signs of the disease (Emery 1963). This is attributed to skewed distribution of X-inactivation (Lyonization) (Azofeifa *et al.* 1995). The proportion of muscle cell nuclei in which the active X-chromosome is the one bearing the dystrophin gene is presumed to be significantly greater by chance than in carriers without such manifestations.

Around 5–10 per cent of carriers have some degree of muscle weakness (Emery 1993). Onset may be in childhood or not become evident until adult life. Weakness may be progressive or relatively static. The distribution of muscle weakness often resembles that seen in limb girdle dystrophy but differs in that it can be asymmetric and is often associated with calf pseudohypertrophy. The SCK is invariably raised though female carriers, may have equally high SCK levels and yet remain symptom-free. There is occasionally familial concordance for such manifestations, mothers and daughters or sisters being similarly affected (Emery 1993; Moser and Emery 1974). Most importantly, the heart may also be affected (Emery 1969; Lane *et al.* 1980) and recent studies indicate that a proportion may develop a dilated cardiomyopathy which can occur in isolation (Grain *et al.* 2001). Clearly all presumed female carriers of DMD should be examined carefully and particular attention paid to the possibility of cardiac involvement.

Muscle histopathology in manifesting carriers, but not usually in symptomless carriers, reveals some variation in fibre size, hypercontracted eosinophilic fibres, and even fibre necrosis and phagocytosis although the latter are only ever found when there is florid muscle weakness. Dystrophin staining reveals a pattern not very dissimilar from that found in males affected with Becker muscular dystrophy: variation in staining both between and within muscle fibres (Hoshino *et al.* 2000) and Western blot may reveal some reduction in abundance of normal-sized dystrophin (Fig. 4.7).

Prevention

For carrier detection and prenatal diagnosis the identification of the specific genetic defect in an affected case in the family is important. Some of the methods available for mutation detection have been mentioned already. In the case of a gene deletion, carrier detection can be possible through a variety of techniques. For example, Southern blot analysis may reveal a *dosage* effect (Abbs and Bobrow 1992), or the presence of a *junctional fragment* (Yamagishi *et al.* 1996). A variety of other laboratory techniques are also available if these methods should prove unhelpful or if a point mutation is involved. When a DNA sample from an affected individual in a family is available then carrier identification (and prenatal diagnosis) is usually straightforward. However, a major problem arises when the affected member of a family is deceased or not available for study. Reliance has then to be on the suspected carrier's SCK level and data from possible linked markers (the data being combined in Bayesian statistics) and the possibility that a junction fragment may be present. A relevant dystrophin gene defect and/or the absence of muscle dystrophin in a fetus (Heckel *et al.* 1999) would confirm that the mother was a carrier.

One other important problem to be considered in genetic counselling is the possibility of *germ-line mosaicism.* That is, a female who by all relevant tests appears *not* to be a genetic carrier yet transmits a mutation to her offspring because she harbors a somatic mutation within a fraction of her ovaries. The frequency of such mosaicism among families with DMD varies in different studies between 12 and 20 per cent. From a practical point of view, it means that it can never be assumed that a male fetus of a mother with an apparently normal genotype will be unaffected. It is therefore advisable to consider prenatal diagnosis in *all* pregnancies in at least the mother and sisters of an isolated case of DMD.

Management and treatment

Until a few years ago there was a general nihilism in the medical profession toward therapy in DMD. But recently there has been a significant change in attitude and most

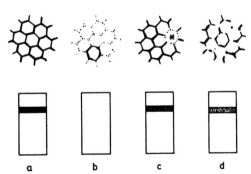

Fig. 4.7 Diagrammatic representation of possible findings on immunohistochemistry and Western blot analysis (a) Control: normal size (427 kDa) and abundance. (b) DMD: occasional positive fibre, virtually no dystrophin. (c) Non-manifesting carrier of DMD: occasional negative fibre (*) and *possible* reduction in abundance of normal size dystrophin. (d) Manifesting carrier of DMD: variation in staining between and within fibres and reduction in abundance of normal size dystrophin.

now have a positive approach to the disease (Emery 2000b). The three most important points now considered in good management of boys with DMD, and for that matter many other forms of muscular dystrophy, are:

- promotion and maintenance of good health in general,
- prevention of deformities through exercises, physiotherapy, orthoses and surgery,
- preservation of respiratory function.

There is also now a more positive approach to finding an effective treatment. Avenues currently being explored include drug treatment, steroids, and the possibilities of gene and stem cell therapy. All these various aspects of management and treatment are considered in detail in subsequent chapters.

References

Abbs, S. and Bobrow, M. (1992). Analysis of quantitative PCR for the diagnosis of deletion and duplication carriers in the dystrophin gene. *Journal of Medical Genetics*, **29**, 191–6.

Austin, R.C., Morris, G.E., Howard, P.L. *et al.* (2000). Expression and synthesis of alternatively spliced variants of Dp 71 in adult human brain. *Neuromuscular Disorders*, **10**, 187–93.

Azofeifa, J., Voit, T., Hubner, C., and Cremer, M. (1995). X-chromosome methylation in manifesting and healthy carriers of dystrophinopathies. *Human Genetics*, **96**, 167–76.

Bakker, E and van Ommen, G.J.B. (1998). Duchenne and Becker muscular dystrophy. In *Neuromuscular disorders: clinical and molecular genetics* (ed. A.E.H. Emery) pp. 59–85. Wiley, Chichester & New York.

Bardoni, A., Sironi, M., Felisari, G., Comi, G.P., and Bresolin, N. (1999). Absence of brain Dp 140 isoform and cognitive impairment in Becker muscular dystrophy. *Lancet*, **353**, 897–8.

Bardoni, A., Felisari, G., Sironi, M. *et al.* (2000). Loss of Dp 140 regulatory sequences is associated with cognitive impairment in dystrophinopathies. *Neuromuscular Disorders*, **10**, 194–9.

Bieber, F.R., Hoffman, E.P., and Amos, J.A. (1989). Dystrophin analysis in Duchenne muscular dystrophy: use in fetal diagnosis and in genetic counseling. *American Journal of Human Genetics*, **45**, 362–7.

Bonsett, C.A. (1969). *Studies of pseudohypertrophic muscular dystrophy*. Thomas, Springfield.

Brown, S.C. and Lucy, J.A. (ed.) (1997). *Dystrophin - gene, protein and cell biology*. Cambridge University Press, Cambridge.

Bushby, K., Hill, A., and Steele, J.G. (1999). Failure of early diagnosis in symptomatic Duchenne muscular dystrophy. *Lancet*, **353**, 557–8.

Chamberlain, J.S., Chamberlain, J.R., Fenwick, R.G. *et al.* (1992). Diagnosis of Duchenne and Becker muscular dystrophy by polymerase chain reaction: a multicentre study. *Journal of the American Medical Association*, **267**, 2609–15.

Chen, Y-W, Zhao, P, Borup, R. and Hoffman, E.P. (2000). Expression profiling in the muscular dystrophies: Identification of novel aspects of molecular pathophysiology. *Journal of Cell Biology*, **151**, 1321–36.

Cohn, R.D. and Campbell, K.P. (2000a). Pathogenetic role of the sarcoglycan–sarcospan complex in cardiomyopathies. *Acta Myologica*, **19**, 171–80.

Cohn, R.D. and Campbell, K.P. (2000b). Molecular basis of muscular dystrophies. *Muscle & Nerve*, **23**, 1456–71.

Crosbie, R.H. (2001). NO vascular control in Duchenne muscular dystrophy. *Nature Medicine*, 7, 27–9.

Cziner, D.G. and Levin, R.I. (1993). The cardiomyopathy of Duchenne's muscular dystrophy and the function of dystrophin. *Medical Hypotheses*, **40**, 169–73.

Duchenne, G.B.A. (1861). *De l'electrisation localisée et son application à la pathologie et à la thérapeutique* (2nd edn.) Baillière et fils, Paris.

Duchenne, G.B.A. (1868). Recherches sur la paralysie musculaire pseudohypertrophique ou paralysie myo-sclérosique. *Archives Génerales de Médecine*, **11**, 5–25, 179–209, 305–21, 421–43, 552–88.

Emery, A.E.H. (1963). Clinical manifestations in two carriers of Duchenne muscular dystrophy. *Lancet*, **1**, 1126–8.

Emery, A.E.H. (1969). Abnormalities of the electrocardiogram in female carriers of Duchenne muscular dystrophy. *British Medical Journal*, **2**, 418–20.

Emery, A.E.H. (1972). Abnormalities of the electrocardiogram in hereditary myopathies. *Journal of Medical Genetics*, **9**, 8–12.

Emery, A.E.H. (1991). Population frequencies of inherited neuromuscular diseases – a world survey. *Neuromuscular Disorders*, **1**, 19–29.

Emery, A.E.H. (1993). *Duchenne Muscular Dystrophy* (2nd edn.) Oxford University Press, Oxford.

Emery, A.E.H. (1994). Some unanswered questions in Duchenne muscular dystrophy. *Neuromuscular Disorders*, **4**, 301–3.

Emery, A.E.H. (2000a). Emery–Dreifuss muscular dystrophy—a 40 year retrospective. *Neuromuscular Disorders*, **10**, 228–32.

Emery, A.E.H. (2000b). *Muscular dystrophy: the facts* (2nd edn.) Oxford University Press, Oxford.

Essex, C. and Roper, H. (2001). Late diagnosis of Duchenne's muscular dystrophy presenting as global developmental delay. *British Medical Journal*, **323**, 37–8.

Ferlini, A., Sewry, C., Melis, M.A., Mateddu, A., and Muntoni, F. (1999). X-linked dilated cardiomyopathy and the dystrophin gene. *Neuromuscular Disorders*, **9**, 339–46.

Górecki, D.C. and Barnard, E.A. (1997). Expression of the dystrophin complex in the brain. In *Dystrophin – gene, protein and cell biology* (eds. S.C. Brown and J.A. Lucy) pp. 105–38. Cambridge University Press, Cambridge.

Grain, L., Cortina-Borja, M., Forfar, C., Hilton-Jones, D., Hopkin, J. and Burch, M. (2001). Cardiac abnormalities and skeletal muscle weakness in carriers of Duchenne and Becker muscular dystrophies and controls. *Neuromuscular Disorders*, **11**, 186–91.

Heckel, S., Favre, R., Flori, J. *et al.* (1999). In utero fetal muscle biopsy: a precious aid for the prenatal diagnosis of Duchenne muscular dystrophy. *Fetal Diagnosis and Therapy*, **14**, 127–32.

Hoshino, S., Ohkoshi, N., Watanabe, M., and Shoji, S. (2000). Immunohistochemical staining of dystrophin on formalin-fixed paraffin-embedded sections in Duchenne/Becker muscular dystrophy and manifesting carriers of Duchenne muscular dystrophy. *Neuromuscular Disorders*, **10**, 425–9.

Kääriäinen, M., Kääriäinen, J., Järvinen, T.L.N. *et al.* (2000). Integrin and dystrophin associated adhesion protein complexes during regeneration of shearing-type muscle injury. *Neuromuscular Disorders*, **10**, 121–32.

Klein, C.J., Coovert, D.D., Bulman, D.E., Ray, P.N., Mendell, J.R., and Burghes, A.H.M. (1992). Somatic reversion/suppression in Duchenne muscular dystrophy (DMD): evidence supporting a frame-restoring mechanism in rare dystrophin-positive fibers. *American Journal of Human Genetics*, **50**, 950–9.

Koenig, M., Monaco, A.P., and Kunkel, L.M. (1988). The complete sequence of dystrophin predicts a rod-shaped cytoskeletal protein. *Cell*, **53**, 219–28.

Kunkel, L.M., Monaco, A.P., Middlesworth, W. *et al.* (1985). Specific cloning of DNA fragments absent from the DNA of a male patient with an X chromosome deletion. *Proceedings of the National Academy of Sciences, USA*, **82**, 4778–82.

Lane, R.J.M., Gardner-Medwin, D., and Roses, A.D. (1980). Electrocardiographic abnormalities in carriers of Duchenne muscular dystrophy. *Neurology*, **30**, 497–501.

Loufrani, L., Matrougui, K., Gorny, D. *et al.* (2001). Flow (shear stress)-induced endothelium-dependent dilation is altered in mice lacking the gene encoding for dystrophin. *Circulation*, **103**, 864–70.

Meryon, E. (1851). On fatty degeneration of the voluntary muscles (Report of the Royal Medical & Chirurgical Society, Dec. 9, 1851) *Lancet*, **2**, 588–9.

Meryon, E. (1852). On granular and fatty degeneration of the voluntary muscles. *Medico-Chirurgical Transactions*, **35**, 73–84.

Monaco, A.P., Bertelson, C.J., Liechti-Gallati, S., Moser, H., and Kunkel, L.M. (1988). An explanation for the phenotypic differences between patients bearing partial deletions of the DMD locus. *Genomics*, **2**, 90–5.

Morton, N.E. and Chung, C.S. (1959). Formal genetics of muscular dystrophy. *American Journal of Human Genetics*, **11**, 360–79.

Moser, H. and Emery, A.E.H. (1974). The manifesting carrier in Duchenne muscular dystrophy. *Clinical Genetics*, **5**, 271–84.

Muntoni, F., Gobbi, P., Sewry, C. *et al.* (1994). Deletions in the 5′ region of dystrophin and resulting phenotypes. *Journal of Medical Genetics*, **31**, 843–7.

Murray, J.M., Davies, K.E., Harper, P.S., Meredith, L., Mueller, C.R., and Williamson, R. (1982). Linkage relationship of a cloned DNA sequence on the short arm of the X chromosome to Duchenne muscular dystrophy. *Nature*, **300**, 69–71.

Nigro, G., Politano, L., Nigro, V. *et al.* (1994). Mutation of dystrophin gene and cardiomyopathy. *Neuromuscular Disorders*, **4**, 371–9.

van Ommen, G.J.B. and Scheuerbrandt, G. (1993). Neonatal screening for muscular dystrophy. *Neuromuscular Disorders*, **3**, 231–9.

Perloff, J.K., Roberts, W.C., De Leon, A.C., and O'Doherty, D. (1967). The distinctive electrocardiogram of Duchenne's progressive muscular dystrophy. *American Journal of Medicine*, **42**, 179–88.

Perloff, J.K., Henze, E., and Schelbert, H.R. (1984). Alterations in regional myocardial metabolism, perfusion, and wall motion in Duchenne muscular dystrophy studied by radionuclide imaging. *Circulation*, **69**, 33–42.

Petrof, B.J., Shrager, J.B., Stedman, H.H. *et al.* (1993). Dystrophin protects the sarcolemma from stresses developed during muscle contraction. *Proceedings of the National Academy of Sciences, USA*, **90**, 3710–14.

Pfister, M.H., Apaydin, F., Turan, O. *et al.* (1998). A second family with nonsyndromic sensorineural hearing loss linked to Xp21.2: refinement of the DFN4 locus within DMD. *Genomics*, **53**, 377–82.

Ray, P.N., Belfall, B., Duff, C. *et al.* (1985). Cloning of breakpoint of an X;21 translocation associated with Duchenne muscular dystrophy. *Nature*, **318**, 672–5.

Roest, P.A.M., Roberts, R.G., Sugino, S. *et al.* (1993). Protein truncation test (PTT) for rapid detection of translation termination mutations. *Human Molecular Genetics*, **2**, 1719–21.

Sander, M., Chavoshan, B., Harris, S. A. *et al.* (2000). Functional muscle ischaemia in neuronal nitric oxide synthase-deficient skeletal muscle of children with Duchenne muscular dystrophy. *Proceedings of the National Academy of Sciences, USA*, **97**, 13818–23.

Sewry, C.A. (2000). Immunocytochemical analysis of human muscular dystrophy. *Microscopy Research Technique*, **48**, 142–54.

Sitnik, R., Campiotto, S., Vainzof, M. *et al.* (1997). Novel point mutations in the dystrophin gene. *Human Mutation*, **10**, 217–22.

Sugita, H., Arahata, K., Ishiguro, T. *et al.* (1988). Negative immunostaining of Duchenne muscular dystrophy (DMD) and mdx muscle surface membrane with antibody against synthetic peptide fragment predicted from DMD cDNA. *Proceedings of the Japan Academy*, **64**, 37–9.

Tkatchenko, A.V., Piétu, G., Cros, N. *et al.* (2001). Identification of altered gene expression in skeletal muscles from Duchenne muscular dystrophy patients. *Neuromuscular Disorders* **11**, 269–77.

Yamagishi, H., Kato, S., Hiraishi, Y. *et al.* (1996). Identification of carriers of Ducehnne/Becker muscular dystrophy by a novel method based on detection of junction fragments in the dystrophin gene. *Journal of Medical Genetics*, **33**, 1027–31.

Zubrzycka-Gaarn, E.E., Bulman, D.E., Karpati, G. *et al.* (1988). The Duchenne muscular dystrophy gene product is localized in sarcolemma of human skeletal muscle. *Nature*, **333**, 466–9.

Chapter 5

Becker muscular dystrophy

Marianne de Visser and Edo M. Hoogerwaard

History

The disease is named after the well-known German geneticist Prof. P.E. Becker. However, as in Duchenne muscular dystrophy (DMD), others gave the first description of this particular muscular dystrophy. In 1934, Kostakow reported on 14 patients from a kindred from an area in the vicinity of Bonn, Germany, who were suffering from an X-linked, progressive proximal myopathy. Six of these also had 'pseudohypertrophic' calves. In 1937, Kostakow and Derix more extensively described the same family. They emphasised that in 5 out of 14 patients the first symptoms of muscle weakness of the pelvic girdle and thighs were noticed between age 3–17 years. Gradually, trunk, shoulder girdle and upper arm muscles became involved. Kostakow and Derix (1937) reported that the disease had a benign course, since 5 of the 14 patients were still able to ambulate after a disease duration of 10–20 years. Nevertheless, they neglected to stress that they had identified a new disease entity. In 1955, Becker and a psychologist, called Kiener, described a benign muscular dystrophy in a family related to Kiener himself and living in southeast Bavaria (Grimm 1995). It was the merit of Becker (1955) to recognize that the disease was distinct from Duchenne muscular dystrophy in as much as affected individuals became unable to walk only after 25 to 30 years of illness and had offspring, which had never been the case in DMD. They referred to the disease as 'eine neue X-Chromosomale Muskeldystrophie' (a new X-chromosomal muscular dystrophy). It has taken some time before Walton and Natrass (1954) who initially considered this disease as a variant of DMD could be convinced after a number of additional families, some in retrospect, had been reported in the fifties and sixties (Becker 1957; 1962; Blyth and Pugh 1959; Rotthauwe and Kowalewski 1966; Walton 1955).

Becker strongly believed that the newly discovered muscular dystrophy was allelic to DMD. For many years Duchenne type and Becker type of muscular dystrophy were considered to be distinct genetic entities. In 1983, Kingston *et al.* with molecular genetic evidence, showed that both disorders segregate with the same Xp21 chromosomal region and that DMD and Becker type muscular dystrophy (BMD) most likely were allelic disorders, possibly caused by mutations in the same gene. With the discovery of the dystrophin gene and its product, the dystrophin protein, Becker eventually proved to be correct. DMD and BMD are allelic disorders, both due to mutations in the dystrophin gene at Xp21 (Burghes *et al.* 1987; Koenig *et al.* 1989; Monaco *et al.* 1988).

Epidemiology

In the pre-dystrophin era, BMD was estimated to have a prevalence of 12.5–40 per cent of that of DMD and an incidence between 6 and 20 per cent of that of DMD. Bushby *et al.* (1991) measured the prevalence and incidence of DNA proven cases in the Northern Health Region of the United Kingdom. The cumulative birth incidence of BMD was at least 1 in 18 450 male live births against 1 in 5618 in DMD. Thus, the incidence of BMD is one-third of that of DMD, a much higher figure than was previously thought implying that BMD has been underdiagnosed in the past. This was confirmed by studies in Slovenia (Peterlin *et al.* 1997) and in North-West Tuscany (Siciliano *et al.* 1999). In another Italian study (Mostacciuolo *et al.* 1993) an even higher incidence (1 in 14 000) was found. The prevalence rate of BMD is approximately 2.5/100 000 in all epidemiological studies.

Molecular genetics

DNA studies

A detailed description of the molecular genetics of the dystrophinopathies is given in Chapter 4.

Dystrophin gene deletions account for approximately 65 per cent of Becker patients (Beggs *et al.* 1990; van Essen *et al.* 1997). Deletions are clustered in two 'hot spots', one proximal at the 5′ end (exons 2–20) and one more distal, comprising exons 45–53. The explanation of the difference between DMD and BMD, was first postulated by Monaco *et al.* (1988). BMD is mostly associated with rearrangements (deletions, point mutations, and rarely duplications) in which the translational reading frame is maintained (Monaco *et al.* 1988). However, rare out-of-frame deletions have been reported in BMD patients (Baumbach *et al.* 1989; Comi *et al.* 1994; Gillard *et al.* 1989; Hodgson *et al.* 1992; Malhotra *et al.* 1988; Winnard *et al.* 1993).

Descriptions of gross alterations of the gene, such as a more than 400 000 bp duplication of the dystrophin gene (Angelini *et al.* 1990) or a large (40–50 per cent of the coding region of dystrophin) in-frame deletion (England *et al.* 1990; Love *et al.* 1991; Mirabella *et al.* 1998; Morandi *et al.* 1993; Passos-Bueno *et al.* 1994) giving rise to a mild muscular dystrophy suggest that in the case of gene therapy for DMD a minigene may suffice.

The reading frame rule holds in about 92 per cent of the cases (Koenig *et al.* 1989). However, exceptions to the reading frame rule have been found, about 50 per cent of which occur in exon 3–7 deletions, which produce a great variety of phenotypes, from severe DMD through intermediate MD to mild BMD (Baumbach *et al.* 1989; Gillard *et al.* 1989; Malhotra *et al.* 1988).

Dystrophin analysis

Dystrophin, the large protein product of the gene that is localized in the surface membrane, was found to be reduced in quantity or with a different molecular weight in muscle of patients with BMD (Hoffman *et al.* 1988; 1989; Nicholson *et al.* 1990; Fig. 5.1) on immunoblots. Immunocytochemical staining shows a patchy and discontinuous, and usually faint appearance in the surface membrane (Arahata *et al.* 1989; Fig. 5.2). However, the interpretation of immunohistochemical staining in some BMD patients can not be distinguished with certainty from non-Xp21-linked muscular dystrophies (Gold *et al.* 1992; Nicholson *et al.* 1990). In addition, dystrophin deficient fibres may be 'false-negative' due to necrosis or regeneration. In these cases, Western blot analysis is far more superior. In case of point mutations, dystrophin analysis may not be conclusive. Rarely, absence of dystrophin, which is by definition compatible with a diagnosis of DMD, has been reported in patients with Becker muscular dystrophy (Hattori *et al.* 1999; Mongini *et al.* 1992).

Clinical features

Presentation and age at onset

Becker (1957, 1962) reported that there is a wide range in age of onset (2–35 years), but in most cases the first symptoms were noticed between the 6th and 18th year of life

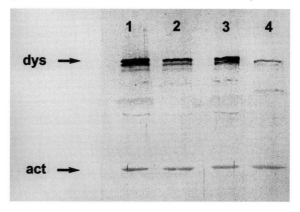

Fig. 5.1 Dystrophin immunoblot analysis of muscle tissue extracts of various patients. Lanes 1 and 3 are controls, lanes 2 and 4 are from BMD patients showing reduction of dystrophin. At the bottom actinin is depicted which serves for standardization. (Courtesy of H.B. Ginjaar).

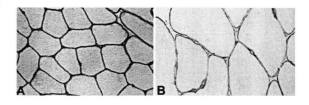

Fig. 5.2 Immuno-histochemical labelling of dystrophin in skeletal muscle of a healthy control (A) and of a 35-year-old patient with Becker muscular dystrophy showing a heterogeneous pattern of expression of dystrophin in every muscle fibre (B). (Courtesy of H.B. Ginjaar).

with a mean age of onset of 11.1 years (Emery and Skinner 1976). Although the time of clinical onset is admittedly an unreliable parameter (Bradley *et al.* 1978) most studies have found a similar mean age at onset. Bushby and Gardner-Medwin (1993) drew attention to the fact that BMD can also present with delayed walking which is related to an earlier age of onset. Usually patients present with symptoms, including frequent falling, difficulty climbing stairs, waddling gait and poor running, which can be ascribed to weakness of the muscles of the lower extremities (Bushby and Gardner-Medwin 1993; Comi *et al.* 1994). There are exceptional cases in which the dystrophinopathy remains asymptomatic for a long time and causes muscle weakness in the seventh decade (Comi *et al.* 1994; England *et al.* 1990; Love *et al.* 1991).

Other reported presenting symptoms are myalgia or cramps, especially in the calf region (Angelini *et al.* 1994; Beggs *et al.* 1991; Bushby *et al.* 1991; Bushby and Gardner-Medwin 1993; Comi *et al.* 1994; Doriguzzi *et al.* 1993; Franz *et al.* 1995; Gold *et al.* 1992; Gotspe *et al.* 1989; Higucchi *et al.* 1993; Hoffmann *et al.* 1989; Kuhn *et al.* 1979; Morandi *et al.* 1995; Siciliano *et al.* 1994; Yoshida *et al.* 1993), toe walking (Bushby and Gardner-Medwin 1993; Comi *et al.* 1994; Morandi *et al.* 1995), rhabdomyolysis, exercise or anaesthesia-triggered (Angelini *et al.* 1994; Beggs *et al.* 1991; Bush and Dubowitz 1991; Bushby and Gardner-Medwin 1993, Doriguzzi *et al.* 1993; Gold *et al.* 1992; Gotspe *et al.* 1989; Hoffmann *et al.* 1989; Morandi *et al.* 1995; Ohkoshi *et al.* 1995; Siciliano *et al.* 1994; 1999), life-threatening arrhythmias and cardiac arrest associated with the use of succinylcholine during induction of anaesthesia or malignant hyperthermia (Hoffmann *et al.* 1989; Sullivan *et al.* 1994), cognitive dysfunction and psychiatric disturbances (North *et al.* 1996), congenital cataract (Mirabella *et al.* 1998), or cardiac failure (Angelini *et al.* 1994; Beggs *et al.* 1991; Doriguzzi *et al.* 1993; Gotspe *et al.* 1989; Kuhn *et al.* 1979; Palmucci *et al.* 1992; Siciliano *et al.* 1994, 1999). Some of these features may be the sole manifestation (Doriguzzi *et al.* 1993; Gold *et al.* 1992; Gotspe *et al.* 1989; Palmucci *et al.* 1992; Siciliano *et al.* 1994).

Skeletal muscle involvement

Muscle weakness

Muscle weakness and wasting is usually symmetric and starts in the proximal muscles of the lower extremities (Fig. 5.3). Becker and Kiener (1955) and Becker (1962) systematically investigated their patients and reported the following order of involvement. The gluteus maximus, medius, and minimus muscles were the first muscles to be affected. Subsequently, the iliopsoas, quadriceps femoris and erector spinae muscles were involved. Gradually, weakness extended to the long dorsal muscles of the trunk and upper extremities. First, the pectoral muscle (especially the sternocostal part), followed by the latissimus dorsi, rhomboids, serratus anterior, trapezius (middle and lower parts), deltoid, biceps and triceps brachii, and the brachioradialis muscles. In due course, the adductors of the thigh, tibialis anterior, toe extensors and peroneal muscles were involved. The calf muscles remained preserved until late stages of the disease, as

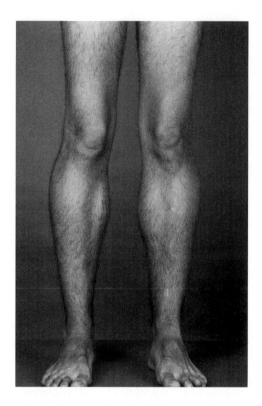

Fig. 5.3 17-year-old male with Becker muscular dystrophy—The calf muscles are hypertrophic, specially when compared to the atrophic thighs.

did the fore arm muscles, intrinsic muscles of the feet and hands, and the sternocleido-mastoids. Facial muscles remain unaffected. We and others found that the hamstrings and hip adductors were also among the first muscles to become affected. The neck flexors showed weakness at the same time as involvement of the upper arm muscles occurred.

By means of muscle imaging, i.e. computed tomography (de Visser and Verbeeten 1985), an even more accurate order of involvement could be made. In the early stages the adductor magnus (Fig. 5.4), gluteus maximus and long head of the biceps femoris muscle showed fatty infiltration, followed by the semimembranosus (Fig. 5.4) and glu-teus medius muscle. Subsequently, abnormalities were found in the vastus muscles, the semitendinosus, gluteus minimus, adductor longus, rectus femoris, tensor fasciae latae, medial head of the gastrocnemius, and the short head of the biceps femoris muscle. Only in the late stages were the tibialis anterior, peroneal, lateral head of the gastrocne-mius, toe extensors, iliac and soleus muscles affected. Interestingly, the sartorius and gracilis muscle were nearly always preserved and often hypertrophic which might be considered compensation for the paretic agonist thigh muscles.

There are cases of molecular genetically proven BMD who manifest with so-called 'quadriceps myopathy,' in whom muscle weakness, and especially wasting, is initially restricted to the quadriceps femoris muscles (Sunohara *et al.* 1990; Wada *et al.* 1990).

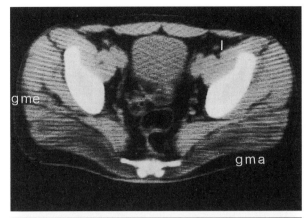

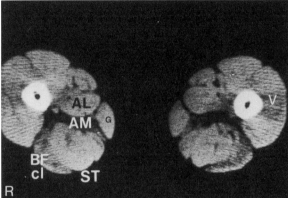

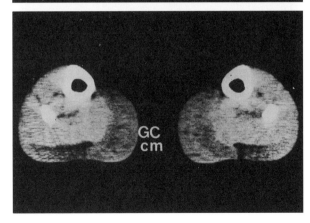

Fig. 5.4 (A) CT scan of the pelvic girdle region: decreased attenuation of the gluteus maximus (Gma) and gluteus medius (Gme) muscles. The m. iliacus (I) is notably spared. (B) CT scan of the thighs: decreased attenuation of the vasti (V) muscles, adductor magnus (AM) and caput longum of the biceps femoris (BFcl), and hypertrophic appearance of the adductor longus (AL), semitendinosus (ST) and gracilis (G) muscles. (C) Twelve-year-old boy with Becker muscular dystrophy - CT scan of the lower legs: decreased attenuation and enlargement (pseudohypertrophy), especially of the medial gastrocnemius (GCcm) muscles. (C) With permission from John Wiley and Sons.

Muscle hypertrophy

Muscle hypertrophy is often present (Fig. 5.3), but not invariably noticed (Becker and Kiener 1955; Bradley *et al.* 1978; Kostakow and Derix 1937; Kuhn *et al.* 1979; Ringel *et al.* 1977; de Visser *et al.* 1990). Muscle hypertrophy may precede muscle weakness

Table 5.1 Clinical characteristics and cardiac data of 27 patients with BMD

Family	Age[a]	ECG 1980[b]	Echo 1980[c]	ECG 1994[d]	Echo 1994[e]	Diagnosis[f]	Death
A-1	43	A	n	R, Qlat	n	a ECG	
2	17	N	n	n	n	N	
3	53	N	n	n	n	N	
4	56	N	n	LBBB, ST	LV dil, FS	CHF	1993
5	53	A	n	LBBB	LV dil, GH	CHF	1989
B-1	39	A	DCM	R, RS, Qlat, ST	LV dil, GH	DCM	
2	21	N	n	NA	LV dil, FS	CHF	1991
3	36	A	DCM	R, RS, Qinf	LV dil, FS	CHF	
4	44	N	n	n	GH	Borderline	
5	46	A	n	Qlat	n	a ECG	
6	47	A	n	R, RS, Qlat	LV dil, GH	DCM	
7	40	A	n	R, Qlat	LV dil, GH	DCM	
8	29	N	n	R, Qlat	LV dil	Borderline	
9	28	N	n	R, RS, Qlat, ST	LV dil	Borderline	
C-1	33	A	DCM	NA	NA	CHF	1984
2	26	A	n	Qlat	n	a ECG	
3	22	A	n	Qlat	n	a ECG	
D-1	60	A	DCM	LBBB	NA	CHF	1984
2	39	N	n	NA	n	N	
E-1	27	N	n	R	n	a ECG	
F-1	37	N	n	n	n	N	
2	40	A	n	R, RS	inf. hypokin.	Borderline	
G-1	32	N	n	LVH, ST	LV dil	Borderline	
2	35	N	n	ST	LV dil	Borderline	
3	37	N	n	n	n	N	
H-1	43	N	n	R, RS, Qinf	n	a ECG	
J-1	33	N	n	Qinf, LVH	n	a ECG	

[a] Age at time of examination or age at death.

[b] ECG examination in 1980. A: abnormal ; N: normal.

[c] Echo; echocardiofgraphic examination in 1980. n: normal investigation; DCM: dilated cardiomyopathy.

[d] ECG examination in 1994 or in the period preceding death. R: high R wave in V1; Qlat: Q waves in lateral leads; n: normal ECG; LBBB: Left Bundle Branch Block; ST: non-specific ST segment; RS: R/S ratio >1 in V1; Qinf: Q waves in inferior leads; NA: Not available; LVH: left ventricle hypertrophy.

[e] Echocardiographic examination in 1994 or in the period preceding death. n: normal echocardiography; LV dil: left ventricle dilatation; FS: diminished fractional shortening; GH: Global Hypokinesia; NA: Not available; inf. hypokin.: infero lateral hypokinesia.

[f] diagnosis. a ECG: abnormal ECG; N: normal investigation; CHF: congestive heart failure; DCM: dilated cardiomyopathy; borderline: borderline abnormal echocardiographic examination.

(Emery and Skinner 1976). In particular the calf muscles are hypertrophic (Becker and Kiener, 1955; Fig. 5.3), but virtually every limb muscle and also the erector spinae muscles can show enlargement (Becker and Kiener 1955; Doriguzzi *et al.* 1993). Muscle imaging revealed that there is often replacement of fat within the enlarged muscle (pseudohypertrophy (Fig. 5.4)).

Contractures

Achilles tendon contractures are an early sign and considered to be compensatory mechanism for weakness of the gluteus maximus muscles, as is also the case in DMD.

Pes cavus was found in patients described by Becker (1962) and Bradley *et al.* (1978).

Other contractures and scoliosis are usually seen in advanced stages of the disease, especially when the patient has become bedridden (Becker and Kiener 1955; Bradley *et al.* 1978; Ringel *et al.* 1977; Rotthauwe and Kowalewski 1966).

Other clinical features

Cardiac features (Table 5.1)

Cardiac involvement is not an exception in BMD as was thought for a long time. As in DMD, it seems more likely that the heart muscle invariably becomes affected (Comi *et al.* 1994; Hoffmann *et al.* 1989; Hoogerwaard *et al.* 1997; Melacini *et al.* 1993; Nigro *et al.* 1983; 1995; Steare and Dubowitz 1992; de Visser *et al.* 1992). The most frequently observed electrocardiographic abnormalities include a high R-wave in V1 and pathological Q-waves. Based on studies in DMD this most likely reflects damage of the posterobasal and inferior wall of the left ventricle (Perloff *et al.* 1967) and is probably the first sign of left ventricular involvement, ultimately leading to DCM. However, there are two reports of patients with either BMD or X-linked dilated cardiomyopathy (X-LDC) who have primary involvement of the right myocardium (Franz *et al.* 1995; Melacini *et al.* 1993). We and others found a marked variability between and within families, as is also the case with skeletal muscle involvement (Beggs *et al.* 1991; Comi *et al.* 1994; Hoogerwaard *et al.* 1997).

Cardiomyopathy may be more pronounced than skeletal muscle involvement (Angelini *et al.* 1994; Melacini *et al.* 1993; 1996; Siciliano *et al.* 1994), and even precede skeletal muscle weakness. There are descriptions of patients who present with cardiomyopathy and do not develop or have only mild skeletal muscle weakness (Ferlini *et al.* 1998; Franz *et al.* 1995; 2000; Milasin *et al.* 1996; Muntoni *et al.* 1993; 1997; Palmucci *et al.* 1992; Piccolo *et al.* 1994; Towbin *et al.* 1993; Yoshida *et al.* 1993). Many but not all (Milasin *et al.* 1996; Muntoni *et al.* 1997) affected patients have an increased serum CK activity. The disease is being referred to as X-linked dilated cardiomyopathy (X-LDC). X-LDC may be caused by the presence of a single point mutation at the first exon-intron boundary or a nonsense mutation in exon 29, by a rearrangement downstream from the 5' end of intron 11 or by a deletion in the mid-rod domain of the dystrophin gene. All these mutations have in common that they show a different pattern of expression in cardiac as compared to skeletal muscle. The skeletal muscle is able to maintain dystrophin synthesis via exon skipping or alternative splicing that the heart is not able to put in place (Ferlini *et al.* 1998).

Cognitive impairment

Mental retardation in DMD is known to occur in about 30 per cent of the cases. Becker (1962) reported that 'feeble-mindedness' of low degree seemed to belong to the clinical picture of BMD. Others have also reported reduced intellectual performance (Beggs *et al.* 1991; Bushby and Gardner-Medwin 1993; Comi *et al.* 1994; Emery and Skinner 1976). However, only recently this was quantified. Intellectual impairment (defined as IQ < 75) was found in 25 per cent of patients with BMD. A correlation was found with the loss of an isoform of dystrophin (Dp 140) with predominant expression during foetal brain development (Bardoni *et al.* 2000), rather than with the duration of the disease as had been previously thought. North *et al.* (1996) described four patients who also had behavioural and emotional disturbances in addition to cognitive disturbances.

Retinal changes

The localization of three isoforms of dystrophin, that is, Dp427, Dp260, and Dp70 are expressed in the outer plexiform layer of the retina. Thus, it is not surprising that abnormal retinal neurotransmission as measured by the b-wave amplitude on electroretinography (ERG) has been looked for and found both in DMD and, to a lesser extent, in BMD and in DMD carriers (Girlanda *et al.* 1997; Pillers *et al.* 1993; 1999). The most important determinant in the ERG b-wave phenotype is the position of the mutation. Pillers *et al.* (1999) found abnormal ERGs in 46 per cent of the patients with mutations 5' of the Dp260 transcript start site as opposed to 94 per cent with more distal mutations.

Course of the disease

Unlike DMD where the course of the disease is quite uniform showing wheelchair dependency at the age of 12, in BMD the clinical picture is variable. As mentioned earlier, many patients can be asymptomatic until their mid sixties, whereas the occasional patient shows rapid progression of muscle weakness comparable to that of DMD. There is not only marked interfamilial variability, but also within families the clinical picture may show considerable variation (Beggs *et al.* 1991; Comi *et al.* 1994; Emery and Skinner 1976; Furukawa and Peter 1977; Ginjaar *et al.* 2000; Hoogerwaard *et al.* 1997; Medori *et al.* 1989; Toscano *et al.* 1995).

The age of loss of ambulation ranges from 12 to over 70 (Becker and Kiener 1955; Becker 1962; Bradley *et al.* 1978; Emery and Skinner 1976; Kostakow 1934; Kostakow and Derix 1937; Markand *et al.* 1969; Rotthauwe and Kowalewski 1966; Zellweger and Hanson 1967).

According to the same authors, age at death is also highly variable (17–74 years). The mean age at death is about 40 years, some 25–30 years after onset of the disease.

The same variability holds true with regard to heart involvement. Some patients die due to a fulminating cardiomyopathy whereas their family members may have marked subclinical left ventricle dilatation for decades. We and others performed longitudinal studies on families with BMD and found that the prevalence of cardiac abnormalities increases over the years (Nigro *et al.* 1995; Hoogerwaard *et al.* 1997). There also seems to be a tendency for cardiomyopathy to occur in ambulatory rather than in wheelchair bound patients, but in both studies this did not reach a statistical significance, and therefore, more follow-up is needed to substantiate this observation which may have important consequences in daily practice.

Genotype–phenotype correlations

As has been described already the reading frame hypothesis holds true in 92 per cent of the cases. Exceptions are reported by Baumbach *et al.* (1989); Gillard *et al.* (1989) and Malhotra *et al.* (1988).

Initially, specific genotypes seemed to correlate with a particular phenotype (Bushby *et al.* 1993). The high incidence of severe cramps and myalgia among patients with mutations in the proximal rod domain (Beggs *et al.* 1991) suggests that this domain is functionally different from the distal portion of the rod. Deletions of exons 45–47 corresponded with preserved ambulation. However, more recent observations refuted this. The same holds true for cardiac complications. Although there are some reports claiming a correlation between site of the mutation, in particular deletions encompassing exons 48–49, and cardiac complications (Melacini *et al.* 1993; Nigro *et al.* 1994), we and others found no association between mutation type and dilated cardiomyopathy (Comi *et al.* 1994; Hoogerwaard *et al.* 1997; Morandi *et al.* 1995; Politano *et al.* 1991). A mutation in the promotor region and exon one, in exon 29, or in the central rod domain is associated with dilated cardiomyopathy without or with only mild muscle weakness (Ferlini *et al.* 1998; Franz *et al.* 1995; 2000; Milasin *et al.* 1998; Muntoni *et al.* 1993; 1997; Palmucci *et al.* 1992; Piccolo *et al.* 1994; Towbin *et al.* 1993; Yoshida *et al.* 1993).

Ginjaar *et al.* (2000) studied a BMD family in which different phenotypes occurred in three males due to a mutation causing skipping of exon 29. It was hypothesized that the differences in phenotype could be related to the level of skipping of exon 29.

Some (Angelini *et al.* 1994; Beggs *et al.* 1991; Hoffmann *et al.* 1989) noticed a correlation between the amount of dystrophin and clinical severity: the lower the dystrophin (between 3 and 10 per cent), the poorer the clinical outcome. However, Comi *et al.* (1994) and Morandi *et al.* (1995) were not able to find this correlation. The observation that the absence of dystrophin may actually be associated with a mild BMD clinical picture (Mongini *et al.* 1992; Hattori *et al*. 1999) seems to corroborate this.

Ancillary investigations

Estimation of serum creatine kinase activity

Serum creatine kinase (CK) activity is almost invariably elevated (Emery and Skinner 1976; Rotthauwe and Kowalewski 1965), usually more than five-fold, except for the odd case presenting late or in an end-stage of the disease. CK is at its highest in early stages and decreases with progression of the disease (Bradley *et al.* 1978; Emery and Skinner 1976; Goebel *et al.* 1979; Rotthauwe and Kowalewski 1966; Zellweger and Hanson 1967). There are patients in whom elevation of CK is the presenting or even the only expression of dystrophinopathy (Emery and Skinner 1976; Hoffmann *et al.* 1989; Melis *et al.* 1998; Morandi *et al.* 1995; Mostacciuolo *et al.* 1993; Siciliano *et al.* 1999; Tachi *et al.* 1992).

Electromyography

Short-duration, low-amplitude motor unit action potential (MUAPs) are consistent with a myopathy. However, in BMD, it is not unusual to find high frequency discharges, positive sharp waves or fibrillations (Bradley *et al.* 1978; Kuhn *et al.* 1979; Sunohara *et al.* 1990) or long-duration polyphasic MUAPs (Uncini *et al.* 1990). These findings were found to correlate with the appearance of regenerating muscle fibres. These apparently 'neurogenic' findings may give rise to confusion with autosomal recessive proximal spinal muscular atrophy (Kugelberg–Welander disease), clinically resembling BMD.

Muscle histology

There is a wide range of histological changes, mostly compatible with a muscular dystrophy. Although the histological picture resembles that encountered in DMD, there are clear differences. Hyaline fibres and necrosis are observed in BMD, but are not as prominent as in DMD (Bradley *et al.* 1978). As in EMG studies so-called 'neurogenic' changes such as small angular muscle fibres, clumped pycnotic nuclei (Bradley *et al.* 1978; Goebel *et al.* 1979; ten Houten and de Visser 1984; Kaido *et al.* 1991; Kuhn *et al.* 1979; McDonald *et al.* 1991; Ohkoshi *et al.* 1995; Sunohara *et al.* 1990) and even type grouping (Kaido *et al.* 1991), may cause diagnostic difficulties. These changes should probably be considered either the result of fibre splitting or as regenerating fibres. Younger patients tend to show more active muscle fibre necrosis and regeneration than do older patients who are found to have more chronic myopathic changes such as moth-eaten fibres, fibre splitting, hypertrophic fibres and marked endomysial fibrosis (Bradley *et al.* 1978; ten Houten and de Visser 1984; Kaido *et al.* 1991; Ringel *et al.* 1977). Unusual histological findings include rimmed vacuoles and small foci of inflammatory cells (Bradley *et al.* 1978; McDonald *et al.* 1991; de Visser *et al.* 1990).

The manifesting carrier

Clinical features (skeletal muscle weakness and cardiac involvement)

BMD carriers manifesting with skeletal muscle weakness were considered to be rare. For a long time only one report of a manifesting BMD carrier existed (Moser 1971) in which the author described a four-year-old daughter of a patient with BMD. This girl had impaired motor development and had problems with walking and climbing stairs. She developed generalized muscular hypotonia with atrophy of pelvic and shoulder girdle muscles. Subsequently, more reports appeared (Aguilar *et al.* 1978; Bushby *et al.* 1993; Glass *et al.* 1992; Haginoya *et al.* 1991; Moser, 1971; Voit *et al.* 1991). In a survey, carried out in the United Kingdom in 1989, four BMD manifesting carriers were detected (Norman and Harper 1989). A recently conducted Dutch survey by Hoogerwaard *et al.* (1999) showed that six out of 43 (14 per cent) definite BMD carriers had mild to moderate muscle weakness as compared to 19 per cent (16 out of 64) DMD carriers. Two out of six BMD carriers with muscle weakness were identified with hand-held dynamometry which is a sensitive method for the detection of muscle weakness. Another 5 per cent complained about exertion-related myalgia or cramps in both carrier groups.

The mean age at onset of symptoms in the BMD carriers was 24 years. In four carriers muscle weakness was asymmetric. One carrier had weakness limited to the upper arms/shoulder girdle, in three it was limited to the pelvic girdle or upper legs and in two carriers both upper and lower limbs were involved.

Although several publications reported DMD carriers presenting with cardiac failure, until recently BMD carriers with cardiac abnormalities have hardly been mentioned. Two case reports mentioned a normal electrocardiography in a BMD carrier (Sunohara *et al.* 1990; Aguilar *et al.* 1978). The same Dutch group of carriers was also screened for cardiac abnormalities. Twelve (27 per cent) BMD carriers had ECG abnormalities, similar to those found in male DMD patients. The most frequently observed abnormalities were increased R-wave (>4 mm in V1) or increased R/S ratio in V2 (Hoogerwaard *et al.* 1999). Fifteen (34 per cent) BMD carriers had abnormal echocardiographic findings. Whereas no actual dilated cardiomyopathy could be detected in BMD carriers as opposed to 8 per cent in the DMD carriers evidence of left ventricle dilatation was found in seven (16 per cent) BMD carriers. In the series of Politano *et al.* (1996) 11 out of 45 BMD carriers (24 per cent) had hypertrophic echocardiographic abnormalities. Six (13 per cent) BMD carriers had dilated cardiomyopathy, of whom one died of heart failure during follow-up.

Ancillary investigations

Estimation of serum creatine kinase activity

In the pre-dystrophin era CK was used for calculations of the risk of carriership. Depending on whether one or more measurements are carried out, serum CK activity is elevated in 30–62 per cent of carriers (Emery *et al.* 1967; Hoogerwaard *et al.* 1999; Kingston *et al.* 1985; Zatz *et al.* 1976).

Muscle histology

Muscle histology in BMD carriers may show changes which are similar to those found in DMD carriers. In symptomatic BMD carriers in which a muscle biopsy was performed the following abnormalities were observed: increased fibre size variability, internal nuclei (Bushby *et al.* 1993; Glass *et al.* 1992; Haginoya *et al.* 1991; Hoogerwaard 2000; Moser 1971) hypertrophic fibres (Haginoya *et al.* 1991), regenerating fibres

(Haginoya *et al.* 1991; Moser 1971), necrotic fibres (Haginoya *et al.* 1991) and increased connective tissue (Bushby *et al.* 1993). Asymptomatic BMD carriers may show mild myopathic alterations (Hoogerwaard 2000; Mora *et al.* 1993; Vainzof *et al.* 1993).

Dystrophin studies

BMD carriers may have abnormally sized and reduced amounts of dystrophin on Western blot (Bushby *et al.* 1993; Chevron *et al.* 1992; Mora *et al.* 1993; Vainzof *et al.* 1993). Immunohistochemical analysis may reveal a mosaic pattern of faintly positive disruptive dystrophin staining (Bushby *et al.* 1993; Chevron *et al.* 1992; Glass *et al.* 1992; Haginoya *et al.* 1991; Vainzof *et al.* 1993) or a proportion of dystrophin negative muscle fibres (Glass *et al.* 1992; Haginoya *et al.* 1991; Mora *et al.* 1993). Two larger series of dystrophin analyses in definite BMD carriers showed that in 8 per cent (1 out of 12) and 50 per cent (5 out of 10), respectively, dystrophin negative fibres could be detected on immunohistochemistry (Hoogerwaard 2000; Mora *et al.* 1993) and 25 per cent and 50 per cent, respectively, had an abnormal protein size on immunoblot.

The clinical and genetic approach to establish the diagnosis in BMD (and related dystrophinopathies, excluding DMD) and in BMD carriers at risk

Consensual diagnostic criteria

In 1997, a consensus meeting report in which Dutch (child)neurologists, geneticists ands paediatricians participated yielded diagnostic criteria that have been published (Bakker *et al.* 1997).

Elements

(1) Clinical signs comprise progressive symmetrical muscular weakness and atrophy: proximal limb muscles more than distal; initially lower limb muscles. Calf hypertrophy is often present. Weakness of quadriceps femoris may be the only manifestation for a long time. Some patients have cramps that are mostly induced by activity. Contractures of the elbows occur late in the course of the disease. Becker-type dystrophy may present with myalgia and cramps, exercise intolerance, asymptomatic hyperCKemia, malignant hyperthermia, cardiomyopathy or cognitive dysfunction.

(2) Exclusions: fasciculations, loss of sensory modalities.

(3) No wheelchair dependency before 16th birthday.

(4) There is a more than 5-fold increase of serum creatine kinase activity (in relation to age and mobility).

(5) Electromyography: short duration, low amplitude, polyphasic action potentials, fibrillations and positive sharp waves. Normal motor and sensory nerve conduction velocities.

(6) Muscle biopsy: dystrophin of abnormal size and/or amount (Fig. 5.1). Exceptionally dystrophin may be absent.

(7) DNA: Becker-type mutation within the dystrophin gene, identical haplotype, involving closely linked markers, as in previous case in the family.

(8) Positive family history, compatible with X-linked recessive inheritance.

Assessment
  The diagnosis is definite when:

(A) The first case in a family:

  (1), 2, 3, 4, 5 and either 8 or 6 and 7 all present.

(B) Another case in the family (according to element 9) complies with the criteria under A:

  a. the case is a first-degree relative: 4 (at least twice) present

  b. in other situations: (1), 2, 3, 4, 5 and either 8 or 6 and 7 all present.
The diagnosis is possible when:

  (1), 2, (3), 4, 5 and 6 all present.

Procedure for genetic analysis (van Essen *et al.* 1997)

In BMD patients detection of large rearrangements by means of polymerase chain reaction (PCR) or Southern blotting is feasible in 65–70 per cent of the cases. Other methods are reverse transcription PCR (RT-PCR) or fluorescent *in situ* hybridization (FISH). Immunohistochemical or immunobiochemical analysis of dystrophin in muscle tissue is, of course, a simple method to detect dystrophin abnormalities in BMD, similar to DMD. In carriers methods to detect microdeletions in the dystrophin gene are possible but usually not on a routine basis in most laboratories. These methods include: single strand confirmation polymorphism (SSCP), heteroduplex analysis (HDA) or protein truncation test (PTT), chemical mismatch cleavage (CMC) or denaturing gradient gel electrophoresis (DGGE).

  Carrier detection is dependent on the availability of patient material. The following approaches are suggested.

Patient DNA available, mutation detectable by PCR and/or Southern blotting. Carrier detection by differences in band intensities should possibly be confirmed by using confirmative polymorphisms in the region corresponding to the deletion which requires availibity of DNA of the carriers parents.

Patient DNA available, mutation not detectable by PCR and/or Southern blotting. When no mutation can be found a diagnosis has to be made on immunohistochemical grounds. As soon as the diagnosis DMD or BMD is certain, single strand confirmation polymorphism (SSCP), heteroduplex analysis (HDA) or protein truncation test (PTT) should be employed for screening the gene for a mutation. When an aberrant band is found this band must be amplified and sequenced for a pathogenic mutation. This also allows for carrier detection. When the mutation produces or abolishes a restriction site, restriction analysis readily confirms a carrier status.

In families where the mutation cannot be found carrier risks have to be calculated on the pedigree, serum CK activities in close female relatives, and linkage data using flanking and intragenic markers. Two notes of concern should be raised. First, possible recombinations remain a drawback in linkage analysis. Second, CK is elevated in only 30–62 per cent of the BMD carriers (Emery *et al.* 1967; Hoogerwaard *et al.* 1999; Kingston *et al.* 1985; Zatz *et al.* 1976).

Patient DNA not available. In patients where DNA from a blood sample is not available, a search for stored muscle tissue, Guthrie spots or decidous teeth may be worth trying. If this search is unfruitful, band intensity can be determined in quantitative PCR blots and/or Southern blots in female relatives. Detection of J-bands in the latter would be most helpful. If not, pulse field gel electrophoresis (PFGE), RT-PCR, SSCP, FISH and PTT can be considered.

Dystrophin analysis in carriers is not a reliable method. Both in manifesting carriers and in asymptomatic carriers dystrophin abnormalities may or may not be present, varying from single dystrophin negative muscle fibres to a mosaic pattern. At any rate, immunohistochemical analysis is much more sensitive than immunoblotting (Arahata *et al.* 1989).

Differential diagnosis

There are two diseases which may mimic BMD: limb girdle muscular dystrophy (Norman *et al.* 1989) and spinal muscular atrophy, type III (Lunt *et al.* 1989; McDonald *et al.* 1991; Zerres *et al.* 1990). For almost a decade rapid molecular genetic developments have expanded the field of limb girdle muscular dystrophies (LGMD) which is the most important disease from which BMD has to be differentiated. The clinical picture of BMD and LGMD can be almost identical. Even cardiac involvement may occur in LGMD, albeit in only a small proportion of patients (van der Kooi *et al.* 1998). Ancillary studies including estimation of CK, EMG and histological examination of a muscle biopsy specimen are not helpful in distinguishing one disease from the other. Immunohistochemical analysis of the dystrophin-related proteins, the sarcoglycans, followed by subsequent identification of the disease-causing mutation, is then the appropriate means to properly establish the diagnosis. (See Chapter 7).

Treatment

Therapeutic interventions are supportive and aimed at optimization of mobility and prevention of cardiac failure. It is recommended that patients be referred to rehabilitation medicine as soon as muscle weakness gives rise to walking difficulties. Physical therapy may prevent contractures that develop in particular when the patient becomes wheelchairbound.

Unlike DMD, there have not been any studies on the effects of prednisone treatment on muscle weakness in BMD. There is, however, one case-report by Higuchi *et al.* (1993) who describe a favourable response to prednisone as regards myalgia.

Since it is convincingly demonstrated that cardiomyopathy is part of dystrophinopathies, regular follow-up of the cardiological function is recommended, including electrocardiography and echocardiography. Cardiac complications can occur at any stage of the disease and may develop rapidly (Casazza *et al.* 1988; personal observation). There have, as yet, not been randomised clinical trials for DCM in dystrophinopathies. Supportive measures, vasodilator therapy and angiotensin converting enzyme inhibitors are indicated for asymptomatic DCM from whatever cause, and are, therefore, also recommended in DMD and BMD patients with this complication. Diuretics have been recommended as adjunctive therapy for DCM in cases with congestive heart failure.

In recent studies beta-blockers reduced mortality, improved left-ventricular function, and reduced hospital admissions in patients with symptomatic ischemic and non-ischemic chronic heart failure (CHF), with unusually high cost-effectiveness. If there is progression despite medical treatment and terminal heart failure is likely, the patient should be referred for assessment for possible heart transplantation (Quinlivan and Dubowitz 1992).

Rhabdomyolysis is a rare but potentially fatal complication of anaesthesia in dystrophinopathy (Bush and Dubowitz 1991). In order to prevent such a catastrophe succinyl choline which seems to trigger this event should be avoided during general anaesthesia (Sullivan *et al.* 1994).

In many countries there are active patient support organizations. These offer the patients information about their disease and, even more important, help them cope through informal get-togethers with other patients.

References

Aguilar, L., Lisker, R., and García Ramos, G. (1978). Unusual inheritance of Becker type muscular dystrophy. *Journal of Medical Genetics*, **15**, 116–8.

Angelini, C., Beggs, A.H., Hoffman, E.P., Fanin, M., and Kunkel, L.M. (1990). Enormous dystrophin in a patient with Becker muscular dystrophy. *Neurology*, **40**, 808–12.

Angelini, C., Fanin, M., Pegoraro, E., Freda, P., Cadaldini, M., and Martinello, F. (1994). Clinical-molecular correlation in 104 mild X-linked muscular dystrophy patients: characterization of sub-clinical phenotypes. *Neuromuscular Disorders*, **4**, 349–58.

Arahata, K., Ishiura, S., Ishiguro, T., Tsukahara, T., Suhara, Y., Eguchi, C. *et al.* (1988). Immunostaining of skeletal and cardiac muscle surface membrane with antibody against Duchenne muscular dystrophy. *Nature*, **333**, 861–3.

Arahata, K. Hoffman, E.P., Kunkel, L.M., Ishiura, S., Tsukahara, T., Ishihara, T. *et al.* (1989). Dystrophin changes: comparison of dystrophin abnormalities by immunofluorescent and immunoblot analyses. *Proceedings of the National Academy of Sciences*, **86**, 7154–8.

Bakker, E., Jennekens, F.G.I., Visser, M. de, and Wintzen, A.R. (1997). Duchenne and Becker muscular dystrophies, In *Diagnostic criteria for Neuromuscular disorders* (ed. A.E.H. Emery), Royal Society of Medicine Press, London.

Bardoni, A., Felisari, G., Sironi, M., Comi, G., Lai, M., Robotti, M. *et al.* (2000). Loss of Dp140 regulatory sequences is associated with cognitive impairment in dystrophinopathies. *Neuromuscular Disorders*, **10**, 194–9.

Baumbach, L.L., Chamberlain, J.S., Ward, P.A., Farwell, N.J., and Caskey, C.T. (1989). Molecular and clinical correlations of deletions leading to Duchenne and Becker muscular dystrophy. *Neurology*, **39**, 465–74.

Becker, P.E. and Kiener, F. (1955). Eine neue X-chromosomale Muskeldystrophie. *Archiv für Psychiatrie und Zeitschrift Neurologie*, **193**, 427–48.

Becker, P.E. (1957). Neue Ergebnisse der Genetik der Muskeldystrophien. *Acta Genetica (Basel)*, **7**, 303–10.

Becker, P.E. (1962). Two new families of benign sex-linked recessive muscular dystrophy. *Revue of Canadian Biology*, **21**, 551–66.

Beggs, A.H., Koenig, M., Boyce, F.M., and Kunkel, L.M. (1990). Detection of 98% of DMD/BMD gene deletions by polymerase chain reaction. *Human Genetics*, **86**, 45–8.

Beggs, A.H., Hoffmann, E.P., Snyder, J.R., Arahata, K., Specht, L., Shapiro, F. *et al.* (1991). Exploring the molecular basis for variability among patients with Becker muscular dystrophy: dystrophin gene and protein studies. *American Journal of Human Genetics*, **49**, 54–67.

Blyth, H. and Pugh, R.J. (1959). Muscular dystrophy in childhood; the genetic aspect. *Annals of Human Genetics*, **23**, 127–63.

Bradley, W.G., Jones, M.Z., Mussini, J.M., and Fawcett, P.R.W. (1978). Becker-type muscular dystrophy. *Muscle & Nerve*, **1**, 111–32.

Burghes, A.H.M., Logan, C., Hu, X., Belfall, B., Worton, R.G., and Ray, P.N. (1987). A cDNA clone from the Duchenne/Becker muscular dystrophy gen. *Nature*, **328**, 434–7.

Bush, A. and Dubowitz, V. (1991). Fatal rhabdomyolysis complicating general anaesthesia in a child with Becker muscular dystrophy. *Neuromuscular Disorders*, **1**, 201–4.

Bushby, K.M.D., Thambyayah, M., and Gardner-Medwin, D. (1991). Prevalence and incidence of Becker muscular dystrophy. *Lancet*, **337**, 1022–4.

Bushby, K.M.D. and Gardner-Medwin, D. (1993). The clinical, genetic and dystrophin characteristics of Becker muscular dystrophy. I. Natural history. *Journal of Neurology*, **240**, 98–104.

Bushby, K.M.D., Goodship, J.A., Nicholson, L.V.B., Johnson, M.A., Haggerty, I.D., and Gardner-Medwin, D. (1993). Variability in clinical, genetic and protein abnormalities in manifesting carriers of Duchenne and Becker muscular dystrophy. *Neuromuscular Disorders*, **3**, 57–64.

Casazza, F., Brambilla, G., Salvato, A., Morandi, L., Gronda, E., and Bonacina, E. (1988). Cardiac transplantation in Becker muscular dystrophy. *Journal of Neurology*, **235**, 496–8.

Chevron, M.P., Tuffery, S., Echenne, B., Demaille, J., and Claustres, M. (1992). Becker muscular dystrophy: demonstration of the carrier status of a female by immunoblotting and immunostaining. *Neuromuscular Disorders*, **2**, 47–50.

Comi, G.P., Prelle, A., Bresolin, N., Moggio, M., Bardoni, A., Gallanti, A. *et al.* (1994). Clinical variability in Becker muscular dystrophy. Genetic, biochemical and immunohistochemical correlates. *Brain*, **117**, 1–14.

Doriguzzi, C., Palmucci, L., Mongini, T., Chiadò-Piat, L., Restagno, G., and Ferrone, M. (1993). Exercise intolerance and recurrent myoglobinuria as the only expression of Xp21 Becker type muscular dystrophy. *Journal of Neurology*, **240**, 269–71.

Emery, A.E., Clack, E.R., Simon, S., and Taylor, J.L. (1967). Detection of carriers of benign X-linked muscular dystrophy. *British Medical Journal*, **4**, 522–3.

Emery, A.E.H. and Skinner, R. (1976) Clinical studies in benign (Becker type) X-linked muscular dystrophy. *Clinical Genetics*, **10**, 189–201.

England, S.B., Nicholson, L.V.B., Johnson, M.A., Forrest, S.M., Love, D.R., Zubrzycka-Gaarn, E.E. *et al.* (1990). Very mild muscular dystrophy associated with the deletion of 46% of the dystrophin. *Nature*, **343**, 180–2.

van Essen, A.J., Kneppers, A.L., van der Hout, A.H., Scheffer, H., Ginjaar, I.B., ten Kate, L.P. *et al.* (1997). The clinical and molecular genetic approach to Duchenne and Becker muscular dystrophy: an updated protocol. *Journal of Medical Genetics*, **34**, 805–12.

Ferlini, A., Galie, N., Merlini, L., Sewry, C., Branzi, A., and Muntoni, F. (1998). A novel Alu-like element rearranged in the dystrophin gene causes a splicing mutation in a family with X-linked dilated cardiomyopathy. *American Journal of Human Genetics*, **63**, 436–46.

Franz, W.M., Muller, M., Muller, O.J., Herrmann, R., Rothmann, T., Cremer, M. *et al.* (2000). Association of nonsense mutation of dystrophin gene with disruption of sarcoglycan complex in X-linked dilated cardiomyopathy. *Lancet*, **355**, 1781–5.

Franz, W.M., Cremer, M., Herrmann, R., Grunig, E., Fogel, W., Scheffold, T. *et al.* (1995). X-linked dilated cardiomyopathy. Novel mutation of the dystrophin gene. *Annals of New York Academic Sciences*, **752**, 470–91.

Furukawa, T. and Peter, J.B. (1977). X-linked muscular dystrophy. *Annals of Neurology*, **2**, 414–6.

Gillard, E.F., Chamberlain, J.S., Murphy, E.G., Duff, C.L., Smith, B., Burghes, A.H. *et al.* (1989). Molecular and phenotypic analysis of patients with deletions within the deletion-rich region of the Duchenne muscular dystrophy (DMD) gene. *American Journal of Human Genetics*, **45**, 507–20.

Ginjaar, I.B., Kneppers, A.L.J., van der Meulen, J.-D.M., Anderson, L.V.B., Bremmer-Bout, M., van Deutekom, J.C.T. *et al.* (2000). Dystrophin nonsense mutation induces different levels of exon 29 skipping and leads to variable phenotypes within one BMD family. *European Journal of Human Genetics*, **8**, 793–6.

Girlanda, P., Quartarone, A., Buceti, R., Sinicropi, S., Macaione, V., Saad, F.A. *et al.* (1997). Extra-muscle involvement in dystrophinopathies: an electroretinography and evoked potential study. *Journal of the Neurological Sciences*, **146**, 127–32.

Glass, I.A., Nicholson, L.V., Watkiss, E., Johnson, M.A., Roberts, R.G., Abbs, S. *et al.* (1992). Investigation of a female manifesting Becker muscular dystrophy. *Journal of Medical Genetics*, **29**, 578–82.

Goebel, H.H., Prange, H., Gullotta, F., Kiefer, H., and Jones, M.Z. (1979). Becker's X-linked muscular dystrophy. Histological, enzyme-histochemical, and ultrastructural studies of two cases, originally reported by Becker. *Acta Neuropathologica* (Berlin), **46**, 69–77.

Gold, R., Kress, W., Meurers, B. Meng, G., Reichmann, H., and Muller, C.R. (1992). Becker muscular dystrophy: detection of unusual disease courses by combined approach to dystrophin analysis. *Muscle & Nerve*, **15**, 214–8.

Gospe, S.M., Lazaro, R.P., Lava, N.S., Grootscholten, P.M., Scott, M.O., and Fischbeck, K.H. (1989). Familial X-linked myalgia and cramps: A nonprogressive myopathy associated with a deletion in the dystrophin gene. *Neurology*, **39**, 1277–80.

Grimm, T. (1995). Peter Emil Becker—a short biography on the occasion of his 85th birthday. *Neuromuscular Disorders*, **5**, 243–7.

Haginoya, K., Yamamoto, K., Linuma, K., Yanagisawa, T., Ichinohasama, Y., Shimmoto, M. *et al.* (1991). Dystrophin immunohistochemistry in a symptomatic carrier of Becker muscular dystrophy. *Journal of Neurology*, **238**, 375–8.

Hattori, N., Kaido, M., Nishikagi, T., Inui, K., Fujimura, H., Nishimura, T. *et al.* (1999). Undetectable dystrophin can still result in a relatively benign phenotype of dystrophinopathy. *Neuromuscular Disorders*, **9**, 220–36.

Higuchi, I., Nakamura, K., Nakagawa, M., Nakamura, N., Usuki, F., Inose, M. *et al.* (1993). Steroid-responsive myalgia in a patient with Becker muscular dystrophy. *Journal of the Neurological Sciences*, **115**, 219–222.

Hodgson, S.V., Abbs, S., Clark, S., Manzur, A., Heckmatt, J.Z.H., Dubowitz, V. *et al.* (1992). Correlation of clinical and deletion data in Duchenne and Becker muscular dystrophy, with special reference to mental ability. *Neuromuscular Disorders*, **2**, 269–76.

Hoffman, E.P., Fischbeck, K.H., Brown, R.H., Johnson, M., Medori, R., Loike, J.D. *et al.* (1988). Characterization of dystrophin in muscle biopsy specimens from patients with Duchenne's and Becker's muscular dystrophy. *New England Journal of Medicine*, **318**, 1363–8.

Hoffman, E.P., Kunkel, L.M., Angelini, C., Clarke, A., Johnson, M., and Harris, J.B. (1989). Improved diagnosis of Becker's muscular dystrophy via dystrophin testing. *Neurology*, **39**, 1011–7.

Hoogerwaard, E.M., de Voogt, W.G., Wilde, A.A.M., van der Wouw, P.A., van Ommen, G.-J. B., and de Visser, M. (1997). Evolution of cardiac abnormalities in Becker muscular dystrophy over a 13-year period. *Journal of Neurology*, **244**, 657–63.

Hoogerwaard, E.M., Bakker, E., Ippel, P.F., Oosterwijk, J.C., Majoor-Krakauer, D.F., Leschot, N.J. *et al.* (1999). Signs and symptoms of Duchenne muscular dystrophy and Becker muscular dystrophy among carriers in the Netherlands: a cohort study. *Lancet*, **353**, 2116–9.

Hoogerwaard, E.M. (2000). *Duchenne & Becker muscular dystrophy. Neurological, cardiological, and genetic studies in carriers and patients*. Tela Thesis, Amsterdam.

Ten Houten, R. and de Visser, M. (1984). Histopathological findings in Becker-type muscular dystrophy. *Archives of Neurology*, **41**, 729–33.

Kaido, M., Arahata, K., Hoffman, E.P., Nonaka, I., and Sugita, H. (1991). Muscle histology in Becker muscular dystrophy. *Muscle & Nerve*, **14**, 1067–73.

Kingston, H.M., Thomas, N.S., Pearson, P.L., Sarfarazi, M., and Harper, P.S. (1983). Genetic linkage between Becker muscular dystrophy and a polymorphic DNA sequence on the short arm of the X chromosome. *Journal of Medical Genetics*, **20**, 255–8.

Kingston, H.M., Sarfarazi, M., Newcombe, R.G., Willis, N., and Harper, P.S. (1985). Carrier detection in Becker muscular dystrophy using creatine kinase estimation and DNA analysis. *Clinical Genetics*, **27**, 383–91.

Koenig, M., Beggs, A.H., Moyer, M., Scherpf, S., Heindrichs, K., Bettecken, T. *et al.* (1989). The molecular basis for Duchenne versus Becker muscular dystrophy: correlation of severity with type of deletion. *American Journal of Human Genetics*, **45**, 498–506.

van der Kooi, A.J., de Voogt, W.G., Barth, P.G., Busch, H.F., Jennekens, F.G., Jongen, P.J. *et al.* (1998). The heart in limb girdle muscular dystrophy. *Heart*, **79**, 73–7.

van der Kooi, A,J,, Barth, P.G., Busch, H.F., de Haan, R., Ginjaar, H.B., van Essen, A.J. *et al.* (1996). The clinical spectrum of limb girdle muscular dystrophy. A survey in The Netherlands. *Brain*, **119**, 1471–80.

Kostakow, St. (1934). Die progressive Muskeldystrophie, ihre Vererbung und Glykokollbehandlung. *Deutsche Archiv für klinischen Medizin*, **176**, 467–74.

Kostakow, St. and Derix, F. (1937). Familienforschung in einer muskeldystrophischen Sippe und die Erbprognose ihrer Mitglieder. *Deutsche Archiv für klinischen Medizin*, **180**, 585–60.

Kuhn, E., Fiehn, W., Schröder, J.M., Assmus, H., and Wagner, A. (1979). Early myocardial disease and cramping myalgia in Becker-type muscular dystrophy. *Neurology*, **29**, 1144–9.

Kunkel, L.M. and co-authors. (1986). Analysis of deletions in DNA from patients with Becker and Duchenne muscular dystrophy. *Nature*, **322**, 73–7.

Love, D.R., Flint, T.J., Genet, S.A., Middleton-Price, H.R., and Davies, K.E. (1991). Becker muscular dystrophy patient with a large intragenic dystrophin deletion: implications for functional minigenes and gene therapy. *Journal of Medical Genetics*, **28**, 860–4.

Lunt, P.W., Cummings, W.J.K., Kingston, H., Read, A.P., Mountford, R.C., Mahon, M. *et al.* (1989). DNA probes in differential diagnosis of Becker muscular dystrophy. *Lancet*, **333**, 46–7.

McDonald, T.D., Medori, R., Younger, D.S., Chang, H.W., Minetti, C., Uncini, A. *et al.* (1991). Becker muscular dystrophy or spinal muscular atrophy?-Dystrophin studies resolve conflicting results of electromyography and muscle biopsy. *Neuromuscular Disorders*, **1**, 195–200.

Malhotra, S.B., Hart, K.A., Klamut, H.J., Thomas N.S., Bodrug, S.E., Burghes, A.H. *et al.* (1988). Frame-shift deletions in patients with Duchenne and Becker muscular dystrophy. *Science*, **242**, 755–9.

Markand, O.N., North, R.R., D'Agosstino, A.N., and Daly, D.D. (1969). Benign sex-linked muscular dystrophy. *Clinical and pathological features. Neurology*, **19**, 617–33.

Medori, R., Brooke, M.H., and Waterston, R.H. (1989). Two dissimilar brothers with Becker's dystrophy have an identical genetic defect. *Neurology*, **39**, 1439–6.

Melacini, P., Fanin, M., Danieli, G.A., Fasoli, G., Villanova, C., Angelini, C. *et al.* (1993). Cardiac involvement in Becker muscular dystrophy. *Journal of American Cardiology*, **22**, 1927–34.

Melacini, P., Fanin, M., Danieli, G.A., Villanova, C., Martinello, F., Miorin, M. *et al.* (1996). Myocardial involvement is very frequent among patients affected with subclinical Becker's muscular dystrophy. *Circulation*, **94**, 3168–75.

Melis, M.A., Cau, M., Muntoni, F., Mateddu, A., Galanello, R., Boccone, L. *et al.* (1998). Elevation of serum creatine kinase as the only manifestation of an intragenic deletion of the dystrophin gene in three unrelated families. *European Journal of Paediatric Neurology*, **2**, 255–61.

Milasin, J., Muntoni, F., Severini, G.M., Bartoloni, L., Vatta, M., Krajinovic, M. *et al.* and the Heart Muscle Disease Study Group (1996). A point mutation in the 5′ splice site of the dystrophin gene first intron responsible for X-linked dilated cardiomyopathy. *Human Molecular Genetics*, **5**, 73–9.

Mirabella, M., Galluzzi, G., Manfredi, G., Bertiniu E., Ricci, E., De Leo, R. *et al.* (1998). Giant dystrophin deletion associated with congenital cataract and mild muscular dystrophy. *Neurology*, **51**, 592–5.

Monaco, A.P., Bertelson, C.J., Liechti-Gallati, S., Moser, H., and Kunkel, L.M. (1988). An explanation for the phenotypic differences between patients bearing partial deletions of the DMD locus. *Genomics*, **2**, 90–5.

Mongini, T., Palmucci, L. Doriguzzi, C., Chiadò-Piat, L., and Restagno, G. (1992). Absence of dystrophin in two patients with Becker type Xp21 muscular dystrophy. *Neuroscience Letters*, **147**, 37–40.

Mora, M., Morandi, L., Piccinelli, A., Gussoni, E., Gebbia, M., Blasevich, F. *et al.* (1993). Dystrophin abnormalities in Duchenne and Becker dystrophy carriers: correlation with cytoskeletal proteins and myosins. *Journal of Neurology*, **240**, 455–61.

Morandi, L., Mora, M., Confalonieri, V., Barresi, R., Di Blasi, C., Brugnoni, R. *et al.* (1995). Dystrophin characterization in BMD patients: correlation of abnormal protein with clinical phenotype. *Journal of the Neurological Sciences*, **132**, 146–55.

Morandi, L., Mora, M., Bernasconi, P., Mantegazza, R., Gebbia, M., Balestrini, M.R. *et al.* (1993). Very small dystrophin molecule in a family with a mild form of Becker muscular dystrophy. *Neuromuscular Disorders*, **3**, 65–70.

Moser, H. (1971). Biochemische, histologische und klinische Befunde bei einer vierjährigen Konduktorin der gutartigen X-chromosomalen Muskeldystrophie (Typ Becker). *Humangenetik*, **11**, 328–35.

Mostacciuolo, M.L., Miorin, M., Pegoraro, E., Fanin, M., Schiavon, F., Vitiello, L. *et al.* (1993). Reappraisal of the incidence rate of Duchenne and Becker muscular dystrophies on the basis of molecular diagnosis. *Neuroepidemiology*, **12**, 326–30.

Muntoni, F., Cau, M., Ganau, A., Congiu, R., Arvedi, G., Mateddu, A. *et al.* (1993). Deletion of the dystrophin muscle-promoter region associated with X-linked dilated cardiomyopathy. *New England Journal of Medicine*, **329**, 921–5.

Muntoni, F., Di Lenarda, A., Porcu, M., Sinagra, G., Mateddu, A., Marrosu, G. *et al.* (1997). Dystrophin gene abnormalities in two patients with idiopathic dilated cardiomyopathy. *Heart*, **78**, 608–12.

Nicholson, L.V., Johnson, M. A., Gardner-Medwin, D., Bhattacharya, S., and Harris, J.B. (1990). Heterogeneity of dystrophin expression in patients with Duchenne and Becker muscular dystrophy. *Acta Neuropathologica*, **80**, 239–50.

Nigro, G., Comi, L.I., Limongelli, F.M., Passamano, L., and Stefanelli, S. (1983). Prospective study of X-linked progressive muscular dystrophy in Campania. *Muscle & Nerve*, **6**, 253–62.

Nigro, G., Politano, L., Nigro, V., Petretta, V.R., and Comi, L.I. (1994). Mutation of dystrophin gene and cardiomyopathy. *Neuromuscular Disorders*, **4**, 371–9.

Nigro, G., Comi, L.I., Politano, L., Limongelli, F.M., Petretta, V.R., Passamano, L. *et al.* (1995). Evaluation of the cardiomyopathy in Becker muscular dystrophy. *Muscle & Nerve*, **18**, 283–91.

Norman, A. and Harper, P. A survey of manifesting carriers of Duchenne and Becker muscular dystrophy in Wales (1989). *Clinical Genetics*, **36**, 31–7.

Norman, A., Thomas, N., Coakley, J., and Harper, P. (1989). Distinction of Becker from limb girdle muscular dystrophy by means of dystrophin cDNA probes. *Lancet*, **i**, 466–8.

North, K.N., Miller, G., Iannacone, S.T., Clemens, P.R., Chad, D.A., Bella, I. *et al.* (1996). Cognitive dysfunction as the major presenting feature of Becker's muscular dystrophy. *Neurology*, **46**, 461–5.

Ohkoshi, N., Yoshizawa, T., Mizusawa, H., Shoji, S., Toyama, M., Iida, K. *et al.* (1995). Malignant hyperthermia in a patient with Becker muscular dystrophy: dystrophin analysis and caffeine contracture study. *Neuromuscular Disorders*, **5**, 53–8.

Palmucci, L., Doriguzzi, C., Mongini, T., Chiado-Piat, L., Restagno, G., Carbonara, A. *et al.* (1992). Dilating cardiomyopathy as the expression of Xp21 Becker type muscular dystrophy. *Journal of the Neurological Sciences*, **111**, 218–21.

Passos-Bueno, M.R., Vainzof, M., Marie, S.K., and Zatz, M. (1994). Half the dystrophin gene is apparently enough for a mild clinical course: confirmation of its potential use for gene therapy. *Human Molecular Genetics*, **3**, 919–22.

Perloff, J.K., De Leon, A.C., Roberts, W.C., and O'Doherty, D.O. (1967). The distinctive electrocardiogram of Duchenne's progressive muscular dystrophy. *American Journal of Medicine*, **42**, 179–88.

Peterlin, B., Zidar, J., Meznaric-Petrusa, M., and Zupancic, N. (1997). Genetic epidemiology of Duchenne and Becker muscular dystrophy in Slovenia. *Clinical Genetics*, **51**, 94–7.

Piccolo, G., Azan, G., Tonin, P., Arbustini, E., Gavazzi, A., Banfi, P. *et al.* (1994). Dilated cardiomyopathy requiring cardiac transplantation as initial manifestation of Xp21 Becker type muscular dystrophy. *Neuromuscular Disorders*, **4**, 143–6.

Pillers, D.M., Bulman, D.E., Weleber, R.G., Sigesmund, D.A., Musarella, M.A., Powell, B.R. *et al.* (1993). Dystrophin expression in the human retina is required for normal function as defined by electroretinography. *Nature Genetics*, **4**, 82–6.

Pillers, D.M., Fitzgerald, K.M., Duncan, N.M., Rash, S.M., White, R.A., Dwinnell, S.J. *et al.* (1999). Duchenne/Becker muscular dystrophy: correlation of phenotype with sites of mutations. *Human Genetics*, **105**, 2–9.

Politano, L., Colonna-Romano, S., Esposito, M.G., Nigro, G.V., Comi, L.I., Passamano, L. *et al.* (1991). Genotype-phenotype correlations in patients with deletions of Duchenne/Becker gene. *Acta Cardiomyologica*, **3**, 239–44.

Politano, L., Nigro, V., Nigro, G., Petretta, V.R., Passamano, L., Papparella, S. *et al.* Development of cardiomyopathy in female carriers of Duchenne and Becker muscular dystrophy. *Journal of American Medical Association*, **275**, 1335–8.

Quinlivan, R.M. and Dubowitz, V. (1992). Cardiac transplantation in Becker muscular dystrophy. *Neuromuscular Disorders*, **2**, 165–7.

Ringel, S.P., Carroll, J.E., and Schold, S.C. (1977). The spectrum of mild X-linked recessive muscular dystrophy. *Archives of Neurology*, **34**, 408–16.

Rotthauwe, H.W. and Kowalewski, S. (1966). Gutartige X-rezessive X-chromosomal vererbte Muskeldystrophie. *Humangenetik*, **3**, 17–40.

Siciliano, G., Fanin, M., Angelini, C., Pollina, L.E., Miorin, M., Saad, F.A. *et al.* (1994). Prevalent cardiac involvement in dystrophin Becker type mutation. *Neuromuscular Disorders*, **4**, 381–6.

Siciliano, G., Tessa, A., Renna, M., Manca, M.L., Mancuso, M., and Murri, L. (1999). Epidemiology of dystrophinopathies in North-West Tuscany: a molecular genetics-based revisitation. *Clinical Genetics*, **56**, 51–8.

Steare, S.E. and Dubowitz, V. (1992). Subclinical cardiomyopathy in Becker muscular dystrophy. *British Heart Journal*, **68**, 304–8.

Sullivan M, Thompson WK, and Hill GD. (1994). Succinylcholine-induced cardiac arrest in children with undiagnosed myopathy. *Canadian Journal of Anaesthesia*, **41**, 497–501.

Sunohara, N., Arahata, K., Hoffman, E.P., Yamada, H., Nishimiya, J., Arikawa, E. *et al.* (1990). Quadriceps myopathy: forme fruste of Becker muscular dystrophy. *Annals Neurology*, **28**, 634–9.

Tachi, N., Wakai, S., Watanabe, Y., Chiba, S., Nagaoka, M., and Minami, R. (1992). Delayed expression of dystrophin on regenerating muscle from two siblings with Becker muscular dystrophy. *Journal of the Neurological Sciences*, **110**, 165–8.

Toscano, A., Vitiello, L., Comi, G.P., Calvagni, F., Miorin, M., Prelle, A. *et al.* (1995). Duplication of dystrophin gene and dissimilar clinical phenotype in the same family. *Neuromuscular Disorders*, **5**, 475–81.

Towbin, J.A., Hejtmancik, J.F., Brink, P., Gelb, B., Zhu, X.M., Chamberlain, J.S. *et al.* (1993). X-linked dilated cardiomyopathy. Molecular genetic evidence of linkage to the Duchenne muscular dystrophy (dystrophin) gene at the Xp21 locus. *Circulation*, **87**, 1854–65.

Uncini, A., Lange, D.J., Lovelace, R.E., Solomon, M., and Hays, A.P. (1990). Long-duration polyphasic motor unit potentials in myopathies: a quantitative study with pathological correlation. *Muscle & Nerve*, **13**, 263–7.

Vainzof, M., Nicholson, L.V., Bulman, D.E., Tsanaclis, A.M., Passos-Bueno, M.R., Pavanello, R.C.M. *et al.* (1993). Sarcolemmal distribution of abnormal dystrophin in Xp21 carriers. *Neuromuscular Disorders*, **3**, 135–40.

de Visser, M. and Verbeeten, M. (1985). Computed tomography of the skeletal musculature in Becker-type muscular dystrophy and benign infantile spinal muscular atrophy. *Muscle & Nerve*, **8**, 435–44.

de Visser, M., Bakker, E., Defesche, J.C., Bolhuis, P.A., and van Ommen, G.J. (1990). An unusual variant of Becker muscular dystrophy. *Annals of Neurology*, **27**, 578–81.

de Visser, M., de Voogt, W.G. and de la Rivière, G.V. (1992). The heart in Becker muscular dystrophy, facioscapulohumeral dystrophy, and Bethlem myopathy. *Muscle & Nerve*, **15**, 591–6.

Voit, T., Stuettgen, P., Cremer, M., and Goebel, H.H. (1991). Dystrophin as a diagnostic marker in Duchenne and Becker muscular dystrophy. Correlation of immunofluorescence and western blot. *Neuropediatrics*, **22**, 152–62.

Wada, Y., Itoh, Y., Furukawa, T., Tsukagoshi, H., and Arahata, K. (1990). "Quadriceps myopathy": a clinical variant form of Becker muscular dystrophy. *Journal of Neurology*, **237**, 310–2.

Walton, J.N. and Natrass, F.J. (1954). On the classification, natural history and treatment of the myopathies. *Brain*, 77, 12–231.

Walton, J.N. (1955). On the inheritance of muscular dystrophies. *Annals of Human Genetics*, 21, 40–58.

Winnard, A.V., Klein, C.J., Coovert, D.D., Prior, T., Papp, A., Snyder, P. *et al.* (1993). Characterization of translational frame exception patients in Duchenne/Becker muscular dystrophy. Human Molecular Genetics, 2, 737–44.

Yoshida, K., Ikeda, S., Nakamura, A., Kagoshima, M., Takeda, S., Shoji, S. *et al.* (1993). Molecular analysis of the Duchenne muscular dystrophy gene in patients with Becker muscular dystrophy presenting with dilated cardiomyopathy. *Muscle & Nerve*, 16, 1161–6.

Zatz, M., Frota-Pessoa, O., Levy, J.A., and Peres, C.A. (1976). Creatine-phosphokinase (CPK) activity in relatives of patients with X-linked muscular dystrophies: a Brazilian study. *Journal de Génétique Humane*, 24, 153–68.

Zellweger, H. and Hanson, J.W. (1967). Slowly progressive X-linked recessive muscular dystrophy (type IIIb). Report of cases and review of the literature. *Archives of Internal Medicine*, 120, 525–35.

Zerres, K., Rudnik-Schöneborn, S., and Rietschel, M. (1990). Heterogeneity in proximal spinal muscular atrophy. *Lancet*, 336, 749–50.

Chapter 6

Emery–Dreifuss muscular dystrophy

Daniela Toniolo

Introduction

Emery–Dreifuss muscular dystrophy (EMD) is an inherited disorder characterized by early onset contractures, progressive weakness in humero-peroneal muscles, and cardiomyopathy with conduction block. The disease may have been described for the first time in 1902 (Cestan and Lejonne 1902). However, in 1966, Emery examined a large Virginian family affected with an X-linked muscular dystrophy (Emery and Dreifuss 1966) whose members had been reported earlier by Dreifuss and Hogan (1961) as having a possible benign form of Duchenne muscular dystrophy (DMD). After detailed clinical, electrophysiological and biochemical analysis, Emery realized that the disease observed in Dreifuss' family was quite distinct from both DMD and BMD (Becker type, the benign form of DMD) because of the unusual elbow and spine contractures, the weakness of proximal arm and distal leg, the essential cardiac abnormalities and the absence of muscle hypertrophy and intellectual impairment (Emery 1989; Emery and Dreifuss 1966; Emery and Emery 1995). Similar symptoms were later described in other families and in 1979 Rowland suggested the term 'Emery–Dreifuss muscular dystrophy (EMD)' for this distinctive disease (Rowland et al. 1979).

In the original reports, most families showed X-linked recessive inheritance (X-EMD: OMIM no.310300), but autosomal dominant (AD-EMD: OMIM no.181350) and autosomal recessive (AR-EMD: OMIM no.604929) forms were also described. The three forms have a striking resemblance of clinical symptoms that makes them indistinguishable and quite distinctive from other forms of muscular dystrophy (Emery 1993; Witt et al. 1988). Diagnostic criteria were established for X-EMD (Yates 1991) and it was later agreed that they could be applied also for AD-EMD (Yates 1997).

The genes responsible for the three genetic forms of EMD were identified (Bione et al. 1994; Bonne et al. 1999; Di Barletta et al. 2000). The X-EMD gene encodes emerin, a ubiquitous protein localized, in most cell types, to the inner nuclear membrane (Cartegni et al. 1997; Manilal et al. 1996; Nagano et al. 1996). AD-EMD and AR-EMD are caused by mutations in the gene LMNA, that encodes two lamins, A and C, by differential maturation of the 3' end of the mRNA (Bonne et al. 1999). The finding that lamin A/C and emerin mutations are responsible for clinically similar disorders showed that, in skeletal muscle and heart, interactions between nuclear membrane components is critical for skeletal and cardiac muscle function and loss of integrity of the nuclear envelope is an underlying cause of muscular dystrophy.

Clinical features

X-linked EMD (X-EMD)

Based on investigation of the large Virginian family (eight cases in three generations), the clinical triad of X-EMD were summarized by Emery as follows; (1) early contractures, often before there is any significant weakness, of the elbows, Achilles tendons and posterior neck (Fig. 6.1). Initially limitation of neck flexion is observed, but later contractures may abolish forward flexion of the entire spine; (2) slowly progressive muscle wasting and weakness with a humero-peroneal distribution early in the course of the disease (Fig. 6.1). Later, weakness also affects the proximal limb girdle musculature; and (3) a cardiomyopathy usually presenting as an atrio-ventricular conduction block ranging from sinus bradycardia, prolongation of the PR interval to complete heart block.

In most patients cardiac abnormalities appear later than the muscle involvement, in general after 20–30 years of age. Voit *et al.* (1988) performed a detailed cardiological follow up study in patients with EMD, and found four main features; (1) impairment of impulse generating cells; (2) conduction defects with atrial preponderance; (3) increased atrial and ventricular heterotopia; and (4) functional impairment of ventricular

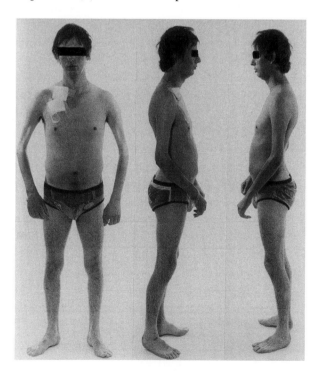

Fig. 6.1 A 17-year-old boy with X-linked muscular dystrophy with early contractures and cardiomyopathy. Note the flexion contractures of the elbows, and wasting of the lower legs. A cardiac pacemaker has been inserted.

myocardium. There is only one report of a male with X-EMD presenting severe cardiac involvement and only very minor muscle involvement (Vohanka *et al.* 2001). The disease associated cardiomyopathy makes early recognition of EMD very important as it is life-threatening but can be cured by implantation of a cardiac pacemaker (Emery 1989).

Serum creatine kinase (CK), lactate dehydrogenase, and aldolase levels increase moderately in affected male patients. They are often in the normal range in EMD carriers (Bialer *et al.* 1990; Merlini *et al.* 1986). The CK activity decreases with age in affected males.

Autosomal dominant EMD (AD-EMD)

In the typical cases, AD-EMD differs little clinically from X-EMD (Emery 1989, 1993; Hauptman and Thannhauser 1941). However, after the identification of the LMNA gene, a careful study of a large French family and of many familial and isolated cases demonstrated that in AD-EMD families, age at onset and degree of severity are more variable (Bonne *et al.* 2000). Moreover isolated cardiac involvement is observed frequently and impaired left ventricular function is not uncommon at later stages. Molecular genetic analysis is essential in distinguishing the two types of EMD.

Autosomal recessive EMD (AR-EMD)

Two possible cases of an autosomal recessive form of EMD have been reported (Takamoto *et al.* 1984; Taylor *et al.* 1998). Di Barletta *et al.* (2000) showed that, in addition to AD-EMD, the LMNA gene is responsible of AR-EMD. One of the patients in their study (MG) was homozygote for the mutation C664T (Fig. 6.2) carried in the heterozygous state by both his parents who were first degree cousins. The patient presented a very severe form of muscular dystrophy that had been previously diagnosed either as an atypical EMD or congenital muscular dystrophy. Walking difficulties became apparent when the patients started walking at 14 months and at 5 years he could no longer stand due to contractures. However, at 40 years, he did not have cardiac problems. The clinical characteristics of patient MG are very similar to those reported for one of the two families previously described (Taylor *et al.* 1998): patients had very early onset of the disease with rapid progression of weakness and normal cardiac function. This findings suggest that AR-EMD may represent a more severe form of the muscle disorder.

Pathology

Skeletal muscle

Skeletal muscle biopsy show mild dystrophic changes with few scattered necrotic and regenerating fibres and a small increase in fatty and fibrous connective tissue (Merlini *et al.* 1986; Takamoto *et al.* 1984). Skeletal muscles show variation in fiber diameter associated with increased number of hypertrophic fibres, splitting fibres, and internal nuclei. Intermyofibrillary networks are often disorganized with a moth-eaten appearance. Both type 1 and type 2 fibres are equally affected (Voit *et al.* 1988). Different and specific muscle involvement has been suggested (Yates 1997).

Cardiac muscle

Few reports of cardiac muscle pathology are available. Myocardial changes with focal degeneration and increased endomysial fatty and fibrous connective tissues have been described (Yoshioka *et al.* 1989). In an autopsy case, marked enlargement and thinning of the atria has been observed, together with fibrosis in the ventricle (Hara *et al.* 1987).

Joint contractures

While in most types of muscular dystrophy, contractures occur in the later stages of the disease, in EMD, they occur prior to significant weakness of muscle. The nature of the early onset contractures of the elbows, Achilles tendons, and posterior neck muscles, is not understood. Whether the contractures occur as a consequence of an abnormality of tissues surrounding the joints, or are secondary to primary dystrophic changes in skeletal muscle, remains to be clarified. Based on CT-scan tests, Merlini pointed out the early role of the primary muscular atrophy that may precede the contractures (Yates 1997).

Other tissues

An autopsy case (50-year-old male) that had typical clinical features of EMD had no morphological abnormalities in the brain, spinal anterior horn cells, and myelinated nerve fibers in the ventral roots (Hara *et al.* 1987). Indeed, no intellectual impairment has been reported in EMD.

Inheritance

The X-linked EMD gene is inherited as a recessive character, with 100 per cent penetrance by the third decade of life. Typical of the X-linked recessive pattern, heterozygous females show no indication of skeletal muscle disorder. Arrythmia and bradychardia are occasionally observed in older carrier women (Bialer *et al.* 1991; Fishbein *et al.* 1993; Merlini *et al.* 1986). There is however no direct demonstration of a correlation with the disease. In one case, studied in the author's laboratory, such correlation was excluded as two older woman from an affected family, carried a pace maker but did not have the mutation in the STA gene segregating in the family. Thus arrhythmia and bradycardia in older women may be just the result of aging.

Mutations in LMNA, responsible for AD-EMD and AR-EMD, show a higher heterogeneity of the pattern of inheritance. Most mutations in LMNA have a dominant effect with 100 per cent penetrance by the third decade of life (Bonne *et al.* 1999; 2000). Some mutations have no phenotypic effect in the heterozygous form and they appear to require either a second mutation in the same gene (AR-EMD) or in a third, still unidentified, gene (Di Barletta *et al.* 2000).

Molecular Genetics

X-EMD

The X-EMD gene was mapped to a 2MB region in the distal part of Xq28 (Consalez *et al.* 1991; Romeo *et al.* 1988) and was identified by a positional candidate approach, among a large number of candidates (Bione *et al.* 1994).

The EMD gene (STA) is 2.1 kb long and it encodes an mRNA of 1.3 kb, ubiquitously expressed in many cell types and, in the mouse, early during development. The gene encodes a 254 amino acids protein, named emerin.

Emerin, shows limited sequence similarity to the lamina associated protein 2 (LAP2) and to few nuclear envelope proteins (Bione *et al.* 1994; Furukawa *et al.* 1995). Antibodies raised against synthetic peptide fragments or to the whole protein as well as mono-clonal antibodies showed positive immunostaining of the nuclear membrane in skeletal, cardiac and smooth muscle cells in normal controls (Cartegni *et al.* 1997; Manilal *et al.* 1996; Nagano *et al.* 1996). By Western blot emerin was identified as a 34 kDa protein slightly larger than the size estimated from the nucleotide sequence (29 kDa) because of heavy phosphorylation (Cartegni *et al.* 1997). Not all cell types show nuclear membrane staining with emerin antibodies (Nagano *et al.* 1996). Many cell types exhibited diffuse cytoplasmic staining of various degrees. On the other hand, by Western blot a 34 kDa protein was always detected confirming that emerin is ubiquitous and suggesting that its subcellullar localization may be restricted by interaction with other proteins.

Most mutations in the X-EMD gene are point mutations or small deletions/insertions. They cause interruption of transcription or translation and a null phenotype (Bione *et al.* 1994; 1995; Klauck *et al.* 1995; Nigro *et al.* 1995; Wulff *et al.* 1997; Yates and Wehnert 1999). As a consequence, emerin immunostaining of muscle fibres nuclear membrane and other cell types in patients with X-EMD was negative. The distribution of the mutations is homogeneous along the gene with no evidence of mutation 'hot spots'. In one case a complex rearrangement with a deletion of 429 bases and an insertion of 103 bases was found (Bione *et al.* 1994). Few large deletions, involving the entire gene, have been reported (Small *et al.* 1997) and it was shown that they may be due to a complex rearrangement related to the presence of two very large (11.3 kb) and highly conserved inverted repeats flanking the X-EMD and the FLN1 genes (Chen *et al.* 1996).

Of special interest are mutations occurring in the last exon and affecting the C-terminal part of the protein, containing the hydrophobic transmembrane domain. Many such mutations have been reported and some patients of this group completely lack emerin (Nagano *et al.* 1996) thus demonstrating the importance of the hydrophobic

C-terminal domain for membrane insertion and protein stability. In a few patients, presenting frameshift mutations in the sixth exon, a new hydrophobic tail was synthesized, compatible in aminoacid composition and length with a nuclear envelope transmembrane domain. In one of these patients, Western blot analysis revealed the presence of the truncated form of the protein and the immmunochemical studies on muscle sections demonstrated the presence, although in reduced amount, of the protein in the correct localization (Cartegni *et al.* 1997). A nuclear localization is then necessary but not sufficient to ensure a normal phenotype.

Only very few missense mutations have been described (Morris and Manilal 1999; Yates *et al.* 1999).

AD-EMD and AR-EMD

Families affected with AD-EMD were definitively identified by analysis of the X-linked gene and by the presence of emerin in skeletal muscle biopsies. Linkage analysis in a large French pedigree mapped the AD-EMD locus to a 8 cM interval between D1S2346 and D1S2125 (Bonne *et al.* 1999). LMNA, the gene encoding two components of the nuclear lamina, lamins A and C, was localized to 1q21.2–q21.3, in the critical interval. Sequence analyses of the LMNA gene in affected and unaffected members of five families demonstrated that LMNA was the gene responsible for AD-EMD (Bonne *et al.* 1999). One mutation in the large pedigree was a C to T transition which changes Q6 to a stop codon. Missense mutations introducing aminoacid changes in the coding sequence were found in most of the other families analyzed and their distribution is shown in Fig. 6.2. They appear to be the most common mutations in the LMNA gene (Bonne *et al.* 1999; 2000; Di Barletta *et al.* 2000). Immunostaining of nuclei of patients showed that both emerin and lamina A/C are present and suggested that AD-EMD may be due to haploinsufficiency for lamin A/C. However a dominant negative effect of the aminoacid changes cannot be ruled out. It is significant that recurrent changes were observed in AD-EMD patients: Di Barletta *et al.* (2000) reported that 11 of the 16 (68 per cent) dominant mutations causing AD-EMD were localized to the central region of the tail domain, and three of the remaining five patients carried the same mutation in the 2A rod domain. There is, however, no relation between the type of mutation and its localization along the protein and the phenotype of patients; patients with identical mutations showed different degree of severity (Bonne *et al.* 2000).

Nuclear lamins are members of the intermediate filament multigene family which form the nuclear lamina, a meshwork of intermediate filaments on the nucleoplasmic side of the nuclear envelope (Stuurman *et al.* 1998). Lamin A/C is absent from early embryos and from undifferentiated and tumor cells. It is present in many differentiated cells where it interacts with chromatin and integral proteins of the inner nuclear membrane (Manilal *et al.* 1999). In addition to a structural function, providing the nuclear cytoskeleton, there is increasing evidence that, by analogy with microtubules and microfilaments, nuclear lamins and inner nuclear membrane proteins (LBR, LAPs

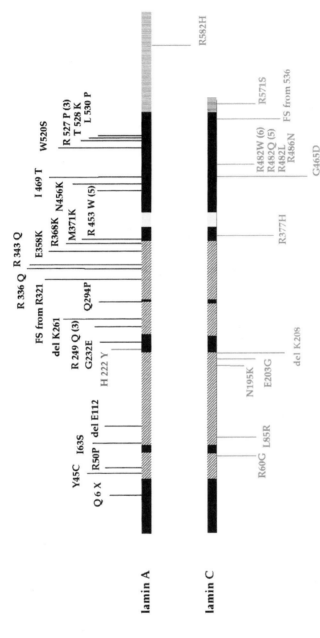

Fig. 6.2 Distribution along the lamins of the mutations in LMNA gene. The molecular organization of lamins A and C is schematically represented. Dashed boxes are the coil coiled domains. In yellow is the chromatin binding domain. Striped are the two alternative N terminal regions. Above, in black, are the mutations in AD-EMD; in red the mutation in AR-EMD. Below are the mutations in the other three disorders, in light blue, mutations in DCM-CD; in orange, mutations in LGMD1B; in green, mutations in OFPLD. Please see four colour plate section between pages 20 and 21.

Fig. 6.3 Schematic representation of the organization of emerin and lamins in the nuclear envelope and nuclear lamina. Lamina A/C, dashed boxes; lamin B dotted boxes; INM, inner nuclear membrane; ONM, outer nuclear membrane; LAP, lamina associated proteins.

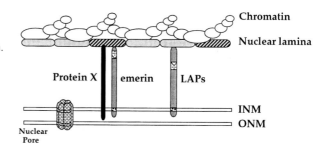

and other) determine the functional diversity and the dynamic properties of the nuclear envelope and are important in regulation of cell division, integrity of nuclei and nuclear pore complex and in chromatin structure (Foisner 1997).

The finding that lamin A and emerin mutations are responsible for very similar disorders demonstrates that, in muscle, specific interactions between the nuclear membrane and nuclear lamina exist which are important either for gene expression or for molecular signalling between nuclei and cytoplasm and eventually for muscle integrity. Lamins A and C, emerin and possibly other integral proteins of the nuclear envelope interacting with lamins and emerin may be involved (Fig. 6.3). In X-linked EMD, lack of emerin, which is responsible for the phenotype, may alter the putative complex. In AD-EMD, emerin is present but its localization or the ratio between nuclear and cytoplasmic emerin could be altered. Moreover, additional components may be directly altered by the mutations in lamin A/C. From this point of view the recently published study of mice, lacking lamin A (Sullivan *et al.* 1999) is of great interest. Soon after birth, the LMNA −/− mice develop a severe muscular dystrophy and cardiomyopathy: their phenotype is associated with ultrastructural perturbations of the nuclear envelope and mislocalization of emerin. Another nuclear envelope protein, LAP2, known to interact with chromatin and B type lamins (Foisner and Gerace 1993) but not with lamin A/C, was found to have a normal association with the nuclear envelope. Study of specific LMNA mutations in the mouse model in the heterozygote and homozygote state may help to clarify the role and the interactions of lamin A/C in the different affected tissues.

LMNA mutations and other pathologies

Fatkin *et al.* described mutations in LMNA in patients affected with dilated cardiomyopathy and conduction system disorder (DCM-CD), but not presenting contractures or skeletal myopathy (Fatkin *et al.* 1999). This group of patients is clinically similar to some of the patients with isolated cardiac involvement described among AD-EMD families (Bonne *et al.* 2000). The LMNA mutations in DCM-CD patients were in the rod domain 1 or in the tail of lamin C (Fig. 6.2). Among the mutations found in EMD families, mutations identified in exon 1 were identical to those in DCM-CD patients, showing that there is no relation between mutations occurring in LMNA in the two groups of patients.

Limb girdle muscular dystrophies (LGMD) are a heterogeneous group of disorders characterized by a limb girdle distribution of weakness. LGMD1B is a form of LGMD inherited as an autosomal dominant trait. It is slowly progressive with age related atri- oventricular cardiac conduction defect and dilated cardiomyopathy (van der Kooi *et al.* 1997). It differs from EMD because of the lack of early contractures and the distribu- tion of affected skeletal muscles. The locus was mapped to 1q11-q21 to the same region as the AD-EMD (van der Kooi *et al.* 1997). Mutations in the LMNA gene were identi- fied in three LGMD1B families (Muchir *et al.* 2000): the mutations segregated with the disease demonstrating that the two disorders, LGMD1B and AD-EMD are allelic. The mutations were not identical to those found in AD-EMD but they were not altering specific regions of the protein (Fig. 6.2).

Together the results described here suggest that the three disorders AD-EMD, DCM- CD and LGMD1B might be one entity with variable expression of symptoms. It is inter- esting to recall here a family recently described where DCM with EMD-like skeletal muscle abnormalities, DCM with LGMD-like skeletal muscle abnormalities and pure DCM with conduction defects were described and were due to a single nucleotide deletion in LMNA exon 6, causing frameshift and premature translation termination (Brodsky *et al.* 2000; Di Barletta *et al.* 2000).

Specific mutations in LMNA were recently found in a fourth disease, Dunnigan-type familial partial lipodystrophy (OFPLD), a disorder of adipocytes associated with insulin resistance and diabetes, but not presenting muscular or cardiac alterations (Cao and Hegele 2000; Shackleton *et al.* 2000; Speckman *et al.* 2000). The disorder is characterized by complete or partial absence of adipose tissue with regional distribution of progressive degeneration of the adipocytes, similar to the distribution of muscle weakness and wasting in EMD. Recurrent mutations in LMNA have been described that seem specific for OFPLD. The mutations were in a very limited portion of the C-terminal tail of the protein and were not found in the other disorders (Fig. 6.2). Thus the region encompassing the codon 482–486 within the tail domain of lamin A/C may determine specific functions in adipocytes. However, further search for mutations has shown overlaps between mutations in OFPLD and AD-EMD: in Fig. 6.2, it is shown that the change I469T causes AD-EMD (Di Barletta *et al.* 2000) while G465D causes OFPLD (Speckman *et al.* 2000). Thus, it is possible that additional factors, to be identified, are involved in determining whether a mutation in LMNA causes OFPLD or a cardiomyopathy and the finding that four different disorders are caused by muta- tions in the same gene, LMNA, strongly supports the hypothesis that a multiprotein complex exists at the nuclear envelope whose alterations are responsible for the differ- ent phenotypes described.

Diagnosis and prevention

Early diagnosis of EMD can be life saving as the insertion of a pacemaker can prevent cardiac conduction problems. However the pace maker only treats bradychardia, and other symptoms can occur after insertion of the pace maker. Anaesthetic considerations for EMD are also of note. The patients show difficulties in tracheal intubation, spinal anaesthetic, and susceptibility to malignant hyperthermia and cardiac block (Jensen 1996). Despite the characteristic features of EMD, the late onset of some of the symptoms and the phenotypic variability within families make diagnosis not always easy. Moreover molecular diagnosis is necessary to distinguish between X-EMD and AD-EMD, and for accurate genetic counselling.

Diagnosis of X-EMD is done at the protein level, using anti-emerin antibodies. Taking into account the ubiquitous presence of emerin in many tissues and cell types and that the majority of the mutations are null, diagnosis of X-EMD can be achieved by immunodetection of emerin from skin biopsies, leukocytes and buccal smear (Manilal *et al.* 1997; Mora *et al.* 1997; Sabatelli *et al.* 1998). Emerin can be also detected by immunoblot of proteins extracted from minute amount of frozen blood (Manilal *et al.* 1997; Mora *et al.* 1997), and most patients can be correctly diagnosed from the lack of the emerin band in Western blots. As carrier may only have a reduced amount of emerin, immunocytochemistry of skin biopsy or buccal smears is a preferable method to detect a mosaic pattern. The reliability of this protein based diagnosis needs to be confirmed by sequence analysis and identification of a mutation, but its simplicity appears a great advantage.

Diagnosis of AD-EMD and AR-EMD can be done by mutation analysis of the LMNA gene. Both SSCP and DHPLC and direct sequencing of specific fragments have been used until now (Bonne *et al.* 1999; Di Barletta *et al.* 2000).

Treatment

No specific treatment of the muscle disorder is available, however physical therapy is recommended to reduce contractures. The cardiac problem can be in part solved with the insertion of a pace maker and in cases where the muscle are moderately affected heart transplantation can be considered. Despite the identification of the genes responsible for the different forms of the disorder and the possibility of a precise diagnosis at the molecular level, the mechanisms responsible for the disease are still elusive. Emerin and lamin A/C seem to participate in a novel pathway, different from those altered in other muscle disorders. Many questions remain to be answered and will have to be answered before new therapies can be considered.

Acknowledgements

The article is dedicated to the memory of Kiichi Arahata an outstanding scientist and a dear friend. In writing this review without him I tried to save some of his ideas and suggestions. I thank Yukiko Hayashi for help and the members of my laboratory who contributed to the work described here. The experiments done in my laboratory were supported by Telethon Italy and by EU grant QLG1-CT-R99-00870.

References

Bialer, M.G., Bruns, D.E., and Kelly T.E. (1990). Muscle enzymes and isoenzymes in Emery–Dreifuss muscular dystrophy. *Clinical Chemistry* **36**, 427–30.

Bialer, M.G., McDaniel, N.L., and Kelly T.E. (1991). Progression of cardiac disease in Emery–Dreifuss muscular dystrophy. *Clinical Cardiology*, **14**, 411–6.

Bione, S., Maestrini, E., Rivella, S., Mancini, M., Regis, S., Romeo, G. *et al.* (1994). Identification of a novel X-linked gene responsible for Emery–Dreifuss muscular dystrophy. *Nature Genetics*, **8**, 323–7.

Bione, S., Small, K., Aksmanovic, V.M., D'Urso, M., Ciccodicola, A., Merlini, L. *et al.* (1995). Identification of new mutations in the Emery–Dreifuss muscular dystrophy gene and evidence for genetic heterogeneity of the disease. *Human Molecular Genetics*, **4**, 1859–63.

Bonne, G., Di Barletta, M.R., Varnous, S., Becane, H.M., Hammouda, E.H., Merlini, L. *et al.* (1999). Mutations in the gene encoding lamin A/C cause autosomal dominant Emery–Dreifuss muscular dystrophy. *Nature Genetics*, **21**, 285–8.

Bonne, G., Mercuri, E., Muchir, A., Urtizberea, A., Becane, H.M., Recan, D. *et al.* (2000). Clinical and molecular genetic spectrum of autosomal dominant Emery–Dreifuss muscular dystrophy due to mutations of the lamin A/C gene. *Annals of Neurology*, **48**, 170–80.

Brodsky, G.L., Muntoni, F., Miocic, S., Sinagra, G., Sewry, C., and Mestroni, L. (2000). Lamin A/C gene mutation associated with dilated cardiomyopathy with variable skeletal muscle involvement. *Circulation*, **101**, 473–6.

Cao, H. and Hegele, R.A. (2000). Nuclear lamin A/C R482Q mutation in Canadian kindreds with Dunnigan- type familial partial lipodystrophy. *Human Molecular Genetics*, **9**, 109–12.

Cartegni, L., di Barletta, M.R., Barresi, R., Squarzoni, S., Sabatelli, P., Maraldi, N. *et al.* (1997). Heart-specific localization of emerin, new insights into Emery–Dreifuss muscular dystrophy. *Human Molecular Genetics*, **6**, 2257–64.

Cestan, R. and Lejonne, P. (1902). Une myopatie avec retraction. *Nouvelle Inconographie de la Salpetriere*, **15**, 38–52.

Chen, E.Y., Zollo, M., Mazzarella, R., Ciccodicola, A., Chen, C.N., Zuo, L. *et al.* (1996). Long-range sequence analysis in Xq28, thirteen known and six candidate genes in 219.4 kb of high GC DNA between the RCP/GCP and G6PD loci. *Human Molecular Genetics*, **5**, 659–68.

Consalez, G.G., Thomas, N.S., Stayton, C.L., Knight, S.J., Johnson, M., Hopkins, L.C. *et al.* (1991). Assignment of Emery–Dreifuss muscular dystrophy to the distal region of Xq28, the results of a collaborative study. *American Journal of Human Genetics*, **48**, 468–80.

Di Barletta, R.M., Ricci, E., Galluzzi, G., Tonali, P., Mora, M., Morandi, L. *et al.* (2000). Different mutations in the LMNA gene cause autosomal dominant and autosomal recessive Emery–Dreifuss muscular dystrophy. *American Journal of Human Genetics*, **66**, 1407–12.

Dreifuss, F.E. and Hogan, R.G. (1961). Survival in X-chromosomal muscular dystrophy. *Neurology*, **11**, 734–7.

Emery, A.E. and Dreifuss, F.E. (1966). Unusual type of benign x-linked muscular dystrophy. *Journal of Neurology, Neurosurgery, and Psychiatry*, **29**, 338–42.

Emery, A.E.H. (1989). Emery Dreifuss syndrome. *Journal of Medical Genetics*, **26**, 637–41.

Emery, A.E.H. (1993). *Duchenne muscular dystrophy.* (2nd ed) Oxford University Press, Oxford.

Emery, A.E.H. and Emery, M.L.H. (1995). *The History of a Genetic Disease.* Royal Society of Medicine Press, London.

Fatkin, D., MacRae, C., Sasaki, T., Wolff, M.R., Porcu, M., Frenneaux, M. *et al.* (1999). Missense mutations in the rod domain of the lamin A/C gene as causes of dilated cardiomyopathy and conduction-system disease (see comments). *New England Journal of Medicine*, **341**, 1715–24.

Fishbein, M.C., Siegel, R.J., Thompson, C.E., and Hopkins, L.C. (1993). Sudden death of a carrier of X-linked Emery–Dreifuss muscular dystrophy. *Annals of Internal Medicine*, **119**, 900–5.

Foisner, R. (1997). Dynamic organization of intermediate filaments and associated proteins during the cell cycle. *BioEssays*, **19**, 297–305.

Foisner, R. and Gerace, L. (1993). Integral membrane proteins of the nuclear envelope interact with lamins and chromosomes, and binding is modulated by mitotic phosphorylation. *Cell*, **73**, 1267–79.

Furukawa, K., Pante, N., Aebi, U., and Gerace, L. (1995). Cloning of a cDNA for lamina-associated polypeptide 2(LAP2) and identification of regions that specify targeting to the nuclear envelope. *Embo J* **14**, 1626–1636.

Hara, H., Nagara, H., Mawatari, S., Kondo, A., and Sato, H. (1987). Emery–Dreifuss muscular dystrophy. An autopsy case. *Journal of Neurological Science*, **79**, 23–31.

Hauptman, A. and Thannhauser, S.J. (1941). Muscular shortening and dystrophy, a heredofamililal disease. *Archives of Neurological Psychiatry*, **46**, 654–64.

Jensen, V. (1996). The anaesthetic management of a patient with Emery–Dreifuss muscular dystrophy. *Canadian Journal of Anaesthetics*, **43**, 968–971.

Klauck, S.M., Wilgenbus, P., Yates, J.R., Muller, C.R. and Poustka A. (1995). Identification of novel mutations in three families with Emery–Dreifuss muscular dystrophy. *Human Molecular Genetics*, **4**, 1853–7.

Manilal, S., Nguyen, T.M., Sewry, C.A., and Morris, G.E. (1996). The Emery–Dreifuss muscular dystrophy protein, emerin, is a nuclear membrane protein. *Human Molecular Genetics*, **5**, 801–8.

Manilal, S., Sewry, C.A., Man, N., Muntoni, F., and Morris, G.E. (1997). Diagnosis of X-linked Emery-Dreifuss muscular dystrophy by protein analysis of leucocytes and skin with monoclonal antibodies. *Neuromuscular Disorders*, **7**, 63–6.

Manilal, S., Sewry, C.A., Pereboev, A., Man, N., Gobbi, P., Hawkes, S., Love, D.R., and Morris, G.E. (1999). Distribution of emerin and lamins in the heart and implications for Emery–Dreifuss muscular dystrophy. *Human Molecular Genetics*, **8**, 353–9.

Merlini, L., Granata, C., Dominici, P., and Bonfiglioli, S. (1986). Emery–Dreifuss muscular dystrophy, report of five cases in a family and review of the literature. *Muscle Nerve*, **9**, 481–5.

Mora, M., Cartegni, L., Di Blasi, C., Barresi, R., Bione, S., Raffaele di Barletta, M. *et al.* (1997). X-linked Emery–Dreifuss muscular dystrophy can be diagnosed from skin biopsy or blood sample. *Annals of Neurology*, **42**, 249–53.

Morris, G.E. and Manilal, S. (1999). Heart to heart, from nuclear proteins to Emery-Dreifuss muscular dystrophy. *Human Molecular Genetics*, **8**, 1847–51.

Muchir, A., Bonne, G., van der Kooi, A.J., van Meegen, M., Baas, F., Bolhuis, P.A. *et al.* (2000). Identification of mutations in the gene encoding lamins A/C in autosomal dominant limb girdle muscular dystrophy with atrioventricular conduction disturbances (LGMD1B). *Human Molecular Genetics*, **9**, 1453–9.

Nagano, A., Koga, R., Ogawa, M., Kurano, Y., Kawada, J., Okada, R. *et al.* (1996). Emerin deficiency at the nuclear membrane in patients with Emery–Dreifuss muscular dystrophy. *Nature Genetics*, **12**, 254–9.

Nigro, V., Bruni, P., Ciccodicola, A., Politano, L., Nigro, G., Piluso, G. *et al.* (1995). SSCP detection of novel mutations in patients with Emery–Dreifuss muscular dystrophy, definition of a small C-terminal region required for emerin function. *Human Molecular Genetics*, **4**, 2003–4.

Romeo, G., Roncuzzi, L., Sangiorgi, S., Giacanelli, M., Liguori, M., Tessarolo, D. *et al.* (1988). Mapping of the Emery–Dreifuss gene through reconstruction of crossover points in two Italian pedigrees. *Human Genetics*, **80**, 59–62.

Rowland, L.P., Fetell, M., Olarte, M., Hays, A., Singh, N., and Wanat F.E. (1979). Emery–Dreifuss muscular dystrophy. *Annals of Neurology*, **5**, 111–7.

Sabatelli, P., Squarzoni, S., Petrini, S., Capanni, C., Ognibene, A., Cartegni, L. *et al.* (1998). Oral exfoliative cytology for the non-invasive diagnosis in X-linked Emery–Dreifuss muscular dystrophy patients and carriers. *Neuromuscular Disorders*, **8**, 67–71.

Shackleton, S., Lloyd, D.J., Jackson, S.N., Evans, R., Niermeijer, M.F., Singh, B.M. *et al.* (2000). LMNA, encoding lamin A/C, is mutated in partial lipodystrophy (see comments). *Nature Genetics*, **24**, 153–6.

Small, K., Iber, J., and Warren, S.T. (1997). Emerin deletion reveals a common X-chromosome inversion mediated by inverted repeats (see comments). *Nature Genetics*, **16**, 96–9.

Speckman, R.A., Garg, A., Du, F., Bennett, L., Veile, R., Arioglu, E. *et al.* (2000). Mutational and haplotype analyses of families with familial partial lipodystrophy (Dunnigan variety) reveal recurrent missense mutations in the globular C-terminal domain of lamin A/C. *American Journal of Human Genetics*, **66**, 1192–8.

Stuurman, N., Heins, S., and Aebi, U. (1998). Nuclear lamins, their structure, assembly, and interactions. *Journal of Structural Biology*, **122**, 42–66.

Sullivan, T., Escalante-Alcalde, D., Bhatt, H., Anver, M., Bhat, N., Nagashima, K., Stewart, C.L., and Burke, B. (1999). Loss of A-type lamin expression compromises nuclear envelope integrity leading to muscular dystrophy. *Journal of Cell Biology*, **147**, 913–20.

Takamoto, K., Hirose, K., Uono, M., and Nonaka, I. (1984). A genetic variant of Emery–Dreifuss disease. Muscular dystrophy with humeropelvic distribution, early joint contracture, and permanent atrial paralysis. *Archives of Neurology*, **41**, 1292–3.

Taylor, J., Sewry, C.A., Dubowitz, V., and Muntoni, F. (1998). Early onset, autosomal recessive muscular dystrophy with Emery–Dreifuss phenotype and normal emerin expression. *Neurology* **51**, 1116–20.

Van der Kooi, A.J., Van Meegen, M., Ledderhof, T.M., McNally, E.M., de Visser, M., and Bolhuis, P.A. (1997). Genetic localization of a newly recognized autosomal dominant limb-girdle muscular dystrophy with cardiac involvement (LGMD1B) to chromosome 1q11–21. *American Journal of Human Genetics*, **60**, 891–5.

Vohanka, S., Vytopil, M., Bednarik, J., Lukas, Z., Kadanka, Z., Schildberger, J. *et al.* (2001). A mutation in the X-linked Emery Dreifuss muscular dystrophy gene in a patient affected with conduction cardiomyopathy. *Neuromuscular Disorders*, **11**, 411–13

Voit, T., Krogmann, O., Lenard, H.G., Neuen-Jacob, E., Wechsler, W., Goebel, H.H. *et al.* (1988). Emery–Dreifuss muscular dystrophy, disease spectrum and differential diagnosis. *Neuropediatrics* **19**, 62–71.

Witt, T.N., Graner, C.G., Pongratz, D., and Baur, X. (1988). Autosomal dominant Emery–Dreifuss syndrome, evidence of a neurogenic variant of the disease. *European Archives of Psychiatry and Neurological Science*, **273**, 230–6.

Wulff, K., Ebener, U., Wehnert, C.S., Ward, P.A., Reuner, U., Hiebsch, W., Herrmann, F.H., and Wehnert, M. (1997). Direct molecular genetic diagnosis and heterozygote identification in X-linked Emery–Dreifuss muscular dystrophy by heteroduplex analysis. *Disease Markers*, **13**, 77–86.

Yates, J.R., Bagshaw, J., Aksmanovic, V.M., Coomber, E., McMahon, R., Whittaker, J.L. *et al.* (1999). Genotype-phenotype analysis in X-linked Emery-Dreifuss muscular dystrophy and identification of a missense mutation associated with a milder phenotype. *Neuromuscular Disorders*, **9**, 159–65.

Yates, J.R. and Wehnert, M. (1999). The Emery–Dreifuss Muscular Dystrophy Mutation Database. *Neuromuscular Disorders*, **9**, 199.

Yates, J.R.W. (1991). European Workshop on Emery Dreifuss muscular dystrophy. *Neuromuscular Disorders*, **1**, 393–6.

Yates, J.R.W. (1997). 43rd ENMC International Workshop on Emery–Dreifuss muscular distrophy. *Neuromuscular Disorders*, **7**, 67–9.

Yoshioka, M., Saida, K., Itagaki, Y., and Kamiya, T. (1989). Follow up study of cardiac involvement in Emery–Dreifuss muscular dystrophy. *Archives of Disease in Childhood*, **64**, 713–5.

Chapter 7

The limb-girdle muscular dystrophies

Katharine M.D. Bushby

Introduction

Literature on any disease is merely a snapshot of the level of understanding of a condition at that time. Since the introduction of the term in the mid 1950s someone reviewing the literature on the limb-girdle muscular dystrophies (LGMD) would recognize immediately that the field has often been confused and controversial over this period, inciting at times quite extreme views and vigorous debate.

Unlike many other forms of muscular dystrophy where a consistent clinical phenotype and reproducible mode of inheritance allowed the definition of a disease entity very early on, the designation "limb-girdle" muscular dystrophy reached widespread acceptance as a term encompassing right from the outset a heterogeneous group of disorders (Walton 1955; 1956). It described those patients in whom there was clearly a muscular dystrophy which affected the large proximal muscles of the arms and legs and who did not appear to have the more readily recognizable facioscapulohumeral muscular dystrophy nor the X-linked types of muscular dystrophy. That within this category, there was room for much clinical and genetic heterogeneity was also highlighted from the outset with the recognition that such patients might have an autosomal dominant or recessive form of disease. Despite its limitations, the term became adopted clinically for many patients in whom an alternative diagnosis could not easily be sought or even at times as an alternative to seeking rigorously for an alternative cause for a patient's problems.

This lack of precision caused controversy which is reflected in the papers published throughout this period. The variability in descriptions of some large families with what could be described as a limb-girdle muscular dystrophy phenotype served to underline the 'broad church' that this represented and some authors proposed the adoption of the term 'limb-girdle syndrome' in recognition of this (Passos-Bueno *et al.* 1991). In the meantime other authors proposed that the condition did not exist at all but that alternative diagnoses should be sought in every case in whom it was considered. These authors advocated that the term limb-girdle muscular dystrophy should be dropped altogether (Walton and Gardner-Medwin 1988; 1991). A further view came from those who preferred a more "pure" designation of LGMD to be applied to a much more clearly defined group of patients (Fardeau *et al.* 1996). From a purely clinical perspective this problem was essentially unresolvable. Progress in diagnostic techniques allowed, for example, the recognition of cases of dystrophinopathy, spinal muscular atrophy or metabolic and mitochondrial myopathies to be diagnosed amongst patients previously thought to have LGMD (Norman *et al.* 1989). Nonetheless, some patients remained who clearly had a muscular dystrophy that involved the proximal musculature and in whom no alternative diagnoses could be achieved. In clinical practice, these patients, almost by default, still found themselves being given a diagnosis of limb-girdle muscular dystrophy. This diagnosis, though, at a personal level for the individual patient and his or her clinician remained extremely unsatisfactory as it carried with it no real indication as to prognosis nor any indication as to likely outcome for offspring. These limitations were due to the recognized extreme heterogeneity of the conditions grouped together under this name. This heterogeneity has been confirmed and to a great extent resolved by the application of molecular biological techniques. Applying molecular biological techniques to families, who in their eyes, fulfilled an "LGMD" pattern, researchers worldwide have identified at least 14 genetically defined subgroups through the technique of linkage analysis followed by the identification of the causative genes either by positional cloning analysis or a candidate gene strategy (Table 7.1). This has allowed a complete classification of the group, the elucidation of a number of novel mechanisms of disease, and most strikingly, has reached the point where in any given patient with a proximal muscular dystrophy a precise diagnosis may indeed be achievable with concomitant gains in the amount of prognostic and genetic counselling information which can be offered to a patient and his or her family.

The burgeoning literature on the limb-girdle muscular dystrophies over the 1990s illustrates a rapid evolution in the development of a new approach to diagnosis in this group of patients (Beckmann 1999; Beckmann *et al.* 1999; Bushby and Beckmann 1995; Jeanpierre *et al.* 1996; Worton 1995). As loci were identified as causing the disease within families or populations with a limb-girdle muscular dystrophy these were listed sequentially, with the autosomal dominant types of limb-girdle muscular dystrophy designated LGMD1A, B, C etc. and the much commoner autosomal recessive limb-girdle muscular dystrophies designated LGMD2A, B, C etc. (Bushby and Beckmann 1995). A summary of the current state of knowledge of the various disease loci, the genes and proteins is provided in Table 7.1. As the gene locus names (LGMD1A, 2A etc.) have in many cases become superseded by a knowledge of the primary gene and protein abnormalities in these disorders, this is the designation which will primarily be used in this chapter to distinguish the various entities within the group.

The identification of different disease types based on genetic locus and now also molecular pathology has allowed the recognition of both shared and distinct properties for the entities within this classification. Application of such molecular biology techniques to diagnosis has shown that most of these disorders are present in populations worldwide. Diagnosis remains fairly specialized, however, due to the extreme complexity and heterogeneity of this group. Clinically, the ability to achieve a precise diagnosis

Table 7.1 The current classification of the limb-girdle muscular dystrophies

Locus name	Disease designation	Gene location (gene symbol if known)	Protein
Autosomal dominant LGMD			
LGMD1A	LGMD1A	5q22-34	myotilin
LGMD1B	Laminopathy (allelic to autosomal dominant Emery Dreifuss muscular dystrophy and partial lipodystrophy)	1q11-21 (LMNA)	Lamin A/C
LGMD1C	Caveolin 3 deficiency	3p25 (CAV3)	Caveolin 3
LGMD1D	LGMD1D, familial dilated cardiomyopathy with conduction defect and muscular dystrophy (FDC-CDM)	6q23	unknown
LGMD1E	LGMD1E	7q	unknown
Autosomal recessive LGMD			
LGMD2A	Calpain 3 deficiency, calpainopathy	15q15-q21 (CAPN3)	Calpain 3
LGMD2B	Dysferlin deficiency, dysferlinopathy, Miyoshi myopathy	2p13 (DYSF)	Dysferlin
LGMD2C	γ-sarcoglycanopathy, previously known as SCARMD	13q12 (SGCG)	γ-sarcoglycan
LGMD2D	α-sarcoglycanopathy, previously known as SCARMD	17q12-q31 (SGCA)	α-sarcoglycan previously known as adhalin
LGMD2E	β-sarcoglycanopathy	4q12 (SGCA)	β-sarcoglycan
LGMD2F	δ-sarcoglycanopathy	5q33-q34 (SGCD)	δ-sarcoglycan
LGMD2G	Telethonin deficiency	17q11-q12 (TCAP)	telethonin
LGMD2H	LGMD2H	9q31-q34	Not known
LGMD2I	LGMD2I	19q13	Not known

(especially outside the inbred groups in whom the initial gene localization studies were performed) has meant that for many of the disease entities at least a good indication of the distinct phenotypes has been possible to achieve. Therefore, for the clinician involved it becomes possible to recognize within the clinic the types of pointers to a particular diagnosis within the limb-girdle muscular dystrophy classification and these clinical distinctions can then be used to direct molecular analysis in order to achieve a precise diagnosis (Fig. 7.1).

It has been argued that such precision of diagnosis is a luxury. For the patients within this group, however, it is not a luxury but rather a right which dictates in many cases future life choices. Understanding why a disease has happened, where it has come from, what it is likely to cause in the future and what the implications are for one's own

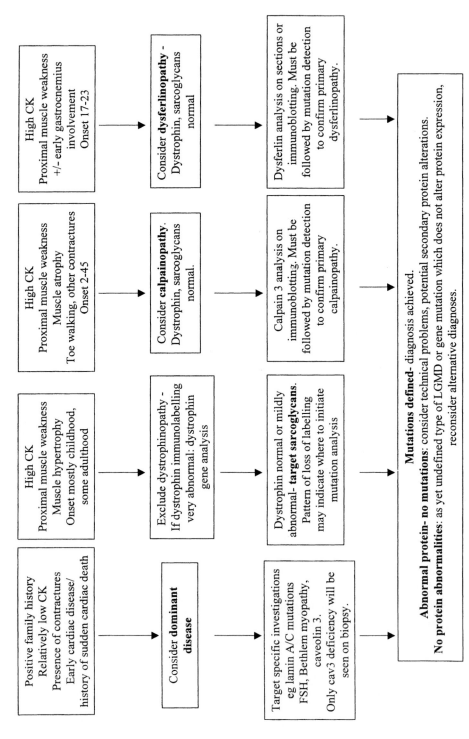

Fig. 7.1 The interplay between clinical, protein and genetic results in achieving a precise diagnosis in LGMD.

children and for relatives in the broader family—all these answers come with precise diagnosis and are all absolutely critical questions in the evolution of a patient coming to terms with one of these chronically disabling disorders.

Autosomal dominant limb-girdle muscular dystrophy

The autosomal dominant forms of limb-girdle muscular dystrophy are individually and overall rarer than the autosomal recessive types. Probably only around 10 per cent of patients presenting to the clinic with a so-called limb-girdle muscular dystrophy diagnosis will have dominant disease. (Bushby 1992; van der Kooi *et al.* 1998). Nonetheless, this proportion is significant enough to require the clinician to be sure that they are not dealing with a dominant disorder before giving a negligible risk of recurrence to their patients. Overall the kinds of indications that one may be dealing with dominant rather than recessive disease include the finding of a relatively lower serum creatine kinase level (within the dominant limb-girdle muscular dystrophy groups CK levels are rarely greater than $10 \times$ normal and are much more often in the range of normal to $3–4 \times$ normal) or the presence of prominent contractures (though this may also be a feature of calpain 3 deficiency, see later). A history of cardiac problems or unexplained cardiac death in relatives may also be a pointer to a dominant form of limb-girdle muscular dystrophy, in particular LGMD1B due to lamin A/C mutations and LGMD1D.

The current autosomal dominant limb-girdle muscular dystrophy classification encompasses types 1A-E, five clinically very disparate disorders which are described briefly below. However, there are other considerations. In patients presenting at the clinic with an apparently autosomal dominant form of "limb-girdle muscular dystrophy?" there are two other diagnoses which are actually probably more likely than any of the disorders within the LGMD classification. The first is facioscapulohumeral muscular dystrophy. In this disorder facial muscle weakness may be relatively mild or even completely absent on formal examination in individual family members and pelvic muscle weakness may at times be detectable at presentation leading to confusion in the diagnosis (Lunt and Harper 1991). On the whole, however, a thorough clinical examination will distinguish these patients and in any case, the DNA based test which is now available and specific in 95 per cent of patients with FSH will eliminate this problem in most families (Upadhyaya *et al.* 1997; van der Maarel *et al.* 1999). The other condition which ought to be considered in the differential diagnosis of families with dominant disease is Bethlem myopathy (Bethlem and Van Wijngaarden 1976; Jobsis *et al.* 1999). Bethlem myopathy is in itself a heterogeneous condition caused by mutations in any of the three collagen 6 genes (collagen 6A1, 6A2, 6A3) (Jobsis *et al.* 1996; Pepe *et al.* 1999; Speer *et al.* 1996). Bethlem myopathy causes a proximal muscle weakness associated usually with serum creatine kinase levels which may be within the normal range or mildly elevated. However, there are usually additional features in these patients or affected family members which point towards this diagnosis. Patients with Bethlem myopathy may present much earlier than is typically seen with a limb-girdle muscular dystrophy: so for example there may be a history of torticollis or contractures present from birth, though such features are highly variable and in fact patients may present at any age. Typically, in older patients with Bethlem myopathy too, joint contractures can be as much, if not more of a problem than the proximal muscle weakness which tends to stabilize in early childhood and be non-progressive for long periods of life, though ultimately deterioration does occur with about half of all patients in time needing a wheelchair (Jobsis *et al.* 1999). Typically, contractures in Bethlem myopathy involve the long finger flexors, elbows and ankles, though contractures may also be present around other joints. However, the contractures in Bethlem myopathy may be fairly subtle and require specific examination in order to be sure that they are not there. For any patient, therefore, with a suspected limb-girdle muscular dystrophy and particularly those in whom there is a possible dominant family history careful examination for contractures is mandatory. The diagnosis of Bethlem myopathy can be suspected clinically once the phenotype is known to the clinician but confirmation of the diagnosis relies on the demonstration of a mutation in one of the collagen 6 genes. In some patients with this diagnosis, there is an unexplained secondary reduction in the muscle protein laminin β1 detectable on muscle biopsy (Merlini *et al.* 1999). This is, however, not specific to Bethlem myopathy (see below).

Finally, patients with a dominant muscular dystrophy may not have a positive family history at all. New dominant mutations and germline mosaicism for new dominant mutations are becoming increasingly well recognized now that molecular biological techniques can distinguish this situation from recessive disorders so that it cannot be assumed that two affected siblings in a family with unaffected parents have a recessive disease. For those patients in whom the clinical features may be suggestive of an auto-somal dominant disorder and in whom no alternative diagnosis can be made it is therefore inappropriate to give a very low risk of recurrence in subsequent generations.

LGMD1A

Clinical and diagnostic considerations

The disorder known as LGMD1A (now known to be caused by mutations in the myotilin gene) was the first form of limb-girdle muscular dystrophy to be linked to a particular locus (on chromosome 5). This study was carried out in a single large North American family of German descent and, to date, this remains the only family in whom this disorder has definitively been seen (Hauser *et al.* 2000; Speer *et al.* 1992a,b; 1994). It had been suggested that the same gene might be involved in this disease as in an autosomal dominant distal myopathy with altered speech and pharyngeal weakness which maps to the same region on chromosome 5 (Feit *et al.* 1998), however this does not appear to be the case. The clinical features in the family with myotilin mutations included a proximal muscular dystrophy of adult onset. In some patients there were tight achilles tendons and others had the additional and unusual feature of dysarthria. Muscle biopsies showed typical dystrophic changes together with a large number of autophagic vacuoles. There was a suggestion in some early reports of anticipation of the disorder with subsequent generations being more severely affected (Speer *et al.* 1994). However, it has subsequently been shown that all affected family members have the same C450T mutation in the myotilin gene which is predicted to result in the conversion of an amino acid from threonine to leucine (Hauser *et al.* 2000). Although, to date, this disease has been seen in only one family worldwide the identification of the myotilin gene as responsible for the disorder in these patients will allow people with a suggestive phenotype to be screened directly for a mutation which may allow the identification of further cases in time.

Molecular biology

Myotilin binds to α actinin and is associated with the Z-line. Its C-terminus contains some homology to the giant muscle protein titin, but its N-terminus is unique. It appears to be a structural component of the sarcomere (Salmikangas *et al.* 1999).

LGMD1B

Clinical and diagnostic considerations

LGMD1B was defined in a group of Dutch families where there was a proximal muscular dystrophy associated with an age-related risk of cardiac rhythm disturbances and cardiomyopathy (van der Kooi *et al.* 1996). The localization of the disease gene in these families to chromosome 1, in a region overlapping with the region already known to show linkage in autosomal dominant Emery–Dreifuss muscular dystrophy caused speculation that this disorder was in fact allelic to this apparently clinically distinct disorder (van der Kooi *et al.* 1997). Subsequent gene cloning efforts proved that this was in fact the case and the phenotype associated with this disorder is now recognized to be relatively broad and variable within and between families (Bonne *et al.* 2000a; Muchir *et al.* 2000). From the strictly "limb-girdle muscular dystrophy" point of view, some patients have been described who have a relatively non-specific proximal muscular dystrophy presenting between the ages of 4 and 35 years without any clear associated features apart from the risk of conduction disturbances present in most patients by the end of the third decade. By contrast other families with mutations in the lamin A/C gene present with an autosomal dominant Emery–Dreifuss muscular dystrophy phenotype with prominent contractures as a major feature of the disease and cardiac complications invariable in this group as well (Bonne *et al.* 2000b). Unrelated to muscular dystrophy, patients with partial lipodystrophy have also been shown to have mutations in the lamin A/C gene (Cao and Hegele 2000; Shackleton *et al.* 2000). These mutations tend to cluster in one region of the gene and therefore may represent a tissue-specific disease process (see Chapter 1).

The diagnosis of LGMD1B is a very important one. Lamin A/C mutations have been reported worldwide, and more commonly than any of the other disorders within the autosomal dominant LGMD categories. It is critical to consider this diagnosis because of the cardiac implications for the patient presenting with muscular dystrophy and potentially affected family members. Cardiac surveillance in this disorder is mandatory for the development of arrhythmias which invariably require pacing and may require the implantation of a pacemaker or even a defibrillator. Even with these types of intervention however, progression may occur to a dilated cardiomyopathy which can be much harder to be treated.

Definitive diagnosis of laminopathy requires mutation detection. Patients have a variably elevated serum creatine kinase level but rarely more than $10\times$ the normal value. Protein analysis of a muscle (or skin) biopsy using antibodies to emerin is useful to exclude the X-linked form of Emery–Dreifuss muscular dystrophy especially in those patients where there are prominent contractures (Nagano et al. 1996; Manilal et al. 1999) but lamin A/C analysis of a muscle biopsy is not abnormal in dominant cases and confirmation of the diagnosis has to be performed via DNA analysis of the lamin A/C gene (Bonne et al. 2000b). As with some patients with Bethlem myopathy, some patients with lamin A/C mutations have a reduction in laminin β1 immunolabelling on their muscle biopsy (Sewry et al. 1999).

Molecular pathology

Both lamin A/C and emerin are components of the nuclear envelope and clearly, despite their widespread tissue distribution, play an important role in the maintenance of muscle fibre integrity. This is further discussed in Chapter 6.

LGMD1C

Clinical and diagnostic considerations

Caveolin 3 deficiency has relatively rarely been described to date. In most cases where descriptions are available the phenotype appears to involve a childhood onset muscular dystrophy which is relatively mild in severity, associated with calf hypertrophy and possibly myalgia (Herrmann et al. 2000; McNally et al. 1998; Minetti et al. 1998). In other children, there has been presentation with hyperCKaemia in the absence of any clear muscle symptoms (Carbone et al. 2000). There do not appear to be any other major associated features and serum creatine kinase in the case reports so far has been only moderately elevated. It appears that protein examination of muscle biopsy using an antibody to caveolin 3 will distinguish at least some cases with this disorder by showing a reduced or absent caveolin 3 immunolabelling pattern. However, confirmation of the diagnosis relies on the demonstration of a caveolin 3 mutation. Intriguingly, it appears that caveolin 3 muscles, may also be responsible for some cases of a non-distropic disorder, rippling muscle disease (Betz et al. 2001).

Molecular pathology

Caveolin 3 is a muscle-specific member of the caveolin protein family. Caveolins are the structural proteins which play a pivotal role in the formation of caveolae, bulb-shaped invaginations of the plasma membrane involved in signal transduction (Engelman *et al.* 1998; Schlegel *et al.* 1998). A proportion of caveolin-3 has been shown to be associated with the DGC (McNally *et al.* 1998a), specifically the C-terminal tail of β-dystroglycan (Sotgia *et al.* 2000). It has also been suggested that caveolin-3 may be involved in the formation of the T-tubule system during myogenesis (Parton *et al.* 1997). Modelling caveolin mutations reported in patients in cell systems showed that these mutations promote the formation of unstable high molecular weight aggregates of caveolin 3 which do not target to the plasma membrane. These mutants behave in a dominant negative fashion (Galbiati *et al.* 1999). Transgenic mice expressing a mutant caveolin 3 allele develop a myopathy associated with an increase in nNOS actively in skeletal muscle. The altered morphology and density in DMD muscle biopsies of caveolae suggests that these proteins may have a broader role in muscular dystrophy than suggested by their involvement in this apparently rare primary dominant disorder (Repetto *et al.* 1999).

Other disorders within the autosomal dominant LGMD classification

Two other conditions are currently classified as autosomal dominant types of LGMD. Both have been reported in small numbers of families and so far only their gene loci are known. LGMD1D (linked to chromosome 6q22) is also known as familial dilated cardiomyopathy with conduction defect and muscular dystrophy, and from this name, the very important cardiac complications of this disorder are obvious. Families typically present with slowly progressive proximal muscle weakness unassociated with facial weakness. Congestive cardiac failure due to dilated cardiomyopathy is typically preceded by conduction disturbances, and a history of sudden cardiac death is common amongst affected family members. Males appear to be affected earlier and more severely from the point of view of both the muscle and cardiac phenotypes (Messina *et al.* 1997). The locus for LGMD1E is on chromosome 7q. The disease has its onset in young adults, and is associated with the development of late contractures and slow progression.

Autosomal recessive limb-girdle muscular dystrophy

The autosomal recessive limb-girdle muscular dystrophies are numerically much more common than the autosomal dominant forms of muscular dystrophy and therefore in a patient presenting with a suggestive phenotype autosomal recessive inheritance is empirically more likely. The various disorders within the autosomal recessive LGMD group can be subdivided into those which involve the sarcoglycan complex (a group of transmembrane proteins which are part of the dystrophin-glycoprotein complex in the muscle fibre membrane (Holt and Campbell 1998; Ozawa *et al.* 1998)) and those which do not (Fig. 7.2). The molecular mechanism by which those proteins not associated with the sarcoglycan complex cause muscular dystrophy are as yet poorly understood though recent insights suggest that there may be a shared pathophysiological mechanism between at least some members of this group as well (Cohn and Campbell 2000).

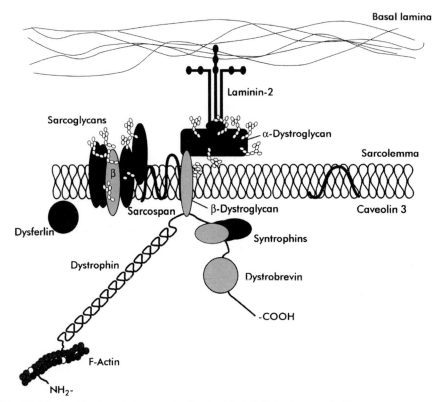

Fig. 7.2 The localization of the proteins involved in LGMD in the muscle fibre.

Sarcoglycanopathies (LGMD2C-2E, α-, β-, γ- and δ-sarcoglycanopathy)

Clinical and diagnostic considerations

Mutations in any of the genes for α, β, γ, or δ sarcoglycan can cause a muscular dystrophy (Bonnemann *et al.* 1995; Mizuno *et al.* 1994; Nigro *et al.* 1996; Piccolo *et al.* 1996). To a great extent, the phenotypes seen in the different sarcoglycanopathies are similar, and maybe unsurprisingly, given the close relationship between the sarcoglycans and dystrophin, muscular dystrophies caused by mutations in the sarcoglycan genes are phenotypically more like the dystrophinopathies than any of the other limb-girdle muscular dystrophies are (Eymard *et al.* 1997). Sarcoglycanopathies in their range of severity also reflect the range of severity seen with different mutations in the dystrophin gene. Presentation of sarcoglycanopathy is most commonly seen in childhood but ranges through to later adult life with a concomitant association with relatively severe or more mildly progressive disease (Beckmann *et al.* 1999). In contrast to patients with dystrophinopathy, patients with sarcoglycanopathy rarely, if ever, have any intellectual impairment which can be attributed to their muscular dystrophy. Perhaps at least partly for this reason the incidence of delayed developmental milestones and late walking in children with sarcoglycanopathy is lower than in dystrophinopathy. From other perspectives it can be hard to distinguish the two. Both will present with weakness in the proximal musculature, often associated with marked muscle hypertrophy. Patients with sarcoglycanopathy have more marked scapular winging and lumbar lordosis than a child with a dystrophinopathy of the same age and one distinction which holds true in many cases is that sarcoglycanopathy predominantly affects the hamstring muscles while in dystrophinopathy the quadriceps muscles are more likely to be more severely affected.

Adults presenting with sarcoglycan deficiency will often give a history of relatively poor performance at school sport before presenting with proximal muscle weakness later on in adult life. Occasionally, they may present with muscle pain. As with the children, muscle hypertrophy is common in this group. For all patients with sarcoglycanopathy there tends to be at presentation a significant elevation of serum creatine kinase levels ($>10–20\times$ normal). With progression of the disease most patients with sarcoglycanopathy will need a wheelchair for mobility at some stage in their lives. Usually, after many years of wheelchair confinement, respiratory impairment becomes important in sarcoglycanopathy just as it does in dystrophin deficiency. Having previously been considered a rarer complication in sarcoglycanopathy than in dystrophinopathy, cardiac involvement is now recognized as a potential problem with these disorders especially with mutations in β- or δ-sarcoglycan (Calvo et al. 2000; Gnecchi-Ruscone et al. 1999; Melacini et al. 1999). It is therefore appropriate that these patients should be offered monitoring for their cardiac status. Cardiomyopathy may have a different mechanism from that seen in dystrophin deficiency with a prominent ischaemic component (see below). Life expectancy in sarcoglycanopathy depends on its severity. For the children with an early onset and rapidly progressive disease the condition shows the same kind of complications as Duchenne dystrophy and lifespan is likely to be restricted, though proper management of cardiac and respiratory complications may help to prolong life. For those patients presenting in adult life with much milder disease, lifespan is not likely to be significantly reduced.

In most populations, dystrophinopathy is much more common than sarcoglycanopathy and in outbred European or US populations sarcoglycanopathy is really very rare. In some populations, founder mutations account for a higher incidence of disease: for example the T151R mutation in β-sarcoglycan seen in the Amish population, the del521T γ-sarcoglycan mutation in the North African population and C283Y (also in γ-sarcoglycan) in the European Gypsies (Jung et al. 1996; Lim et al. 1995b; Piccolo et al. 1996). Few studies have attempted to address the prevalence of sarcoglycan deficiency in outbred populations since the definition of the new diagnostic tools. These suggest that sarcoglycanopathy may represent up to 20 per cent of childhood muscular dystrophy but only about 6 per cent of adult limb-girdle muscular dystrophy (Duggan and Hoffman 1996). Other studies are really necessary in different populations in order to confirm these impressions.

Diagnosis of sarcoglycanopathy relies first of all on the examination of a muscle biopsy (Jones *et al.* 1998; Sewry *et al.* 1996). The diagnosis should be considered in any patient in whom the muscle biopsy is dystrophic with either normal or patchily abnormal dystrophin where molecular genetic analysis has not defined a deletion or other mutation in the dystrophin gene (Fig. 7.1). The importance of using a full range of sarcoglycan antibodies to study these muscle biopsies cannot be overstated. Just as immunolabelling for other complex members may be lost or reduced in dystrophinopathy, patients with a minor reduction in dystrophin may have a primary sarcoglycanopathy. In these cases, there is likely to be a much more marked reduction in one or all of the sarcoglycans than an alteration in dystrophin. The problem of determining the relevance of a reduction in dystrophin is particularly pertinent in female patients in whom a diagnosis of manifesting carrier of Duchenne muscular dystrophy might be considered and also in those patients thought to have Becker muscular dystrophy where there is a reduction in the abundance but not the size of the dystrophin molecule detected by Western blotting.

Use of antibodies to all four sarcoglycans can help to indicate which sarcoglycan is primarily involved. In δ- and β-sarcoglycanopathy immunolabelling for all four sarcoglycans is commonly lost (Bonnemann *et al.* 1995; Lim *et al.* 1995a; Nigro *et al.* 1996; Vainzof *et al.* 1996). In γ- and α-sarcoglycan deficiency the pattern may be much more patchy and the other sarcoglycans may be normal or nearly normal. These general rules can be used to direct mutation analysis to the various sarcoglycan genes. Apart from the founder mutations specific to defined population groups, mutations in the sarcoglycan genes are rarely recurrent, with the exception of the R77C mutation in α-sarcoglycan which accounts for up to 40 per cent of the reported mutations in this gene (Carrie *et al.* 1997; Piccolo *et al.* 1995). Definition of the mutation is necessary in order to give a precise diagnosis of the type of sarcoglycanopathy and also to allow prenatal diagnosis or carrier testing should this be sought by the family. However, there undoubtedly exist some patients in whom the muscle biopsy findings are indicative of a reduction in one or more members of the sarcoglycan complex but in whom a primary mutation cannot be found. Such cases may represent a failure of the techniques used to search for mutations, or alternatively may suggest that mutations in another gene may also cause secondary loss of sarcoglycan immunolabelling.

Molecular biology

The sarcoglycan complex comprises one of the components of the dystrophin-glycoprotein complex (DGC) which acts as a structural link between the F-actin cytoskeleton and the extracellular matrix (Fig. 7.2) (Cohn and Campbell 2000; Ozawa *et al.* 1998). The sarcoglycan complex is associated with an additional protein, sarcospan. No sarcospan mutations have yet been described (Crosbie *et al.* 1997; Lebakken *et al.* 2000). The behaviour of the sarcoglycan complex as a whole has been modelled in cell culture where it has been shown that the presence of a mutant sarcoglycan blocks formation of the complex and its insertion into the plasma membrane (Holt and Campbell 1998). It has also been suggested that the exact composition of the sarcoglycan complex may vary in different tissues. In skeletal and cardiac muscle, the complex consists of α-, β-, γ- and δ-sarcoglycan and sarcospan (Barresi *et al.* 2000b; Straub *et al.* 1999). ε-sarcoglycan (mutations of which have not yet been described) appears to replace α-sarcoglycan in smooth muscle, where α-sarcoglycan is not expressed. ε-sarcoglycan is expressed broadly while α-sarcoglycan expression is limited to skeletal and cardiac muscle (McNally *et al.* 1998b).

The definition of distinct sarcoglycan complexes in different tissues has pathogenic implications which have been further elucidated by the study of the various animal models of sarcoglycanopathy now available. The first identified animal model of sarcoglycanopathy was the so-called cardiomyopathic hamster, where the disease is now known to represent a δ-sarcoglycanopathy (Nigro *et al.* 1997). Targeted disruption of β-, δ-, or γ-sarcoglycan in mice also causes cardiomyopathy, as well as muscular dystrophy, while α-sarcoglycan deficient mice develop a muscular dystrophy only (Allamand and Campbell 2000). Analysis of the vascular musculature in these various mouse models confirmed perturbed microvascular function in β- and δ-sarcoglycan deficient animals, a finding reflected in some sarcoglycanopathy patients (Gnecchi-Ruscone *et al.* 1999). It is therefore likely that there is a complex pathogenetic mechanism in β- and δ-sarcoglycanopathy causing disruption of the sarcoglycan complexes in both skeletal and smooth muscle, and that in these diseases intermittent ischaemia due to microvascular disease may be a part of the pathogenesis, especially of cardiomyopathy (Barresi *et al.* 2000a; Durbeej *et al.* 2000). Meanwhile, specific additional roles for individual sarcoglycans also add to the potential multiplicity of the mechanisms of disease causation in this group: such as for example a role in signalling pathways as suggested for α-sarcoglycan with its apparent ecto-adenosine triphosphate activity (Betto *et al.* 1999). While the DGC clearly has a structural role in the maintenance of muscle fibre integrity, it may be oversimplistic to treat this complex of proteins too much as a whole while the roles of the individual members are more thoroughly elucidated.

Calpain 3 deficiency—LGMD2A

Clinical and diagnostic considerations

Calpainopathy is likely to be one of the more common types of limb-girdle muscular dystrophy though once again a definitive idea of its incidence is not yet possible, with estimates of its frequency ranging from 9 to 40 per cent of LGMD in outbred populations (Chou *et al.* 1999; Richard *et al.* 1999). It has a much higher prevalence in some populations including Reunion Island, with founder mutations also described in the Basque region of Spain and in Turkey (Dincer *et al.* 1997; 2000; Fardeau *et al.* 1996). Clinically calpain 3 deficiency typically does not resemble sarcoglycanopathy or dystrophinopathy being a predominantly atrophic disease in contradistinction to the hypertrophy more commonly seen in the disorders affecting the DGC. Patients with calf hypertrophy have rarely been reported with calpain 3 deficiency: muscle hypertrophy elsewhere has not been reported and there is a much more general pattern of muscle atrophy and wasting in most patients with this disorder. The pattern of muscle involvement in calpain 3 deficiency tends to be very highly selective with the posterior thigh muscles being especially affected from early on and a characteristic sparing of the hip abductors which leads to the typical adoption of a relatively wide based stance. Scapular winging can be a prominent feature at onset and in some patients this may have led to a confusion in diagnosis with facioscapulohumeral muscular dystrophy. Most patients with calpainopathy present between 8 and 15 years but onset between 2 and 45 years has been reported. Together with the proximal limb-girdle muscle weakness contractures are a well recognized feature of calpain 3 deficiency and typically affect the achilles tendons in most patients; in some patients this leads to toe walking being the presenting complaint. Muscle pain is also reported infrequently as an early symptom. Most patients with calpain 3 deficiency will require a wheelchair for mobility as their disease progresses though progression may be very variable. Respiratory failure is a late complication in association with progressive muscle weakness. Cardiac complications have not yet been reported in this disorder.

Diagnosis of calpain 3 deficiency can be suggested clinically but confirmation of the diagnosis may be relatively complex. Serum creatine kinase levels at onset tend to be elevated to around $20\times$ the upper limit of normal. Examination of a muscle biopsy using antibodies to calpain 3 at present is possible only using immunoblotting as available antibodies do not work on muscle biopsy sections (Anderson *et al.* 1998) (Fig. 7.1). Another factor emphasizing the need for the use of multiple antibodies in diagnosis of these types of limb-girdle muscular dystrophy is the fact that in at least half of all patients with dysferlin deficiency (dysferlinopathy or LGMD2B, see below) there is a secondary reduction in calpain 3 levels (Anderson *et al.* 2000). So while loss or reduction of calpain 3 immunolabelling on Western blotting can give a good indication of the diagnosis of calpainopathy, confirmation of the diagnosis using molecular genetic techniques to define the relevant mutation needs to be performed as a follow up to this analysis. The calpain 3 gene is large and multi-exonic and many different mutations have been reported in this gene in association with a muscular dystrophy phenotype (Richard *et al.* 1999). The assessment of the possible pathogenicity of specific sequence changes is another problem in achieving a definitive molecular diagnosis in all cases.

Molecular biology

The involvement of calpain 3 mutations in LGMD2A remains unexplained in terms of a clear hypothesis relating to its molecular pathology. Calpain 3 is the muscle specific member of a family of calcium dependent proteases (Sorimachi *et al.* 1994). Calpains typically have many substrates and the physiological target of calpain 3 in skeletal muscle is as yet undefined. Use of monoclonal antibodies to calpain 3 show that homozygous frameshift mutations of the calpain 3 gene cause complete absence of the protein: missense mutations cause a much more variable pattern of calpain 3 reduction (Anderson *et al.* 1998). Human mutations modelled in cell systems show loss of proteolysis (Ono *et al.* 1998) while other potentially important functions of calpain 3, including its association with titin (Kinbara *et al.* 1997), were not uniformly lost in the presence of these mutations. Transgenic mice with targetted disruption of the so-called active site develop a myopathic phenotype (Tagawa *et al.* 2000). Calpain 3 activity may be involved in the control of muscle specific transcription factors as has previously been suggested, more generally, for the ubiquitous calpains. In keeping with this hypothesis it has been suggested that calpain 3 deficient muscle may be susceptible to apoptosis due to a perturbation of the IκBα/NF-κB pathway (Baghdiguian *et al.* 1999). This finding has yet to be corroborated and its potential significance to this type of muscular dystrophy confirmed. Meantime, the finding of a secondary calpain 3 reduction in some patients with primary dysferlinopathy (Anderson *et al.* 2000) leads to the intriguing possibility that both of these proteins may have a role in a similar pathway resulting in muscular dystrophy.

LGMD2B—Dysferlin deficiency

Clinical and diagnostic considerations

The disease initially linked to the LGMD2B locus on chromosome 2p13 was a form of limb-girdle muscular dystrophy with relatively late onset and slow progression, described in Palestinian and subsequently also in Brazilian families (Bashir *et al.* 1994; Mahjneh *et al.* 1996; Passos-Bueno *et al.* 1995.). However, it quickly became clear that families with a distal muscular dystrophy usually predominantly affecting the gastrocnemius muscles initially with difficulty standing on tip-toe a characteristic early symptom (Miyoshi myopathy) also linked to this locus (Bejaoui *et al.* 1995). A hallmark of the disease associated with dysferlinopathy is therefore that of clinical variability with presentation involving either the proximal or the distal musculature. Having said this, there are some features of dysferlinopathy which to date appear to be fairly typically seen independent of the pattern of muscle involvement at presentation. These include a relatively defined and narrow age at onset in the late teens or early 20s following normal early motor development and even good muscle prowess. Occasional reports of transient calf pain and swelling before the presentation of muscle weakness are intriguing, but not well understood (Argov *et al.* 2000). Following presentation, progression of the disease in dysferlin deficiency is relatively slow though there can be some inter and intrafamilial variability seen and some patients do have a more rapidly progressive course of the disease requiring a wheelchair within 10 years of diagnosis (Weiler *et al.* 1996). No definite association with cardiac or respiratory problems in dysferlinopathy has yet been established. In some families with dysferlin deficiency there is a clear tendency towards variability of the phenotype whereas in others there is a very much more uniform disease. An additional phenotype involving the anterior tibial rather than the gastrocnemius muscles has also been described (Liu *et al.* 1998). The variability in presentation may be seen even in the presence of a homozygous dysferlin mutation, and the pattern of dysferlin immunolabelling in muscle does not distinguish a limb-girdle or Miyoshi type of presentation (Argov *et al.* 2000; Weiler *et al.* 1999). It would appear, therefore, that in dysferlinopathy additional factors as well as the primary mutation are operating to modify the final phenotype, in particular with respect to the exact pattern of muscles involved.

Estimates of the frequency of dysferlinopathy are hard to obtain. In the Brazilian population, it is a relatively common form of LGMD within this very well-defined patient group (Passos-Bueno *et al.* 1999). A survey of undiagnosed LGMD patients found dysferlin abnormalities in around half the muscle biopsies examined of around half (Piccolo *et al.* 2000). However, these patients had not been studied for mutations and so how many represented a primary dysferlinopathy is not known. A particularly high incidence in the Libyan Jewish population can be explained by the presence of a founder mutation in nearly 10 per cent of the population (Argov *et al.* 2000). Apart from this founder mutation, and one seen in the Canadian aboriginal population (Weiler *et al.* 1999), mutations in dysferlin are highly variable, and may affect any part of this large gene (Illarioshkin *et al.* 2000; Matsumura *et al.* 1999). It is therefore logical to approach mutation detection following examination of a muscle biopsy using antibodies to dysferlin. Patients with dysferlinopathy appear to show reduction or absence of dysferlin immunolabelling on muscle biopsy sections or Western blotting (Fig. 7.1). Emphasizing once again the need to follow up this kind of analysis by the detection of the causative mutation, around half of all dysferlinopathy patients studied to date have also had a secondary reduction in calpain 3. Ancillary investigations in dysferlinopathy can be relatively helpful in suggesting the diagnosis, especially as typically serum creatine kinase at presentation is extremely high (up to 100 × normal) and inflammatory features may be prominent in the muscle biopsy (Argov *et al.* 2000; McNally *et al.* 2000). These features may have led to an erroneous diagnosis of polymyositis which is unresponsive to immunosuppression. The phenotype of Miyoshi myopathy appears itself to be genetically heterogeneous, with a second locus on chromosome 10 (Linssen *et al.* 1998).

Molecular biology

At the time of its identification, dysferlin showed no homology to any human nucleotide or protein sequences in the databases, but did show homology to a *C elegans* protein FER-1 (Achanzar and Ward 1997). This protein is expressed only in primary spermatocytes in *C elegans*, and mutations cause failure of spermatogenesis through loss of fusion of membranous organelles. Sequence analysis of dysferlin shows that it is a type II transmembrane protein, with a C-terminal transmembrane domain and the majority of the protein cytoplasmic. The use of specific antibodies to dysferlin have defined plasma membrane localization in muscle, and have also shown that dysferlin is expressed very early in human development (Anderson *et al.* 1999; Matsuda *et al.* 1999). Dysferlin has another interesting structural characteristic predicted from sequence analysis in the presence of 6 C2 domains, distributed along the length of the protein (Britton *et al.* 2000). Since the cloning of dysferlin, two further homologous human proteins have been identified which share the characteristics of a C terminal transmembrane domain and multiple C2 domains. Otoferlin encodes a protein expressed in the inner ear, and mutations of this gene have been shown to cause non-syndromic deafness in the Lebanese population (Yasunaga *et al.* 1999). The third Fer1-like gene, variously designated myoferlin or FER1-L3 is highly homologous to dysferlin (Britton *et al.* 2000), and one study has suggested that it may be upregulated in some forms of muscular dystrophy (Belt Davis *et al.* 2000). The existence of further genomic sequences with homology to dysferlin suggest that additional members of this human gene family remain to be characterized.

The SJL mouse (a commonly used "stock" mouse strain previously widely used as a model for immune myositis) is now known to be a naturally occurring model for dys-ferlinopathy. The mouse has a complex genomic rearrangement in the murine dysfer-lin gene, which results in the production of an in-frame deletion of a very highly conserved C-terminal C2 domain in the RNA (Vafiadaki *et al.* 2001). Antibody studies confirm that the SJL mouse is not a complete knockout for dysferlin, producing some residual levels of protein. The SJL mouse develops a progressive muscle weakness from around three weeks of age, which is accompanied by dystrophic changes in its muscle. In parallel to the situation seen in some patients, the SJL mouse also has a prominent inflammatory infiltrate in its muscles.

Dysferlin is not related to any muscular dystrophy causing proteins so far identified, and the molecular mechanism by which mutations in this gene cause muscular dystro-phy remains unknown. The only secondary protein deficiency so far identified in dysferlinopathy patients has been a secondary deficiency of calpain 3, as described above (Anderson *et al.* 2000). As already discussed, the mechanism by which calpain deficiency itself causes muscular dystrophy is also unknown: this apparently secondary change in dysferlin deficient muscle may point towards the elucidation of some shared common pathological mechanisms. So a definitive function for dysferlin and its role in the pathogenesis of muscular dystrophy is not known. Despite its sarcolemmal local-ization, dysferlin is not associated with the dystrophin–glycoprotein complex (DGC) (Piccolo *et al.* 2000). Dysferlin labelling is lost from the sarcolemma in patients pre-senting with LGMD2B or MM, consistent with a role in development and/or mainte-nance of the sarcolemma, and it has recently been suggested that intracellular vesicles may accumulate in the cytoplasm in dysferlin-deficient muscle (Piccolo *et al.* 2000). The presence of these vesicles links into a common theme which emerges from the often only speculative functions of the FER-1 like gene family, relating to the presence of multiple C2 domains (Rizo and Sudhof 1999). The majority of C2 containing proteins operate in signal transduction, although many are also involved in membrane trafficking. FER-1 is involved in the fusion of membranous vesicles during spermato-genesis (Achanzar and Ward 1997). Based on the fact that its absence causes a non-syndromic sensorineural deafness, it has been suggested that otoferlin may operate in synaptic vesicle fusion in the inner ear (Yasunaga *et al.* 1999; 2000). The function of the

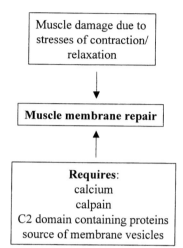

Fig. 7.3 A possible mechanism to link the non-sarcoglycan proteins involved in LGMD in a pathway relating to membrane repair.

FER-1 like protein which is most closely related to dysferlin, FER-1L3 or myoferlin, is not known, and to date no mutant phenotype has been associated with it. However, one study has suggested that this protein may operate in a membrane repair function within myocytes (Belt Davis *et al.* 2000). Extrapolating from these hypotheses, it is therefore possible that dysferlin itself could be involved in membrane fusion events such as those involved in sarcolemmal repair within muscle cells and that deficiency of this process might be the underlying cause of LGMD2B and MM. Such a mechanism may even have a broader pathophysiological role, as suggested by the finding of an altered pattern of dysferlin expression in a range of different muscular dystrophies (Piccolo *et al.* 2000). In model systems of neuronal membrane repair, this exocytotic pathway is mediated by the same family of proteins that are involved in synaptic vesicle exocytosis (Detrait *et al.* 2000a;), the process suggested to be defective in otoferlin deficiency (Yasunaga *et al.* 1999). In addition, such vesicle fusion mediated repair pathways have been shown to be calcium dependent (Eddleman *et al.* 1997), mediated by calpain (Godell *et al.* 1997; Howard *et al.* 1999) and dependent upon membrane fusion proteins including synaptotagmin (Detrait *et al.* 2000a, b) a C2 domain containing protein (Rizo and Sudhof 1999). By extrapolation from this discussion therefore, calpain 3 and caveolin 3 might also be considered candidates for involvement in this pathway, which could present a unifying hypothesis for the mechanism by which muscular dystrophy results from mutations in these diverse genes (Fig. 7.3).

Telethonin—LGMD2G

The seventh mapped form of autosomal recessive LGMD was defined in Brazilian families shown to be excluded from other LGMD loci. Mutations in the telethonin gene on chromosome 17q11–12 are now known to underlie this apparently rare form of LGMD, which has not to date been reported outside Brazil (Moreira *et al.* 1997,

2000). Affected individuals had a mean age of onset of 12.5 years with calf hypertrophy, early foot drop and inability to walk on their heels as well as proximal muscle weakness at onset. Serum CK was 3–17× normal and some muscle fibres showed the presence of rimmed vacuoles. Progression of the disease in the affected families was variable.

Diagnosis can be suggested by loss of labelling with anti-telethonin antibodies in muscle, followed by mutation detection. Telethonin is a sacromeric protein, expressed at high levels in skeletal muscle and also in heart. It is a substrate of titin kinase and may provide binding sites for other proteins important in the assembly of the sarcomere (Valle *et al.* 1997).

Other autosomal recessive forms of LGMD

Two other loci exist for forms of LGMD. LGMD2H was localized to chromosome 9q31–33 in the Manitoba Hutterite population of Canada (Weiler *et al.* 1998). Affected individuals typically have relatively mild disease, with presentation in the late twenties with a proximal pattern of muscle weakness. Serum CK was in the range of 2–20× normal. This disease has not been reported in other populations. Similarly, to date, the latest mapped form of LGMD has been reported only in Tunisia. LGMD2I maps to chromosome 19q13.3 based on results in a single large family (Driss *et al.* 2000). These patients had a relatively slowly progressive proximal pattern of muscular dystrophy, especially involving the pelvic girdle. Serum CK was markedly elevated. For both of these loci, linkage analysis is the only tool for diagnosis available to date, awaiting the identification of the causative genes.

Management principles

The knowledge of the molecular basis for so many forms of LGMD opens up the possibility of specific gene-based treatment being developed in this group, and the various animal models available offer an invaluable resource to test these various treatment options. In the meantime, the proper management of these disorders remains very important for ensuring the quality of life of affected patients. Provision of genetic counselling, prognostic information and practical and emotional support are all basic tenets of management in this group. Prevention and management of complications, such as contractures, respiratory failure and cardiac involvement varies from disorder to disorder but overall cannot be neglected. Even in the absence of a curative treatment, such therapeutic interventions may be life saving and certainly life-enhancing.

Limb-girdle muscular dystrophies – the overall perspective

Quite clearly the disorders which fall within the LGMD category are a heterogeneous group both clinically and at the level of their molecular pathology. The disorders described in this chapter are those which are most likely to be diagnosed in a patient presenting with a proximal muscular dystrophy. However, other muscular dystrophies also come into the differential diagnosis and in some cases a diagnosis may only be inferred from secondary protein abnormalities. Some patients with a laminin α2 deficiency (either primary or secondary) have been described with a limb-girdle muscular dystrophy phenotype (See Chapter 2). In other patients use of a range of antibodies on a muscle biopsy sample may define patterns of secondary protein abnormalities which may be informative as to the type of primary abnormality to look for. So for example, a reduction in laminin β1 has been described in each of Bethlem myopathy, laminopathy (LGMD1B or ADEDMD) and facioscapulohumeral muscular dystrophy though its secondary deficiency is probably associated with other as yet unknown muscular dystrophies as well. Other patients remain undiagnosable with the current level of knowledge even with all of the tools available. A diagnostic scheme relying on protein analysis to direct mutation detection is a logical and time efficient process, but will miss those patients in whom a mutation alters the function of the protein without altering its expression. The development of more exhaustive and efficient mutation screening techniques applied to this group will determine how often this might be the case. For the patients in whom a precise diagnosis is still impossible, careful attention to proper storage of muscle and DNA samples will ensure that in the future a more precise diagnosis should be achievable as our knowledge and techniques improve.

It is tempting to speculate at what point the molecular pathological background to these disorders may at some stage converge to elucidate a final common pathway arriving at a muscular dystrophy. Clearly the diseases caused by the components of the sarcoglycan group share at least some features of molecular pathology as the genes encode proteins which form a tight complex in the muscle fibre membrane. More intriguing perhaps is the observation that dysferlin is also abnormal in some patients with a dystrophinopathy or sarcoglycanopathy indicating perhaps a more widespread role for dysferlin in the production of a muscular dystrophy phenotype than would be suggested from its role in primary dysferlinopathies. Similarly, a secondary reduction in calpain 3 deficiency in those patients with a primary dysferlin deficiency indicates the possibility of a common pathway in these disorders as well. Experiments in cell culture systems and in the various animal models now available in this group should help to determine the primary molecular pathology involved in these disorders, as well as modifying factors which are likely to become of increasing importance as our understanding improves.

This snapshot of the current state of our knowledge about LGMD incorporates the many gains in knowledge accumulated in the 1990s about the molecular basis of these diseases and the advances this has brought about in diagnosis and genotype–phenotype correlations. But by no means has the final statement on LGMD been reached. Other disease entities with this broad group undoubtedly remain to be identified. Equally, the full interrelationship between the different types of disease, the role of modifying genes and the complete elucidation of the underlying molecular pathology all indicate that many more insights are required before the definitive portrait of this intriguing group of muscular dystrophies can be achieved.

References

Achanzar, W.E. and Ward, S. (1997). A nematode gene required for sperm vesicle fusion. *Cell Science*, **110**, 1073–81.

Allamand, V. and Campbell, K.P. (2000). Animal models for muscular dystrophy: valuable tools for the development of therapists. *Human Molecular Genetics*, **9**(16), 2459–67.

Anderson, L.V.B., Davison, K., Moss, J.A., Richard, I., Fardeau, M., Tomé, F.M.S. *et al.* (1998). Characterisation of monoclonal antibodies to calpain 3 and protein expression in muscle from patients with limb-girdle muscular dystrophy type 2A. *American Journal of Pathology*, **153**, 1169–79.

Anderson, L.V.B., Davison, K., Moss, J.A., Young, C., Cullen, M.J., Walsh, J. *et al.* (1999). Dysferlin is a plasma membrane protein and is expressed early in human development. *Human Molecular Genetics*, **8**(5), 855–61.

Anderson, L.V.B., Harrison, R.M., Pogue, R., Vafiadaki, E., Pollitt, C., Davison, K. *et al.* (2000). Secondary reduction in calpain 3 expression in patients with limb-girdle muscular dystrophy type 2B and Miyoshi myopathy (primary dysferlinopathies). *Neuromuscular Disorders*, **10**, 553–9.

Argov, Z., Sadeh, M., Mazor, K., Soffer, D., Kahana, E., Eisenberg, I. *et al.* (2000). Muscular dystrophy due to dysferlin deficiency in Libyan Jews. Clinical and genetic features, *Brain*, **123**, 1229–37.

Baghdiguian, S., Martin, M., Richard, I., Pons, F., Astier, C., Bourg, N. *et al.* (1999). Calpain 3 deficiency is associated with myonuclear apoptosis and profound perturbation of the IxB /NF-kB pathway in limb-girdle muscular dystrophy type 2A. *Nature Medicine*, **5**, 503–11.

Barresi, R., di Blasi, C., Negri, T., Brugnoni, R., Vitali, A., Felisari, G. *et al.* (2000a), Disruption of heart sarcoglycan complex and severe cardiomyopathy caused by β-sarcoglycan mutations. *Journal of Medical Genetics*, **37**, 102–7.

Barresi, R., Moore, S.A., Stolle, C.A., Mendell, J.R., and Campbell, K.P. (2000b), Expression of gamma-sarcoglycan in smooth muscle and its interaction with the smooth muscle sarcoglycan-sarcospan complex. *Journal of Biological Chemistry*, **275**.

Bashir, R., Strachan, T., Keers, S., Stephenson, A., Mahjneh, I., Marconi, GP. *et al.* (1994). A gene for autosomal recessive limb-girdle muscular dystrophy maps to chromosome 2p. *Human Molecular Genetics*, **3**, 455–7.

Beckmann, J.S. (1999). Disease taxonomy-monogenic muscular dystrophy. *British Medical Bulletin*, **55**, 340–57.

Beckmann, J.S., Brown RH, Muntoni, F., Urtizberea, A., Bonnemann, C.G., and Bushby, K.M.D. (1999). 66th/67th ENMC sponsored international workshop: the limb-girdle muscular dystrophies, 26–28th March (1999). Naarden, the Netherlands. *Neuromuscular Disorders*, **9**, 436–45.

Bejaoui, K., Hirabayashi, K., Hentati, F., Haines, J.L., Ben Hamida, C., Belal, S. *et al.* (1995). Linkage of Miyoshi Myopathy (distal autosomal recessive muscular dystrophy) locus to chromosome 2p12–14. *Neurology*, **45**, 768–72.

Belt Davis, D., Delmonte, A.J., Ly, C.T., and McNally, E.M. (2000). Myoferlin, a candidate gene and potential modifier of muscular dystrophy. *Human Molecular Genetics*, **9**(2), 217–26.

Bethlem, J. and Van Wijngaarden, GK. (1976). Benign myopathy with autosomal dominant inheritance: a report of three pedigrees. *Brain*, **99**, 91–100.

Betto, R., Senter, L., Ceoldo, S., Tarricone, E., Biral, D., and Salviati, G. (1999). Ecto-ATPase Activity of α-sarcoglycan (adhalin). *Biological Chemistry*, **274**(12), 7907–12.

Betz, R.C, Scheser, B.G.H., Kasper, D, Thicker, K, Ramirez, A, Stein, V, *et al.* (2001). Mutcher, in cav3 cause mechanical hyper irritability of skeletal muscle in crippling muscle disease nature genetres, **28**, 216–17.

Bonne, G., Mercuri, E., Muchir, A., Urtizberea, A., Becane, H.M., Recan, D. *et al.* (2000a). Clinical and molecular genetic spectrum of autosomal dominant Emery-Dreifuss muscular dystrophy due to mutations of the lamins A/C gene. *Annals of Neurology,* **48**, 170–80

Bonne, G., Mercuri, E., Muchir, A., Urtizberea, A., Becane, H.M., Recan, D. *et al.* (2000b). Clinical and molecular genetic spectrum of autosomal dominant Emery-Dreifuss muscular dystrophy due to mutations of the lamin A/C gene. *Annals of Neurology,* **48**, 170–80.

Bonnemann, C.G., Modi, R., Noguchi, S., Mizuno, Y., Yoshida, M., Gussoni, E. *et al.* (1995). β-sarco-glycan (A3b) mutations cause autosomal recessive muscular dystrophy with loss of the sarcogly-can complex. *Nature Genetics,* **11**, 266–73.

Britton, S., Freeman, T., Keers, S., Vafiadaki, E., Harrison, R., Bushby, K., and Bashir, R. (2000). The third human FER-1 like protein is highly homologous to dysferlin. *Genomics,* **68**, 313–21.

Bushby, K. (1992). Report on the 12th ENMC sponsored international workshop – the limb-girdle muscular dystrophies. *Neuromuscular Disorders,* **2**, 3–5.

Bushby, K.M.D. and Beckmann, J.S. (1995). Report of the 30th and 31st ENMC international work-shop- the limb girdle muscular dystrophies, and proposal for a new nomenclature. *Neuromuscular Disorders,* **5**, 337–44.

Calvo, F., Teijeira, S., Fernandez, J.M., Teijeiro, A., Fernandez-Hojas, R., Fernandez-Lopez, X.A. *et al.* (2000). Evaluation of heart involvement in gamma-sarcoglycanopathy (LGMD2C). A study of ten patients. *Neuromuscular Disorders,* **10**, 560–6.

Cao, H. and Hegele, R.A. (2000). Nuclear lamin A/C R482Q mutation in Canadian kindreds with Dunnigan-type familial partial lipodystrophy. *Human Molecular Genetics,* **9**(1), 109–12.

Carbone, I., Bruno, C., Sotgia, F., Bado, M., Broda, P., Masetti, E. *et al.* (2000). Mutation in the CAV3 gene causes partial caveolin-3 deficiency and hyperCKemia. *Neurology,* **54**(6), 1373–6.

Carrie, A., Piccolo, F., Leturcq, F., de Toma, C., Azibi, K., Beldjord, C. *et al.* (1997). Mutational diver-sity and hot spots in the α-sarcoglycan gene in autosomal recessive muscular dystrophy (LGMD2D). *Journal of Medical Genetics,* **34**, 470–5.

Chou, F.-L., Angelini, C., Daentl, D., Garcia, C., Greco, C., Hausmanowa-Petrusewicz, I., *et al.* (1999). Calpain III mutation analysis of a heterogeneous limb-girdle muscular dystrophy population. *Neurology,* **52**, 1015–20.

Cohn, R.D. and Campbell, K.P. (2000). Molecular basis of muscular dystrophies. *Muscle & Nerve,* **23**, 1456–71.

Crosbie, R.H., Heighway, J., Venzke, D.P., Lee, J.C., and Campbell, K.P. (1997). Sarcospan, the 25-kDa transmembrane component of the dystrophin-glycoprotein complex. *Journal of Biological Chemistry,* **272**(50), 31221–4.

Detrait, E.R., Eddleman, C.S., Yoo, S.M., Fukuda, M., Nguyen, P.N., Bittner, G.D., and Fishman, H.M. (2000a). Axolammal repair requires proteins that mediate synaptic vesicle fusion. *Journal of Neurobiology,* **44**, 382–91.

Detrait, E.R., Yoo, S., Eddleman, C.S., Fukuda, M., Bittner, G.D., and Fishman, H.M. (2000b). Plasmalemmal repair of severed neurites of PC12 cells requires Ca^{2+} and synaptotagmin. *Journal of Neuroscience Research,* **62**(4), 566–73.

Dincer, P., Akcoren, Z., Demir, E., Richard, I., Sancak, O., Kale, G. *et al.* (2000). A cross section of autosomal recessive limb-girdle muscular dystrophies in 38 families. *Journal of Medical Genetics,* **37**, 361–7.

Dincer, P., Leturcq, F., Richard, I., Piccolo, F., Yalnizoglu, D., de Toma, C., Akcoren, Z., Broux, O., Deburgrave, N., Brenguier, L., Roudaut, C., Urtizberea, A., Jung, D., Tan, E., Jenapierre, M.,

Campbell, K.P., Kaplan, J.-C., Beckmann, J.S., and Topaloglu, H. (1997). A Biochemical, Genetic and Clinical Survey of autosomal recessive limb girdle muscular dystrophy in *Turkey. Annals of Neurology*, **42**(2), 222–9.

Driss, A., Amouri, R., Ben Hamida, C., Souilem, S., Gouider-Khouja, N., Ben Hamida, M., and Hentati, F. (2000). A new locus for autosomal recessive limb-girdle muscular dystrophy in a large consanguineous Tunisian family maps to chromosome 19q13.3. *Neuromusc. Disorders*, **10**, 240–6.

Duggan, D.J. and Hoffman, E.P. (1996). Autosomal recessive muscular dystrophy and mutations of the sarcoglycan complex. *Neuromusc. Disorders*, **6**(6), 475–82.

Durbeej, M., Cohn, R.D., Hrstka, R.F., Moore, S.A., Allamand, V., Davidson, B.L. *et al.* (2000). Disruption of the β-sarcoglycan gene reveals pathogenetic complexity of limb-girdle muscular dystrophy type 2E. *Molecular Cell*, **5**, 141–51.

Eddleman, C.S., Ballinger, M.L., Smyers, M.E., Godell, C.M., Fishman, H.M., and Bittner, G.D. (1997). Repair of plasmalemmal lesions by vesicles. *Proceedings of the National Academy of Sciences, USA*, **94**, 4745–50.

Engelman, J.A., Zhang, X., Galbiati, F., Volonte, D., Sotgia, F., Pestell, R.G. *et al.* (1998). Molecular genetics of the caveolin gene family: implications for human cancers, diabetes, Alzheimers Disease and muscular dystrophy. *American Journal of Human Genetics*, **63**, 1578–87.

Eymard, B., Romero, N.B., Leturcq, F., Piccolo, F., Carrie, A., Jenapierre, M. *et al.* (1997). Primary adhalinopathy (α-sarcoglycanopathy): clinical, pathologic and genetic correlation in 20 patients with autosomal recessive muscular dystrophy. *Neurology*, **48**, 1227–34.

Fardeau, M., Hillaire, D., Mignard, C., Feingold, N., Feingold, J., Mignard, D. *et al.* (1996). Juvenile limb-girdle muscular dystrophy. Clinical, histopathological and genetic data on a small community living in the Reunion Island. *Brain*, **119**, 295–308.

Feit, H., Silbergleit, A., Schneider, L.B., Gutierrez, J.A., Fitoussi, R.-P., Reyes, C. *et al.* (1998). Vocal cord and pharyngeal weakness with autosomal dominant distal myopathy: clinical description and gene localisation to 5q31. *American Journal of Human Genetics*, **63**, 1732–42.

Galbiati, F., Volonte, D., Minetti, C., Chu, J.B., and Lisanti, M.P. (1999). Phenotypic behaviour of caveolin-3 mutations that cause autosomal dominant limb-girdle muscular dystrophy (LGMD1C). *Biological Chemistry*, **274**(36), 25632–41.

Gnecchi-Ruscone, T., Taylor, J., Mercuri, E., Paternostro, G., Pogue, R., Bushby, K. *et al.* (1999). Cardiomyopathy in Duchenne, Becker, and sarcoglycanopathies: a role for coronary dysfunction?. *Muscle & Nerve*, **22**, 1549–56.

Godell, C.M., Smyers, M.E., Eddleman, C.S., Ballinger, M.L., Fishman, H.M., and Bittner, G.D. (1997). Calpain activity promotes the sealing of severed giant axons. *Proceedings of the National Academy of Sciences, USA*, **94**, 4751–6.

Hauser, M.A., Horrigan, S.K., Salmikangas, P., Torian, U.M., Viles, K.D., Dancel, R. *et al.* (2000). Myotilin is mutated in limb-girdle muscular dystrophy 1A. *Human Molecular Genetics*, **9**(14), 2141–7.

Herrmann, R., Straub, V., Blank, M., Kutzick, C., Franke, N., Jacob, E.N. *et al.* (2000). Dissociation of the dystroglycan complex in caveolin-3-deficient limb-girdle muscular dystrophy. *Human Molecular Genetics*, **9**(15), 2335–40.

Holt, K.H. and Campbell, K.P. (1998). Assembly of the sarcoglycan complex: insights for muscular dystrophy. *Biological Chemistry*, **273**(52), 34667–70.

Howard, M.J., David, G., and Barrett, J.N. (1999). Resealing of transected myelinated mammalian axons in vivo: evidence for involvement of calpain. *Neuroscience*, **93**(2), 807–15.

Illarioshkin, S., Ivanova-Smolenskaya, I.A., Greenberg, C.R., Nylen, E., Sukhorukov, V.S., Poleshchuk, V.V. *et al.* (2000). Identical dysferlin mutation in limb-girdle muscular dystrophy type 2B and distal myopathy. *Neurology*, **55**, 1931–3.

Jeanpierre, M., Carrie, A., Piccolo, F., Leturcqu, F., Azibi, K., Toma, C. *et al.* (1996). From adhalinopathies to alpha-sarcoglycanopathies: an overview. *Neuromuscular Disorders*, **6**(6), 463–6.

Jobsis, G.J., Boers, J.M., Barth, P.G., and de Visser, M. (1999). Bethlem myopathy: a slowly progressive congenital muscular dystrophy with contractures. *Brain*, **122**, 649–55.

Jobsis, G.J., Keizers, H., Vreijling, J.P., de Visser, M., Speer, M.C., Wolterman, R.A. *et al.* (1996). Collagen VI mutations in Bethlem myopathy, an autosomal dominant myopathy with contractures. *Nature Genetics*, **14**, 113–5.

Jones, K.J., Kim, S.S., and North, K.N. (1998). Abnormalities of dystrophin, the sarcoglycans, and laminin α2 in the muscular dystrophies. *Journal of Medical Genetics*, **35**, 379–86.

Jung, D., Leturcqu, F., Sunada, Y., Duclos, F., Tome, F.M.S., Moomaw, C. *et al.* (1996). Absence of y-sarcoglycan (35 DAG) in autosomal recessive muscular dystrophy linked to chromosome 13q12. *FEBS Lett*, **381**, 15–20.

Kinbara, K., Sorimachi, H., Ishiura, S., and Suzuki, K. (1997). Muscle-specific calpain, p94, interacts with the extreme C-terminal region of connectin, a unique region flanked by two immunoglobulin C2 motifs. *Archives of Biochemistry and Biophysics*, **342**(1), 99–107.

Lebakken, C.S., Venzke, D.P., Hrstka, R.F., Consolino, C.M., Faulkner, J.A., Williamson, R.A., and Campbell, K.P. (2000). Sarcospan-deficient mice maintain normal muscle function. *Molecular Cell Biology*, **20**(5), 1669–77.

Lim, L.E., Duclos, F., Broux, O., Bourg, N., Sunada, Y., Allamand, V. *et al.* (1995a). β-sarcoglycan: characterisation and role in limb-girdle muscular dystrophy linked to 4q12. *Nature Genetics*, **11**, 257–65.

Lim, L.E., Duclos, F., Broux, O., Bourg, N., Sunada, Y., Allamand, V. *et al.* (1995b). β-sarcoglycan: characterisation and role in limb-girdle muscular dystrophy linked to 4q12. *Nature Genetics*, **11**, 257–65.

Linssen, W.H.J.P., de Visser, M., Notermans, N.C., Vreyling, J.P., van Doorn, P.A., Wokke, J.H.J. *et al.* (1998). Genetic heterogeneity in Miyoshi-type distal muscular dystrophy. *Neuromuscular Disorders*, **8**, 317–20.

Liu, J., Aoki, M., Illa, I., Wu, C., Fardeau, M., Angelini, C. *et al.* (1998). Dysferlin, a novel skeletal muscle gene, is mutated in Miyoshi myopathy and limb girdle muscular dystrophy. *Nature Genetics*, **21**(1), 31–6.

Lunt P.W. and Harper P.S. (1991). Genetic counselling in facioscapulohumeral muscular dystrophy. *Journal of Medical Genetics*, **28**, 655–64.

Mahjneh, I., Passos-Bueno, M.R., Zatz, M., Vainzof, M., Marconi, G., Nashef, L. *et al.* (1996). The phenotype of chromosome 2p-linked limb-girdle muscular dystrophy. *Neuromuscular Disorders*, **6**(6), 483–90.

Manilal, S., Sewry, C.A., Pereboev, A., Man, N.T., Gobbi, P., Hawkes, S. *et al.* (1999). Distribution of emerin and lamins in the heart and implications for Emery-Dreifuss muscular dystrophy. *Human Molecular Genetics*, **8**(2), 353–9.

Matsuda, C., Aoki, M., Hayashi, Y.K., Ho, M.F., Arahata, K., and Brown, R.H. (1999). Dysferlin is a surface membrane-associated protein that is absent in Miyoshi myopathy. *Neurology*, **53**, 1119–22.

Matsumura, T., Aoki, M., Nagano, A., Hayashi, Y.K., Asada, C., Ogawa, M. *et al.* (1999). Molecular genetic analysis of dysferlin in Japanese patients with Miyoshi myopathy. *Proceedings of the Japan Academy*, **75**(7), 207–12.

McNally, E.M., de Sa Moreira, E., Duggan, D.J., Bonnemann, C.G., Lisanti, M.P., Lidov, H.G.W. *et al.* (1998a), Caveolin-3 in muscular dystrophy. *Human Molecular Genetics*, **7**(5), 871–7.

McNally, E.M., Ly, C.T., and Kunkel, L.M. (1998b). Human ε-sarcoglycan is highly related to α-sarcoglycan (adhalin) the limb girdle muscular dystrophy 2D gene. *FEBS Lett*, **422**, 27–32.

McNally, E.M., Ly, C.T., Rosenmann, H., Mitrani, R.S., Jiang, W., Anderson, L.V. *et al.* (2000). Splicing mutation in dysferlin produces limb-girdle muscular dystrophy with inflammation. *American Journal of Medical Genetics*, **91**(4), 305–12.

Melacini, P., Fanin, M., Duggan, D.J., Freda, M.P., Berardinelli, A., Danieli, G.A. *et al.* (1999). Heart involvement in muscular dystrophies due to sarcoglycan gene mutations. *Muscle and Nerve*, **22**, 473–9.

Merlini, L., Villanova, M., Sabatelli, P., Malandrini, A., and Maraldi, N.M. (1999). Decreased expression of laminin β-1 in chromosome 21-linked Bethlem myopathy. *Neuromuscular Disorders*, **9**, 326–9.

Messina, D.L., Speer, M.C., Pericak-Vance, M.A., and McNally, E.M. (1997). Linkage of familial dilated cardiomyopathy with conduction defect and muscular dystrophy to chromosome 6q23. *American Journal of Human Genetics*, **61**, 909–17.

Minetti, C., Sotgia, F., Bruno, C., Scartezzini, P., Broda, P., Bado, M. *et al.* (1998). Mutations in the caveolin-3 gene cause autosomal dominant limb-girdle muscular dystrophy. *Nature Genetics*, **18**, 365–8.

Mizuno, Y., Noguchi, S., Yamamoto, H., Yoshida, M., Suzuki, A., Hagiwara, Y. *et al.* (1994). Selective defect of sarcoglycan complex in severe childhood autosomal recessive muscular dystrophy muscle. *Biochemical and Biophysical Research Communications*, **203**(2), 979–83.

Moreira, E.S., Vainzof, M., Marie, S.K., Sertie, A.L., Zatz, M., and Passos-Bueno, M.R. (1997). The seventh form of autosomal recessive limb-girdle muscular dystrophy is mapped to 17q11-12. *American Journal of Human Genetics*, **61**, 151–9.

Moreira, E.S., Wiltshire, T.J., Faulkner, G., Nilforoushan, A., Vainzof, M., Suzuki, O.T. *et al.* (2000). Limb-girdle muscular dystrophy type 2G is caused by mutations in the gene encoding the sarcomeric protein telethonin. *Nature Genetics*, **24**, 163–6.

Muchir, A., Bonne, G., van der Kooi, A.J., van Meegen, M., Baas, F., Bolhuis, P.A. *et al.* (2000). Identification of mutations in the gene encoding lamins A/C in autosomal dominant limb-girdle muscular dystrophy with atrioventricular conduction disturbances (LGMD1B). *Human Molecular Genetics*, **9**(9), 1453–9.

Nagano, A., Koga, R., Ogawa, M., Kurano, Y., Kawada, J., Okada, R. *et al.* (1996). Emerin deficiency at the nuclear membrane in patients with Emery-Dreifuss muscular dystrophy. *Nature Genetics*, **12**, 254–9.

Nigro, V., Moreira, E.S., Piluso, G., Vainzof, M., Belsito, A., Politano, L. *et al.* (1996). Autosomal recessive limb-girdle muscular dystrophy, LGMD2F, is caused by a mutation in the δ-sarcoglycan gene. *Nature Genetics*, **14**, 195–8.

Nigro, V., Okazaki, Y., Belsito, A., Piluso, G., Matsuda, Y., Politano, L. *et al.* (1997). Identification of the Syrian hamster cardiomyopathy gene. *Human Molecular Genetics*, **6**(4), 601–7.

Norman, A.M., Hughes, H.E., Gardner-Medwin, D., and Nicholson, L.V.B. (1989). Dystrophin analysis in the diagnosis of muscular dystrophy. *Archives of Disease in Childhood*, **64**, 1501–3.

Ono, Y., Shimada, H., Sorimachi, H., Richard, I., Saido, T.C., Beckmann, J.S. *et al.* (1998). Functional defects of a muscle-specific calpain, p94, caused by mutations associated with limb-girdle muscular dystrophy type 2A. *Biological Chemistry*, **273**(27), 17073–8.

Ozawa, E., Noguchi, S., Mizuno, Y., Hagiwara, Y., and Yoshida, M. (1998). From dystrophinopathy to sarcoglycanopathy: evolution of a concept of muscular dystrophy. *Muscle & Nerve*, **21**, 421–38.

Parton, R.G., Way, M., Zorzi, N., and Stang, E. (1997). Caveolin-3 associates with developing T-tubules during muscle differentiation. *Journal of Cell Biology*, **136**(1), 137–54.

Passos-Bueno, M.R., Bashir, R., Moreira, E.S., Vasquez, L., Marie, S.K., Vainzof, M. *et al.* (1995). Confirmation of the 2p locus for late-onset autosomal recessive limb-girdle muscular dystrophy and refinement of the candidate region. *Genomics*, **27**, 192–5.

Passos-Bueno, M.R., Vainzof, M., Moreira, E.S., and Zatz, M. (1999). Seven autosomal recessive limb-girdle muscular dystrophies in the Brazilian population: form LGMD2A to LGMD2G. *American Journal of Medical Genetics*, **82**, 392–8.

Passos-Bueno, M.R., Vainzof, M., Pavanello, R.C.M., Pavanello-Filho, I., Lima, M.A.B.O., and Zatz, M. (1991). Limb-girdle syndrome: a genetic study of 22 large Brazilian families – comparison with X-linked Duchenne and Becker dystrophies. *Journal of Neurological Science*, **103**, 65–75.

Pepe, G., Giusti, B., Bertini, E., Brunelli, T., Saitta, B., Comeglio, P. *et al.* (1999). A heterozygous splice site mutation in COL6A1 leading to an in-frame deletion of the α1(VI) collagen chain in an Italian family affected by Bethlem myopathy. *Biochemical and Biophysical Research Communications*, **258**(3), 802–7.

Piccolo, F., Jeanpierre, M., Leturcq, F., Dode, C., Azibi, K., Toutain, A. *et al.* (1996). A founder mutation in the γ-sarcoglycan gene of Gypsies possibly predating their migration out of India. *Human Molecular Genetics*, **5**(12), 2019–22.

Piccolo, F., Moore, S.A., Ford, G.C., and Campbell K.P (2000). Intracellular accumulation and reduced sarcolemmal expression of dysferlin in limb-girdle muscular dystrophies. *Annals of Neurology*, **48**, 902–12.

Piccolo, F., Roberds, S.L., Jeanpierre, M., Leturcq, F., Azibi, K., Beldjord, C. *et al.* (1995). Primary adhalinopathy: a common cause of autosomal recessive muscular dystrophy of variable severity. *Nature Genetics*, **10**, 243–5.

Repetto, S., Bado, M., Broda, P., Lucania, G., Masetti, E., Sotgia, F. *et al.* (1999). Increased number of caveolae and caveolin-3 overexpression in Duchenne muscular dystrophy. *Biochemical and Biophysical Research Communications*, **261**, 547–50.

Richard, I., Roudaut, C., Saenz, A., Pogue, R., Grimbergen, J.E.M.A., Anderson, L.V.B. *et al.* (1999). Calpainopathy - a survey of mutations and polymorphisms. *American Journal of Human Genetics*, **64**(6), 1524–40.

Rizo, J. and Sudhof, T.C. (1999). C2-domains, structure and function of a universal Ca^{2+}-binding domain. *Journal of Biological Chemistry*, **273**, 15879–82.

Salmikangas, P., Mykkanen, O.-M., Gronholm, M., Heiska, L., Kere, J., and Carpen, O. (1999). Myotilin, a novel sarcomeric protein with two lg-like domains, is encoded by a candidate gene for limb-girdle muscular dystrophy. *Human Molecular Genetics*, **8**(7), 1329–36.

Schlegel, A., Volonte, D., Engelman, J.A., Galbiati, F., Mehta, P., Zhang, X.-L. *et al.* (1998). Crowded little caves: structure and function of caveolae. *Cellular Signalling*, **10**(7), 457–63.

Sewry, C.A., Anderson, L.V.B., Ozawa, E., Taylor, J., Pogue, R., Piccolo, F. *et al.* (1996). Abnormalities in α-, β- and γ-sarcolgycan in patients with limb-girdle muscular dystrophy. *Neuromuscular Disorders*, **6**(6), 467–74.

Sewry, C.A., Mercuri, E., and Muntoni, F. (1999). Reduced laminin beta 1 expression in dominant myopathies. *Neuromuscular Disorders*, **6**/7, 510–1.

Shackleton, S., Lloyd, D.J., Jackson, S.N.J., Evans, R., Niermeijer, M.F., Singh, B.M. *et al.* (2000). LMNA, encoding lamin A/C, is mutated in partial lipodystrophy. *Nature Genetics*, **24**, 153–6.

Song, K.S., Scherer, P.E., Tang, Z., Okamoto, T., Li, S., Chafel, M. *et al.* (1996). Expression of caveolin-3 in skeletal, cardiac and smooth muscle cells. *Journal of Biological Chemistry*, **271**(25), 15160–5.

Sorimachi, H., Saido, T.C., and Suzuki, K. (1994). New era of calpain research: Discovery of tissue-specific calpains. *FEBS Lett.*, **343**, 1–5.

Sotgia, F., Lee, J.K., Das, K., Bedford, M., Petrucci, T.C., Macioce, P. *et al.* (2000). Caveolin-3 directly interacts with the C-terminal tail of beta-dystroglycan. Identification of a central WW-like domain within caveolin family members [In Process Citation]. *Journal of Biological Chemistry*, **275**(48), 38048–58.

Speer, M.C., Gilchrist, J.M., Stajich J.M., Yamaoka, L.H., Westbrook, C., and Pericak-Vance, M.A. (1994). Anticipation in autosomal dominant limb-girdle muscular dystrophy (LGMD1A). *American Journal of Human Genetics*, **55**, A7.

Speer, M.C., Tandan, R., Rao, P.N., Fries, T., Stajich, J.M., Bolhuis, P.A. *et al.* (1996). Evidence for locus heterogeneity in the Bethlem myopathy and linkage to 2q37. *Human Molecular Genetics*, **5**(7), 1043–946.

Speer, M.C., Yamaoka, L.H., Gilchrist, J.M., Gaskell, C.P., Stajich, J.M., Vance, J.M. *et al.* (1992a). Confirmation of genetic heterogeneity in limb-girdle muscular dystrophy: linkage of an autosomal dominant form of chromosome 5q. *American Journal of Human Genetics*, **50**, 1211–7.

Speer, M.C., Yamaoka, L.H., Gilchrist, J.M., Gaskell, C.P., Stajich, J.M., Weber, J.L. *et al.* (1992b). Localisation of an autosomal dominant form of limb-girdle muscular dystrophy to chromosome 5q. *HGM11 Abstract No.* 26929.

Straub, V., Ettinger, A.J., Durbeej, M., Venzke, D.P., Cutshall, S., Sanes, J.R., and Campbell, K.P. (1999). ε-sarcoglycan replaces α-sarcoglycan in smooth muscle to form a unique dystrophin-glycoprotein complex. *Biological Chemistry*, **274**(39), 27989–96.

Tagawa, K., Taya, C., Hayashi, Y., Nakagawa, M., Ono, Y., Fukuda, R. *et al.* (2000). Myopathy phenotype of transgenic mice expressing active site-mutated inactive p94 skeletal muscle-specific calpain, the gene product responsible for limb-girdle muscular dystrophy type 2A. *Human Molecular Genetics*, **9**, 1393–402.

Upadhyaya, M., Maynard, J., Rogers, M.T., Lunt, P.W., Jardine, P., Ravine, D., and Harper, P.S. (1997). Improved molecular diagnosis of facioscapulohumeral muscular dystrophy (FSHD): validation of the differential double digestion for FSHD. *Journal of Medical Genetics*, **34**, 476–9.

Urtasun, M., Saenz, A., Roudaut, C., Poza, J.J., Urtizberea, J.A., Cobo, A.M. *et al.* (1998). Limb-girdle muscular dystrophy in Guipuzcoa (Basque Country, Spain). *Brain*, **121**, 1735–47.

Vafiadaki, E., Reis, A., Keers, S., Harrison, R., Anderson, L., Raffelsburger, T. *et al.* Cloning of the mouse dysferlin gene and genomic characterisation of the SJL-dysf mutation. NeuroReport. 2001, **12**, 625–29.

Vainzof, M., Passos-Bueno, M.R., Canovas, M., Moreira, E.S., Pavanello, R.C.M., Marie, S.K. *et al.* (1996). The sarcoglycan complex in the six autosomal recessive limb-girdle muscular dystrophies. *Human Molecular Genetics*, **5**(12), 1963–9.

Valle, G., Faulkner, G., De Antoni, A., Pacchioni, B., Pallavicini, A., Pandolfo, D. *et al.* (1997). Telethonin, a novel sarcomeric protein of heart and skeletal muscle. *FEBS Lett*, **415**, 163–8.

van der Kooi, A.J., Ginjaar, H.B., Busch, H.F.M., Wokke, J.H.J., Barth, P.G., and de Visser, M. (1998). Limb girdle muscular dystrophy: a pathological and immunohistochemical reevaluation. *Muscle & Nerve*, May.

van der Kooi, A.J., Ledderhof, T.M., de Voogt, W.G., res, J.C.J., Bouwsma, G., Troost, D. *et al.* (1996). A newly recognised autosomal dominant limb girdle muscular dystrophy with cardiac involvement. *Annals of Neurology*, **39**, 636–42.

van der Kooi, A.J., van Meegen, M., Ledderhof, T.M., McNally, E.M., de Visser, M., and Bolhuis, P.A. (1997). Genetic localisation of a newly recognised autosomal dominant limb-girdle muscular dystrophy with cardiac involvement (LGMD1B) to chromosome 1q11-21. *American Journal of Human Genetics*, **60**, 891–5.

van der Maarel, S., Deidda, G., Lemmers, R.J.L.F., Bakker, E., Van der Wielen, M.J.R., Sandkuijl, L. *et al.* (1999). A new dosage test for subtelomeric 4;10 translocations improves conventional diagnosis of facioscapulohumeral muscular dystrophy (FSHD). *Journal of Medical Genetics*, **36**, 823–8.

Walton JN (1955). On the Inheritance of Muscular Dystrophy. *Annals of Human Genetics*, **20**, 1–38.

Walton JN (1956). The Inheritance of muscular dystrophy: Further Observations. *American Journal of Human Genetics*, **21**, 40–60.

Walton, J.N. and Gardner-Medwin, D. (1988). The muscular dystrophies, in *Disorders of voluntary muscle*. (5th edn). ed. J.N. Walton, 519–68. Churchill Livingstone, Edinburgh.

Walton, J.N. and Gardner-Medwin, D. (1991). The muscular dystrophies, in *Disorders of voluntary muscle* (5th edn). ed. J.N. Walton, 519–68. Churchill Livingston, Edinburgh.

Weiler, T., Bashir, R., Anderson, L.V.B., Davison, K., Moss, J.A., Britton, S. *et al.* (1999). Identical mutation in patients with limb girdle muscular dystrophy type 2B or Miyoshi myopathy suggests a role for modifier gene(s). *Human Molecular Genetics*, **8**(5), 871–7.

Weiler, T., Greenberg, C.R., Nylen, E., Halliday, W., Morgan, K., Eggertson, D., and Wrogemann, K. (1996). Limb-girdle muscular dystrophy and Miyoshi myopathy in an Aboriginal Canadian kindred map to LGMD2B and segregate with the same haplotype. *American Journal of Human Genetics*, **59**, 872–8.

Worton, R.G. (1995). Muscular dystrophies: diseases of the dystrophin-glycoprotein complex. *Science*, **270**, 755–6.

Yasunaga, S., Grati, M., Cohen-Salmon, M., El-Amraoui, A., Mustapha, M., Salem, N. *et al.* (1999). A mutation in OTOF, encoding otoferlin, a FER-1-like protein, causes DFNB9, a nonsyndromic form of deafness. *Nature Genetics*, **21**, 363–9.

Yasunaga, S., Grati, M., Chardenoux, S., Smith, T.N., Friedman, T.B., Lalwani, A.K. *et al.* (2000). OTOF encodes multiple long and short isoforms: genetic evidence that the lone ones underlie recessive deafness DFNB9. *American Journal of Human Genetics*, **67**, 591–600.

Chapter 8

Facioscapulohumeral muscular dystrophy

Meena Upadhyaya and David N. Cooper

Clinical features

Facioscapulohumeral muscular dystrophy (FSHD) is the third most common form of inherited neuromuscular disorder following the Duchenne and myotonic dystrophies. It is inherited in an autosomal dominant manner and was first recognized by Landouzy and Dejerine in 1885. FSHD usually progresses in a descending manner with the facial muscles involved first, followed by scapular and humeral muscle and finally by pelvic girdle muscle. The progression of weakness is typically slow, with patients often describing prolonged periods of relatively stable function. This disorder affects about 1 person in every 20 000 worldwide (Lunt and Harper 1991; Padberg 1982). At least a fifth of all cases of FSHD are sporadic and presumably result from new mutations of the FSHD gene.

The defining clinical features include the onset of weakness of the facial or shoulder girdle muscles, leading eventually to the wasting of these muscles (Fig. 8.1). Significant facial weakness is evident in more than half of all affected FSHD patients. As the disease progresses, the muscles of the shoulder girdle, the scapula fixators, and the upper arm muscles (especially the biceps and triceps) may become affected. Weakness and atrophy may eventually involve many other skeletal muscles, including the musculature of the pelvic girdle and the foot extensor (Munsat 1986; Padberg 1982; Padberg et al. 1998). Asymmetry of muscle involvement is also often observed in apparently affected patients. In many cases, muscle involvement remains restricted to the facial, scapular, and proximal upper limb musculature, whereas in others, the anterior tibial and peroneal muscles may become involved, resulting in footdrop. Some patients may display involvement of the proximal muscles of the lower limb prior to any evidence of weakness of the distal muscles. Involvement of the musculature of the pelvic girdle is observed infrequently. However, patients who exhibit pelvic girdle muscle weakness before the age of 20 years are more likely to become wheelchair-bound, and at an earlier age. Studies have indicated that although 10–20 per cent of all FSHD gene carriers will require a wheelchair by their fourth decade, a further 22–30 per cent of carriers will only be mildly affected, or may even remain virtually asymptomatic throughout their lives.

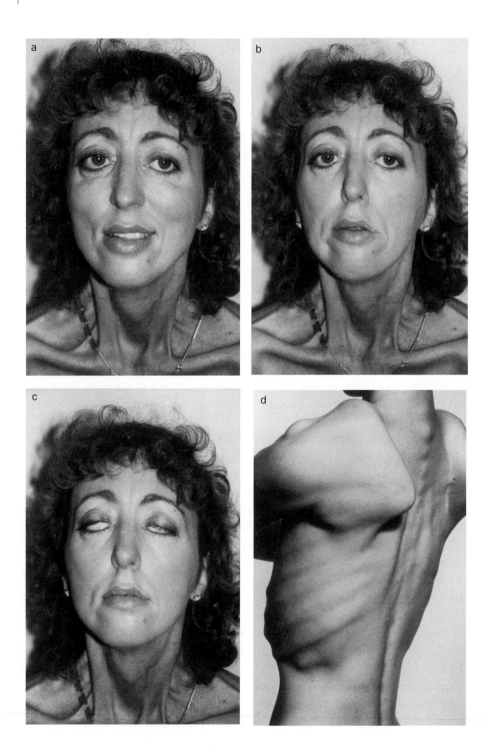

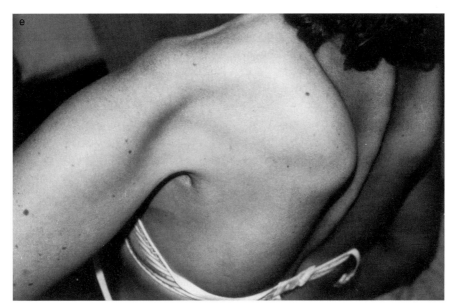

Fig. 8.1 a) Classical mid facial wasting, smile exhibits slight asymmetry; b) Patient attempting to whistle; c) Patient attempting to close eyes, note white sclera below the iris; d) Marked scapular winging; e) Marked scapular winging with wasting of deltoid. This patient also has relative preservation of sterno-mastroid muscle. Reproduced by kind permission of the patient and Dr Mark Rogers.

Thus, FSHD may result in devastating incapacity early in life, or it may be barely detectable even in old age (Fitzsimons 1999). The early onset of disease is usually associated with the most severe forms of the disorder. However, whilst disease onset before the age of 10 is observed in fewer than five per cent of patients, it always involves significant facial weakness (Brouwer *et al.* 1995). The majority of symptomatic cases develop only later, during the second decade of life. Both retinal vasculopathy and high tone deafness (Brouwer *et al.* 1991) may be seen as part of FSHD. However, clinically significant deafness is rare in adult FSHD. Conversely, moderate to severe sensorineural deafness (at times profound) is common in childhood-onset FSHD when there is early involvement of the limbs. The combination of mental retardation and 'Coates syndrome' (exudative retinopathy with telangiectasis, sometimes causing blindness) is seen occasionally in severe childhood cases (Rogers *et al.* 2000). Recent reports have indicated that the clinical expression of FSHD is much broader than perhaps previously recognized (Felice *et al.* 2000; van der Kooi *et al.* 2000). Although FSHD may exhibit a variable clinical picture, in terms of both disease severity and age of onset, the disorder has been shown to manifest almost complete penetrance (>95 per cent) by the age of 20 years (Lunt and Harper 1991). The considerable inter- and intra-familial variability, apparent in both age at onset and clinical severity, make genetic counselling difficult. A further potential complication is genetic anticipation (increasing severity or earlier age of onset in successive generations) but the evidence for this phenomenon is scanty and the topic is somewhat contentious (Lunt *et al.* 1995b; Tawil *et al.* 1996; Zatz *et al.* 1995).

The histopathological changes in FSHD muscle are very variable; although the picture is generally that of a myopathy, there may also be changes more typically seen in neuropathic disorders. Muscle biopsy is necessary to exclude other primary muscle diseases that can present with the FSHD phenotype. The biopsy-based diagnosis is dependent upon the type of muscle sampled; histological changes in the deltoid muscle may be minimal whereas the biceps muscle can be severely affected. Epilepsy and mental retardation have also been noted in some patients, especially in those with the most severe form of FSHD (Funakoshi *et al.* 1998). A small proportion of patients with FSHD may also exhibit cardiac involvement (Laforet *et al.* 1998). Recent studies indicate low penetrance in three per cent of apparently non-symptomatic FSHD gene carriers (van Overveld *et al.* 2000).

In some families, the affected individuals share many of the clinical features of FSHD but show no evidence of facial muscle involvement, even in the most severely affected patients. These 'scapulohumeral muscular dystrophy' families display an autosomal dominant mode of inheritance, and it has been suggested that they may form part of the FSHD disease spectrum (Lunt and Harper 1991).

Gene mapping studies

Extensive linkage studies were undertaken as part of an international collaboration to determine the location of the FSHD gene (Fisher and Upadhyaya 1997). By 1989, the location of the FSHD locus had been excluded from almost 80 per cent of the human genome (Sarfarazi *et al.* 1989). Linkage was finally reported between the disease locus and D4S171, a polymorphic marker locus located in distal 4q (Wijmenga *et al.* 1990). A tightly linked set of markers was subsequently defined from within the 4q35 region (Sarfarazi *et al.* 1992; Upadhyaya *et al.* 1990; 1991; 1992; Wijmenga *et al.* 1990). Further studies positioned the FSHD locus to within a 2–6 CM region that was located distal of the linkage group cen-D4S171-*F11*-D4S163-D4S139. To date, no genetic markers located distal to the FSHD locus have been definitely identified. A restriction map of the 4q35 telomeric region has been constructed and all the closely linked physical and genetic marker loci, D4S139, D4F35S1, D4F104S1 and D4Z4, are confined to a 250 kb genomic region. The significant discrepancy that exists between the genetic and physical maps for this region is almost certainly due to an increased rate of recombination characteristic of subtelomeric regions and possibly resulting from their highly repetitive nature. The order of the various genes and genetic marker loci identified within the overall 4q35 region are: cent- *ANT1*-D4S171- *F11*- *KLK3*- D4S187- D4S130- *HSP-CAL2*-D4S163- *FRG1*- *FRG2*- D4F104S1- D4Z4 - 4q telomere (see Fig. 8.2 for details). The FSHD disease locus (*FSHMD1A*) maps to chromosome 4q35 and is tightly linked

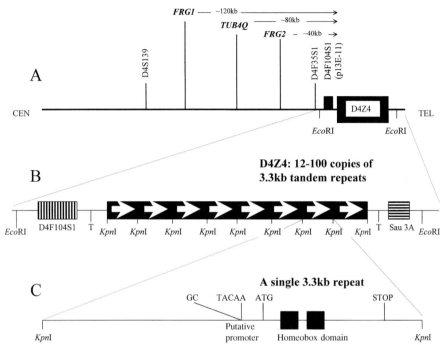

Fig. 8.2 (a) Restriction map of 4q35 region: Relative positions of *FRG1*, *TUB4Q*, *FRG2*, D4F104S1 (p13E11) and D4Z4 (b) *Eco*RI fragment detected by probe p13E11 predominantly comprises an array of 3.3 kb tandem repeats which have a copy number of 12–100 in normal controls and usually 10 in FSHD patients. (c) Each 3.3 kb repeat comprises two home-odomains (shaded boxes) encompassing an ORF with an in-frame start codon (ATG) and a stop codon. It encodes the *DUX4* gene. The positions of the GC and TACAA boxes in the pro-moter-like sequence of *DUX4* gene are indicated.
T – *Tru*91

to the marker locus D4F104S1 as defined by the DNA probe p13E-11 (Wijmenga *et al.* 1992).

Genetic heterogeneity

There is some tentative evidence for genetic heterogeneity in FSHD. Although the vast majority of FSHD families are demonstrably linked to 4q35, linkage in a small number of families has been excluded from this location. A position for this second disease locus, already optimistically designated *FSHD1B*, has, however, still to be identified (Gilbert *et al.* 1995).

Physical map of the FSHD candidate region

A physical map of the genomic region distal to locus D4S163 has been constructed using a panel of rare-cutter restriction enzymes and pulsed-field gel electrophoresis

(PFGE) (Wijmenga *et al.* 1994; Wright *et al.* 1993). This initial physical map information was confirmed and extended by mapping studies of two overlapping yeast artificial chromosomes (YACs), Y25C2E and D4S1093. Although the physical map distances were somewhat shorter than expected from inspection of the genetic map, the order of loci was in good agreement. The PFGE-based studies also identified several CpG islands in the 4q35 region. These largely unmethylated, GC-rich genomic regions are well known as landmarks for the presence of genes. Two CpG-islands were identified in the relevant region, one situated about 150 kb proximal to, and one 5 kb distal to, locus D4F104S1. The physical map of the genes in the 4q35 region is as follows: *ANT1-ARGBP2- SMT7 -ALP- TLR3- F11/KLK3- FAT -MTNR1A- HSPCAL2- FRG1- TUB4Q-FRG2-* Tel.

The DNA rearrangements detected by D4F104S1 and D4Z4 repeats

Probe p13E-11(D4F104S1) identifies an *Eco*RI restriction fragment, from both 4q35 and 10q26. In FSHD patients, one fragment is usually smaller than 35 kb. This restriction fragment contains tandem repeats and probe p13E11 is located proximal to the repeats in the *Eco*RI fragment.

During a genome-wide search for homeobox-like genes (with especial emphasis placed on the genomic region distal of marker D4S139), a cosmid, 13E, was identified and a plasmid subclone, p13E-11 (D4F104S1 or D4S810), was isolated. Probe p13E-11 was found to identify a number of different cross-hybridizing loci; two closely-related polymorphic elements situated at 4q35 and 10q26, and a monomorphic locus located at Yq11. The highly informative variable number tandem repeat (VNTR) polymorphism, observed when *Eco*RI-digested genomic DNA is hybridized to probe p13E-11, actually comprises polymorphic sequences derived from both 4q35 and 10q26 (Wijmenga *et al.* 1992). This whole complex locus, containing both 4q35- and 10q26-derived alleles has been designated D4F104S1, which reflects its initial identification as a 4q35-localized marker. Studies in suitably informative FSHD families have demonstrated the 4q35 component of the D4F104S1 locus to be the closest marker to the disease gene.

Sequence analysis of the entire D4F104S1 locus has shown that p13E-11 identifies a single copy genomic sequence that is located immediately proximal to an array of tandem repeat units (Wijmenga *et al.* 1992). It is variation in the exact number of the individual repeats, in each of the 4q35- and 10q26-derived repeat arrays, that constitutes the polymorphic elements of the D4F104S1 VNTR and of the two specific *Eco*RI restriction sites which define this VNTR; one site is located proximal to the sequence homologous to the p13E-11 probe, whereas the second is situated immediately distal to the tandem repeat array (see Fig. 8.2). Each (virtually identical?) repeat unit is 3.3 kb in size and has been designated D4Z4, regardless of whether the repeat is located within the 4q35- or the 10q26-derived repeat array. The sizes of the variable fragments seen on Southern blots, containing *Eco*RI-digested high-molecular weight genomic DNA derived from normal individuals and hybridized with probe p13E-11, ranges from ~35 kb (10 repeat units) to more than 300 kb (100 repeat units) whereas in FSHD patients, it ranges from 7–35 kb (Fig. 8.3). However, since it is difficult to resolve fragment sizes over 50 kb with conventional Southern blots, pulsed field gel electrophoresis (PFGE) has been employed to increase resolution. Since the majority of people carry two copies of each homologous chromosome, in an informative situation, there is the potential to observe four differently sized *Eco*RI fragments when the DNA from one individual is analysed. Each fragment represents a different D4F104S1 allele, with two alleles coming from the 4q35 locus and two alleles from the 10q26 locus (both loci produce *Eco*RI fragments with the same size range). Following such analyses in a number of FSHD families, it was soon realized that the size of at least one of the four D4F104S1 alleles seen in the affected members of these families, differed significantly from the normal size range with patients having an *Eco*RI fragment from ~35 kb down to ~10 kb (Fig. 8.4).

This potential disease association was confirmed and strengthened by demonstrating the *de novo* occurrence of a smaller *Eco*RI fragment in the majority of sporadic FSHD patients studied, that was not present in either of the unaffected parents

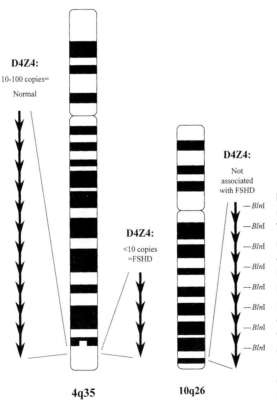

D4Z4:

10-100 copies= Normal

D4Z4:

<10 copies =FSHD

D4Z4:

Not associated with FSHD

—*Bln*I
—*Bln*I
—*Bln*I
—*Bln*I
—*Bln*I
—*Bln*I
—*Bln*I
—*Bln*I

4q35

10q26

Fig. 8.3 Location of D4Z4 repeats at 4q35 and 10q26. The 10q-derived D4Z4 repeats differ from the 4q-derived repeats in having an internal restriction site for *Bln*I. Deletion of D4Z4 repeats at 4q35 is associated with FSHD whereas reduction in the copy number of 10q-derived D4Z4 repeats does not result in any specific phenotype.

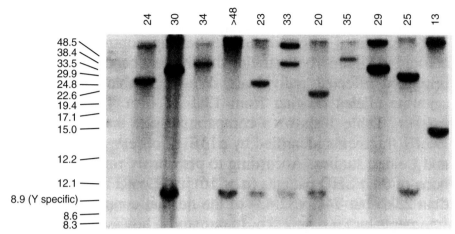

Fig. 8.4 The length of the smallest *Eco*RI fragment associated with the disease in unrelated FSHD individuals. 10 μg DNA was digested with *Eco*RI, fractionated on a 0.5 per cent agarose gel for 48 h at 0.5 volts/cm and Southern blotted onto Hybond N (Amersham). The DNA on the membrane was hybridized with radiolabelled DNA probe p13E-11. Lane 1 contains high molecular weight markers. Lanes 2–12 contain DNA samples from unrelated FSHD patients. The corresponding smallest *Eco*RI fragment size is written at the top of each lane. The 8.9 kb fragment represents a Y-specific sequence.

(Upadhyaya *et al.* 1993; Wijmenga *et al.* 1992). A small proportion of FSHD patients, of both sporadic and familial origin, do not exhibit a small *Eco*RI fragment; this could either be because such cases arise via a different mutational mechanism, or because they represent families unlinked to the *FSHD1A* locus at 4q35, or because they simply represent the result of clinical misdiagnosis.

Attention then turned to the question of exactly how the large deletion of D4F104S1 could be associated with disease expression. Clearly, the range of *Eco*RI fragment sizes observed in affected FSHD patients merely represented the lower end of a continuous range of fragment sizes. What pathognomic process could turn this apparently normal variation into a disease-causing mutation? It was then noted that the severity of disease expression in FSHD patients could be correlated with the size of their disease-associated D4F104S1 alleles (Fig. 8.5). Thus, patients with the smallest *Eco*RI fragments manifested the severe form of the disorder and presented with an earlier age of onset (Lunt *et al.* 1995b).

If the possession of one small D4F104S1 allele is sufficient to confer the disease phenotype (FSHD is a dominant disorder, and hence, only requires mutation of one of the two copies of the FSHD gene), then one might infer that the complete loss of one of the D4F104S1 alleles would yield a still more severe phenotype. A number of individuals have been identified who carry small cytogenetically detectable deletions involving specifically the 4q region and, as a result, are monosomic for one copy of their 4q35-derived D4F104S1 loci. Surprisingly, none of these individuals show any evidence of an

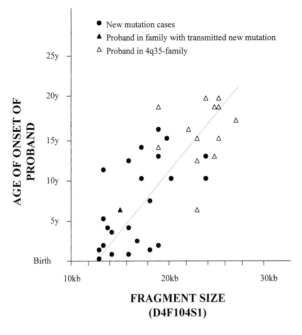

Fig. 8.5 Correlation of age of onset in new mutation cases and probands of 4q35-linked FSHD families, with fragment size at locus D4F104S1. Correlation coefficient: $r = 0.56 + 0.11$; $t_{37} = 4.10$; $p > 0.001$ (Lunt et al. 1995b).

FSHD-like disorder, and indeed most of them appear to be phenotypically normal (Tupler et al. 1996). These findings indicate that FSHD most probably results from a dominant negative ('gain-of-function') mutational mechanism rather than the reduction or loss of a gene product (haploinsufficiency) from within the 4q-deleted region. These observations served to focus the search for the FSHD gene back onto the D4F104S1 locus itself, and in particular to the D4Z4 repeats therein.

The D4Z4 repeat units are members of a large family of 3.3 kb tandem repeat loci that are spread across the genome. These repeats are often situated within, or adjacent to, heterochromatic regions, such as the short arm of the acrocentric chromosomes, the pericentromeric regions (especially on chromosome 1), and the telomeric regions of the long arms of chromosomes 4 and 10 (Lyle et al. 1995). Several 4q35- and 10q26-derived D4Z4 3.3 kb repeat units from normal individuals have now been cloned and sequenced. Each repeat unit, whether from the 4q35 or the 10q26 tandem arrays, is virtually identical and defined by flanking *Kpn*I restriction sites (Fig. 8.2). The internal sequence organization of each 3.3 kb repeat unit is quite complex; each repeat contains a number of known repeat sequence motifs, including *LSau*, a repetitive element often found associated with heterochromatic regions, and *hhspm3*, a highly GC-rich low-copy repeat. However, what really caught the attention of scientists was the presence, in each repeat unit, of a large open reading frame (ORF) that possessed the potential to encode two homeobox-like sequences, situated downstream of a putative promoter region (Fig. 8.2) (Gabriels et al. 1999; Hewitt et al. 1994; Lee et al. 1995).

The size variation observed at the D4F104S1 locus is due to the loss of individual D4Z4 repeat units and does not involve internal deletions within the body of the repeat itself (van Deutekom *et al.* 1993). Thus the normal range of D4F104S1 allele sizes, from about 35 kb to more than 300 kb, represents D4Z4 repeat arrays containing from 10–100 repeats. By contrast, the FSHD-associated D4F104S1 allele size range, from 10 kb to ~35 kb, represents arrays containing between only 1 and 10 D4Z4 repeat units. Large-scale physical mapping and sequencing studies of the entire D4F104S1 genomic region have demonstrated that (i) the 4q35 D4Z4 arrays are located immediately adjacent to the 4q telomere; and (ii) a copy of a single D4Z4 repeat-like sequence is located about 30 kb proximal to the p13E-11 homologous sequence, and that this repeat sequence is oriented in the opposite direction to the D4Z4 repeats in the distally located tandem arrays. From comparative genomic studies, we know that D4Z4-related sequences are present in the genome of many vertebrates, including monkeys, pigs, cows, goats and chickens, although there are apparently no D4Z4-like sequences in rodents (Hewitt *et al.* 1994). A detailed analysis of various primates indicates that multiple tandem copies of the D4Z4 repeats are only found in humans and the great apes, in contrast to Old World monkeys which have two D4Z4-like loci, one of which maps to a region syntenic with human chromosome 4q35 (Clark *et al.* 1996; Winokur *et al.* 1996).

Sequence homology and genetic recombination between 4q35 and 10q26

Various physical mapping studies, cytogenetic fluorescent *in situ* hybridization (FISH)-based analyses and detailed genomic sequencing experiments have now clearly demonstrated that a duplicate (virtually identical) copy of the D4F104S1 locus is located at 10q26, within the heterochromatic subtelomeric region of chromosome 10 (Deidda *et al.* 1995) (See Fig. 8.3). Detailed sequence analysis of D4Z4 repeats from both the 4q35 and 10q26 D4F104S1 loci confirmed their high level of sequence homology (98–100 per cent) and, perhaps more importantly, identified a unique *Bln*I restriction site that is present within each copy of the 10q26-derived repeat units, but which is absent from the 4q35-derived D4Z4 repeats (Deidda *et al.* 1996).

The high degree of sequence homology between the 4q35 and 10q26 D4F104S1 regions appears to have resulted in the occurrence of 'interchromosomal exchanges' between these two loci. During these subtelomeric exchanges, complete repeat arrays (either of 4q35-derived *Bln*I-resistant D4Z4 repeats, or of 10q26-derived *Bln*I-sensitive repeats) may be transferred from one chromosomal location to the other. Owing to the sizes of the genomic fragments involved, these interchromosomal exchange events are best visualized with PFGE; such studies have shown that entire repeat arrays are 'translocated' in the majority of cases (van Deutekom *et al.* 1996a) (Fig. 8.6). In some reports, authors speak blithely of 'translocations'. It should be realized that there is as yet no direct evidence for the physical translocation of genetic material and that other mechanisms such as interchromosomal gene conversion would appear to be more plausible.

Perhaps surprisingly, these dynamic subtelomeric interchanges do not appear to be involved in any way with expression of the FSHD phenotype, since such 4q35/10q26 exchanges are evident in about 20 per cent of normal individuals (Fig. 8.6) (van Deutekom *et al.* 1996a). It should be emphasized, however, that FSHD only occurs when the D4Z4 repeats that are deleted (whether originally chromosome 4q35- or 10q26-derived) are chromosome 4 located (van Deutekom *et al.* 1996a). The transfer

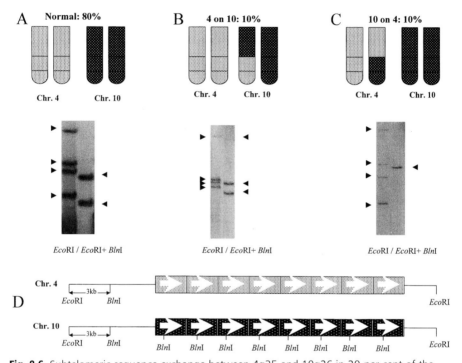

Fig. 8.6 Subtelomeric sequence exchange between 4q35 and 10q26 in 20 per cent of the normal population (adapted from van der Maarel *et al.* 2000). In the control population, 80 per cent of individuals carry a standard configuration, with 4-type repeats on chromosome 4, and 10-type repeats on chromosome 10 (A). In 10 per cent of individuals, 4-derived repeats are also present on one of their chromosomes 10 (B). Likewise, 10 per cent of the control population carry 10-derived repeats on one of their chromosomes 4 (C). 5 μg high molecular weight DNA digested sequentially with *EcoRI* and *EcoRI*/ *BlnI* and hybridized with probe p13E11. In an informative situation, four different sized *EcoRI* fragments are produced following a single digest, two derived from chromosome 4 and two from 10q. Digestion with enzyme *BlnI* will cleave two chromosome 10 specific fragments. Chromosome 4-specific fragments will be reduced by 3 kb owing to the presence of a *BlnI* site proximal to the first repeat but distal to the *EcoRI* site (D). However, in 10 per cent of individuals (B), 4-type repeats (*BlnI* resistant) are translocated to chromosome 10 and therefore with *EcoRI*/*BlnI* digestion, 3 alleles are seen instead of the expected 2 fragments. Similarly, 10 per cent of control individuals (C) carry *BlnI*-sensitive repeats on one of their chromosomes 4; therefore, with a *EcoRI*/*BlnI* double digest, one allele (monosomy) is observed.

of *Bln*I-resistant repeat arrays from 4q35 to 10q26 appears to be more frequent than the transfer of *Bln*I-sensitive repeats from 10q26 to 4q35 (Cacurri *et al.* 1998). Although the significance of this difference is not understood, the apparent lack of reciprocity with respect to the exchange mechanism is consistent with some form of interchromosomal gene conversion being responsible for these exchanges (Campbell *et al.* 1997). The internal structural elements of the *Bln*I-resistant and *Bln*I-sensitive repeats may also undergo further reorganization as a result of these exchanges.

The restriction enzyme *Tru*9I (T, Fig 8.2) has been shown to cut within the D4F104S1 genomic region at a point immediately adjacent to both the proximal and distal ends of each repeat array, whether located at 4q35 or at 10q26 (Cacurri *et al.* 1998). A detailed restriction analysis of individual D4Z4 repeat arrays using various combinations of *Eco*RI, *Bln*I and *Tru*9I enzymes, has identified hybrid repeat arrays, comprising, in normal individuals, a complex mixture of both 4q35-derived and 10q26-derived repeat units (Lemmers *et al.* 1998). The use of the D4Z4 repeat-specific probe 9B6A is required to visualize these repeat arrays since the region normally identified by p13E-11, is lost from the repeat array-containing fragment following digestion with *Tru*9I.

The majority of FSHD patients have D4F104S1-derived *Eco*RI fragments with the expected *Bln*I restriction patterns: they are either completely fragmented (from 10q26), or are merely reduced in size by 3 kb (from 4q35), thereby confirming that it is usually entire repeat arrays that are exchanged. In a few rare cases, D4F104S1 *Eco*RI fragments that are reduced in size by more than the expected 3 kb following *Bln*I digestion have been observed, indicating the probable presence of a hybrid *Eco*RI fragment that contains a number of *Bln*I-sensitive repeat units.

We now know from sequencing studies that 4q35 and 10q26 genomic sequence homology ends at the position of the single D4Z4 repeat-like sequence that is oriented in the opposite direction, and located 30 kb proximal to the p13E-11 homologous sequences on chromosomes 4 and 10. All genes and genomic sequences located proximal of this point are specific to their particular chromosome (Deidda *et al.* 1995).

The molecular mechanism(s) underlying these subtelomeric exchanges has still to be elucidated, as has their potential role or effect (if any) on FSHD disease expression.

Somatic mosaicism

In 20 per cent of cases of *de novo* FSHD, somatic mosaicism, evidenced by the presence of faint bands representing a low number of additional, small *Eco*RI or *Eco*RI/*Bln*I fragments alongside fragments of normal intensity within the normal size range, has been reported in one parent of the affected individual (Kohler *et al.* 1996; Upadhyaya *et al.* 1995a). In these studies, the mosaicism results were based on conventional Southern blots with probe p13E-11; the mosaicism was predominantly maternally derived.

van der Maarel *et al.* (2000) identified mosaicism in *de novo* FSHD families by the detection of a fifth restriction fragment (either *Eco*RI/*Hind*III or *Eco*RI/*Bln*I) by

PFGE followed by Southern blotting with the probe p13E11. They detected somatic mosaicism in 40 per cent of *de novo* FSHD families (14 per cent in an unaffected parent and on 26 per cent of the *de novo* FSHD patients themselves). Interestingly, an excess of mosaic affected males was found in their dataset. To determine whether inter-chromosomal exchanges (either 4-type repeats on chromosome 10 or 10-type repeats on chromosome 4) might play a role in the deletion of repeats on chromosome 4, they examined the repeat array constitutions of 13 mosaic individuals (that is, those with 5 restriction fragments) (Fig. 8.7). Interestingly, 6/13 (46 per cent) carried 4-type repeats on chromosome 10, whereas 10-type repeats on chromosome 4 were not identified in a single mosaic case (0/13). This frequency of exchange differs from the Dutch control population (van Deutekom *et al.* 1996a) in which 10 per cent of individuals carry 4-type repeats on chromosome 10 and 10 per cent carry 10-type repeats on chromosome 4. The high frequency of 4-type repeats on chromosome 10 in mosaic cases compared to the control population (46 per cent cf. 10 per cent), and the absence of 10-type repeats on chromosome 4 suggests that interchromosomal interactions between chromosome 4 and 10 may be ultimately responsible for bringing about the disease-causing mutations, and that the increase in 4-type repeat clusters may be a major predisposing factor.

Genotype/phenotype relationship

The association between the size of the deleted *Eco*RI fragment and the age at disease onset (smaller *Eco*RI fragments are always associated with the most severe form of the disease) has now been observed in patients from a number of ethnic groups (Goto *et al.* 1995; Hsu *et al.* 1997; Lunt *et al.* 1995b; Tawil *et al.* 1996; Zatz *et al.* 1995). The D4F104S1 *Eco*RI fragment size ranges noted in severe childhood cases are 10–18 kb, in typical teenage onset cases between 18 and 34 kb, and in the oldest late-onset patients larger than 30 kb (see Fig. 8.5). Two recent Japanese studies have confirmed these observations; a number of very early onset patients, with a severe form of FSHD often accompanied by epilepsy and mental retardation, manifested short *Eco*RI/*Bln*I fragments, the smallest being 10 kb in size (Funakoshi *et al.* 1998; Muira *et al.* 1998). It is important to stress, however, that it is still impossible to predict accurately the likely severity of disease expression in any one individual. This is due to the high degree of inter- and intra-familial variability of disease expression observed in this disorder, regardless of the fact that all affected members of any particular family exhibit the same sized D4F104S1 allele. As an example, the clinical picture presented by a typical three-generation FSHD family can be used to illustrate the spectrum of clinical variability often observed between affected individuals from the same family. In this family, the grandfather was only very mildly affected whereas the father was moderately affected. The grandchild, the propositus, was the most severely affected and had been confined to a wheelchair since the age of 10 years. Molecular diagnosis established that an identically sized 18 kb *Eco*RI/*Bln*I fragment was present in *all three* affected members of this family (Upadhyaya *et al.* 1999).

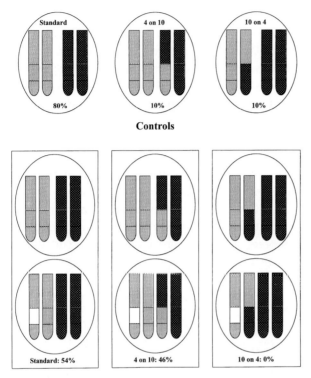

Fig. 8.7 Subtelomeric exchange of the repeat sequences on chromosomes 4 and 10 in the control and FSHD population. Chromosomes 4 are shaded grey whereas chromosomes 10 are blackened. Top: In the control population, 80 per cent individuals have 4-type repeat on chromospme 4 and 10-type repeat on chromosome 10 (adapted from van der Maarel *et al.* 2000). Bottom: the repeat-array constitutions of mosaic individuals from *de novo* FSHD families (adapted from van der Maarel *et al.* 2000). The deletion is indicated by an open bar. These individuals carry two cell populations indicated within a box. In the original population, no FSHD-associated rearrangement is present, whereas, in the other population, a deletion has occurred on chromosome 4. van der Maarel *et al.* (2000) identified mosaicism in *de novo* FSHD families by the detection of a fifth restriction fragment (either *Eco*RI/*Hind*III or *Eco*RI/*Bln*I) by pulsed-field gel electrophoresis (PFGE) followed by Southern blotting with the probe p13E11. They detected somatic mosaicism in 40 per cent of *de novo* FSHD families (14 per cent in an unaffected parent and on 26 per cent of the *de novo* FSHD patients themselves). To determine whether inter-chromosomal exchanges (either 4-type repeats on chromosome 10 or 10-type repeats on chromosome 4) might play a role in the deletion of repeats on chromosome 4, they examined the repeat array constitutions of 13 mosaic individuals (that is, those with 5 restriction fragments). Interestingly, 6/13 (46 per cent) carried 4-type repeats on chromosome 10, whereas 10 type repeats on chromosome 4 were not identified in a single mosaic case (0/13). This frequency of exchange differs from the Dutch control population (van Deutekom *et al.* 1996a) in which 10 per cent of individuals carry 4-type repeats on chromosome 10 and *vice versa*. In mosaic individuals, 54 per cent carry a standard allele configuration, whereas in 46 per cent of cases, 4-derived alleles are transferred to chromosome 10.

Whether FSHD exhibits anticipation, the phenomenon in which disease severity increases in successive generations, has still not really been determined (Lunt *et al.* 1995b; Tawil *et al.* 1996; Zatz *et al.* 1995). However, in a small proportion of FSHD families, the *Eco*RI/*Bln*I fragment size lies in the normal range (Felice *et al.* 2000; Upadhyaya *et al.* 1997).

In addition, a family with a scapulohumeral form of muscular dystrophy but without any associated facial weakness has been reported to exhibit linkage to 4q35 (Jardine *et al.* 1994). However, in this family, the smallest *Eco*RI fragment that co-segregated with the disease was about 38 kb, which is within the normal size range. It is possible that a different type of mutational lesion is responsible for altered FSHD gene expression in this family. In a few families, unaffected parents of *de novo* FSHD individuals share their disease fragment size in full dosage with the affected child (Upadhyaya *et al.* 1993). Similarly, mosaic normal parents of sporadic FSHD patients also have fragment sizes in the disease range but with reduced dose (Kohler *et al.* 1996; Upadhyaya *et al.* 1995b).

Monosomy of FSHD candidate region

Cytogenetic data indicate that monosomy of the distal 4q35 region, resulting in complete haploinsufficiency of the D4Z4 locus, is not associated with FSHD (Tupler *et al.* 1996). These workers reported a three-generation Italian family in which an unbalanced translocation of the terminal 4q region segregated through three phenotypically normal individuals, each of whom was found to be monosomic for the 4q35 subtelomeric region. The complete absence of any clinical phenotype in the translocation carriers indicates that the simple loss of the D4Z4 repeats is insufficient to cause FSHD. FSHD may thus result from some 'gain-of-function' process that is consequent to a large decrease in the number of D4Z4 repeats, but not to their complete loss.

Monozygotic twins

Several studies have reported considerable variation in the clinical expression of FSHD in pairs of affected monozygotic twins (Griggs *et al.* 1995; Tawil *et al.* 1993). Hsu *et al.* (1997) identified monozygotic twins who presented with significantly different levels of disease severity, but who manifested an identically sized D4F104S1 *Eco*RI fragment. This fragment was not found in either asymptomatic parent. Tupler *et al.* (1998) also reported monozygotic twins with identical DNA deletions; one of the twins was virtually asymptomatic whereas the other was severely affected. That the more severely affected twin had had a rabies vaccination raised in the authors' minds the question as to whether the severity of this condition might have an immunological dimension.

Gender bias

There appears to be a gender-specific influence on the degree and rate of disease progression in FSHD. The age of disease onset is invariably later in female gene carriers who are also more likely to exhibit a less severe form of the disease (Zatz *et al.* 1998). It has been suggested that female hormonal status somehow confers a mild protective effect. Consistent with this view, disease progression is markedly accelerated in female patients following the menopause at which time a general decline in muscle strength becomes apparent (Padberg 1998). Other gender effects include the finding that individuals exhibiting mosaicism for small FSHD alleles are usually male (van der Maarel *et al.* 2000) and the marked reduction in disease penetrance evident in female gene carriers (Zatz *et al.* 1998).

Molecular diagnosis of FSHD

Molecular diagnosis of FSHD was potentiated as a direct result of the establishment of the chromosomal location of the FSHD gene (Wijmenga *et al.* 1990). The majority of known closely linked markers were identified at this time (Sarfarazi *et al.* 1992; Upadhyaya *et al.* 1990), as was the D4F104S1 *Eco*RI VNTR. This polymorphism was found to be the nearest marker to the FSHD locus and identified small (<35 kb) *Eco*RI alleles in most affected FSHD patients (Wijmenga *et al.* 1992). It was then recognized that the D4F104S1 locus actually consisted of two polymorphic loci, located at 4q35 and 10q26.3 respectively, both of which were capable of producing a similarly sized range of *Eco*RI alleles (Upadhyaya *et al.* 1993; Wijmenga *et al.* 1992). These findings led to the suggestion that only FSHD families, which could definitely be linked to 4q35, or in whom a small (<35 kb) D4F104S1 *Eco*RI fragment tracked the disease phenotype, should be considered for genetic testing (Lunt *et al.* 1995a).

Despite these misgivings, molecular diagnoses in those sporadic FSHD families in whom a *de novo* D4F104S1 rearrangement was identified were considered to be accurate and reliable. The subsequent identification of a unique *Bln*I restriction site present only in the 10q26-derived D4Z4 repeats (Deidda *et al.* 1995), and its introduction into routine DNA analysis as the differential *Eco*RI/*Bln*I double digest, dramatically improved the applicability of molecular diagnosis for the majority of FSHD families (Bakker *et al.* 1996; Galluzzi *et al.* 1999; Upadhyaya *et al.* 1997; 1999). Whilst the overall specificity and sensitivity of this *Eco*RI-*Bln*I double-digest based test for accurate FSHD diagnosis is now well accepted, an additional diagnostic complication arose when it was realized that dynamic subtelomeric chromosomal exchanges between the 4q35 and 10q26 D4Z4 repeat loci have occurred in some 20 per cent of the population (van Deutekom *et al.* 1996a). This indicated that about 10 per cent of normal individuals might be expected to have a *Bln*I-resistant fragment (interpreted as a 4q35-derived element) present on one of their chromosomes 10, and conversely, another 10 per cent of people will have a *Bln*I-sensitive fragment (interpreted as a 10q26-derived array) on one of their chromosomes 4. FSHD only occurs however when the D4F104S1 located on chromosome 4 is truncated, regardless of whether this array is composed of *Bln*I-resistant repeats, *Bln*I-sensitive repeats, or a hybrid of both types. It is expected that about five per cent of FSHD cases may be associated with a shortened *Eco*RI fragment that is sensitive to *Bln*I.

Diagnostic complexity was further increased when it was recognized that the subtelomeric exchanges may result not simply in the formation of hybrid D4F104S1 loci, composed of a mixture of 4q35 and 10q26 D4Z4 repeat units. Additionally, these exchanges may also give rise to the deletion both of a variable number of the D4Z4 repeats, and the genomic region proximal to the repeats, resulting in the complete loss of the p13E-11 homologous sequences (Lemmers *et al.* 1998).

Although the effect of such complex interchromosomal exchanges on FSHD disease expression is largely unknown, it is estimated that these DNA rearrangements may lead to interpretational difficulties in about five per cent of FSHD cases studied (Bakker *et al.* 1996; van Deutekom *et al.* 1996a). In order to overcome the diagnostic problems associated with the deletion of p13E-11 homologous sequences, an appropriately modified Southern hybridisation-based restriction assay has been developed (van der Maarel *et al.* 1999). This new method is suitable for the identification of 4q35/10q26 repeat array exchanges, with or without the concomitant deletion of the p13E-11 genomic region. The method does not require PFGE, which is often not readily available in the diagnostic laboratory. Genomic DNA is digested with *Bgl*II and *Bln*I, which generates a *Bgl*II/*Bln*I restriction fragment containing both the p13E-11 region and the first, most proximally located D4Z4 repeat unit of the tandem repeat array (Fig. 8.8). The presence of a *Bln*I site in each 10q26-derived repeat yields a 1.8 kb *Bgl*II/*Bln*I fragment, while a 4.0 kb *Bgl*II fragment is produced from each 4q35-derived repeat array. Following hybridization of duplicate filters to either p13E-11 or to probe 9B6A (D4Z4), a comparison of signal intensities for each of the various fragments derived from both chromosomes 4 and 10, permits the identification of exchanged D4Z4 alleles, or of deletions involving the p13E-11 homologous region since this *Bgl*II/*Bln*I dosage test can also identify the chromosomal origin of each repeat array (van der Maarel *et al.* 1999); it is now being introduced as an additional standard in Southern blot analysis to complement the routine *Eco*RI/*Bln*I based analyses with probe p13E-11.

A recent study has found that the restriction enzyme *Xap*I cleaves only within the 4q35-specific repeat units (Lemmers *et al.* 2000). This enzyme, when used in combination with *Eco*RI and *Eco*RI/*Bln*I to digest high molecular weight genomic DNA, has been shown to permit the characterization of each D4F104S1array comprising a mixture of both repeat units. This modification will be particularly useful in helping to resolve whether co-migrating repeat arrays are homogeneous or are instead hybrids. Introduction of a *Xap*I digestion step into routine FSHD diagnosis is now highly recommended and should further help to optimize this diagnostic process.

The demonstration of linkage to 4q35 markers and identification of large D4F104S1 deletions associated with the disease, have successfully been used for molecular diagnosis of scapuloperoneal and scapulohumeral families (Jardine *et al.* 1994). These studies helped both to expand the clinical spectrum associated with FSHD locus mutations and highlighted the need to extend molecular diagnosis to families with much milder forms of the disease. Several families with scapuloperoneal dystrophy are not linked to 4q35 (Tawil *et al.* 1995; Wilhelmsen *et al.* 1996).

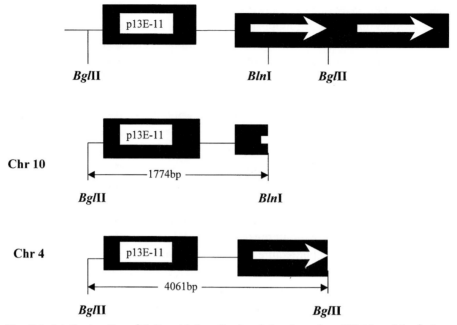

Fig. 8.8 Relative location of *Bgl*II restriction sites in relation to probe p13E-11 and the first D4Z4 repeat. Digestion with *Bgl*II/*Bln*I will result in two fragments; the 4061 bp fragment is derived from chromosome 4. Owing to the presence of an internal *Bln*I restriction site in each of the 10q-derived D4Z4 repeats, a 1774 bp fragment will be derived from chromosome 10. Signal intensities from fragments of both chromosomes can be compared to evaluate the presence of translocated 4 alleles or deletions of the region spanning the probe p13E 11.

The possibility of genetic mosaicism in FSHD, whether germline or somatic, ought to be carefully considered by any diagnostic laboratory, since this mutational mechanism can lead to the recurrence of the disease in a family whose disease was initially thought to be due to a new mutation. This mechanism may also account for the proportion of those FSHD families in which a severely affected child is born to a mother previously classified on clinical grounds as being only very mildly affected, or unaffected. Indeed, the overall risk of underlying parental mosaicism being present in any *de novo* sporadic case is estimated to be up to 40 per cent with an apparent predominance of female carriers in such families (Kohler *et al.* 1996; van der Maarel *et al.* 2000).

The search for the FSHD gene

An extensive use of both conventional gene mapping strategies and standard positional cloning experiments has consistently failed to identify the FSHD gene (Altherr *et al.* 1995; Hewitt *et al.* 1994; Lyle *et al.* 1995; van Deutekom *et al.* 1995; Upadhyaya *et al.* 1995b). Following on from the recognition of the close association between large D4F104S1 locus deletions and disease expression, it was anticipated that the FSHD gene would be quickly identified and characterized. However, despite extensive efforts worldwide, the FSHD gene has not yet been identified. Although D4F104S1-associated deletions are closely associated with FSHD in some way, the exact nature and location of the FSHD gene (or genes?) still remains elusive, as does the mechanistic basis of the association.

Initial attempts to demonstrate that the homeobox-like sequences associated with each D4Z4 repeat were functional have been somewhat equivocal. These studies involved using this ORF sequence as a probe to screen various complementary DNA (cDNA) libraries and expressed sequence tag (EST) databases. Although a number of apparently homologous cDNA clones were identified, none of these could be mapped back to either 4q35 or 10q26. Since no transcribed sequences could be identified from within the D4Z4 repeat units, the *FSHD* gene search was then focused upon the genomic region located proximal to the repeat arrays. An extensive sequence analysis and the application of basic local alignment search tool (BLAST) (Altschul *et al.* 1990) to this genomic region was undertaken to search for possible genes and the locations of any expressed sequences identified in EST database screens. This genomic region was found (i) to be enriched in several types of repetitive element, and (ii) to contain a number of gene-like sequences homologous to loci dispersed across the genome, and which appear to represent pseudogenes (van Deutekom *et al.* 1995).

The highly repetitive nature of the 4q35 region has seriously hampered the search for a possible FSHD candidate gene; particularly difficult has been the identification of suitable single-copy DNA probes required for use in many hybridization-based gene identification methods, such as cDNA selection. Several successful exon trapping and cDNA library screens have been carried out with specific genomic subclones, but the results have generally been disappointing. The close proximity of the FSHD region to the 4q telomere has probably also hindered many cloning studies; similar subtelomeric regions are known to contain few functional genes (Flint *et al.* 1996). Another possible problem could be if the *FSHD* gene normally functioned only at some specific point during development; such a developmental stage-specific gene might only be transiently expressed, and then only in certain tissues. Thus, cDNA libraries screened to date may either simply not contain the *FSHD* gene transcript, or the transcript has been present at too low a level to be detected by the relatively insensitive gene selection methodologies so far employed.

The functional genes identified within the FSHD candidate region are the somewhat intriguingly named FSHD Region Genes 1 and 2 (*FRG1*, *FRG2*). *FRG1* is situated almost 100 kb proximal to the D4Z4 repeat array, within the genomic region that is specific to chromosome 4. *FRG2* is located 37 kb proximal to the D4Z4 repeat array. Complete sequencing of the region between *FRG1* and the 4q telomere has, however, failed to identify other functional genes (van Geel *et al.* 1999), although a number of processed and unprocessed pseudogenes are present. It is possible that additional inactive genes or pseudogenes may be concealed within the subtelomeric heterochromatin. One of these genes (or pseudogenes?) might somehow be released from heterochromatic inactivation (perhaps as a direct result of the deletion of a large number of the D4Z4 repeats) and would then be aberrantly expressed resulting in the production of a protein product that is exclusive to FSHD patients. Some of the gene loci in the vicinity of the FSHD locus will now be described in the belief that they may represent either candidate loci or are more indirectly or peripherally involved in the FSHD phenotype.

Potential gene sequences within the FSHD candidate region

The 161 kb genomic region situated proximal of the D4Z4 repeats has been sequenced and the sequence analysed with a number of gene prediction programs (van Geel *et al.* 1999). Almost half (45 per cent) of this subtelomeric region is made up of repeat sequences, of which LINE-1 elements form the bulk. Several retrotransposed genes have also been identified in this genomic sequence region (van Geel *et al.* 1999). In addition to the known genes and pseudogenes from the region (*FRG1*, *FRG2* and *TUB4Q*), a number of potential coding regions were identified, although none of these potential gene sequences have been confirmed by RT-PCR or cDNA library screening. Further studies are clearly required to assess the functionality of these potential coding regions.

FRG1

Screening a skeletal muscle cDNA library with a CpG island-containing, 4q35 genomic subclone, identified a number of overlapping cDNA clones that mapped within the FSHD candidate region; the complete *FRG1* gene was constructed from some of these clones (van Deutekom *et al.* 1996b). *FRG1* is a member of an evolutionarily conserved multi-gene family with related sequences located on several other chromosomes. Analysis of human *FRG1*-homologous ESTs demonstrated that many of these loci represented non-processed pseudogenes dispersed across the genome. FISH analysis with an *FRG1* probe revealed positive hybridization signals over the pericentromeric region of chromosome 9, on the centromeric region of chromosome 20 and along the short arms of the acrocentric chromosomes. Comparative sequence analysis demonstrated that *FRG1*-related sequences are present in the great apes (chimpanzee, gorilla, the orangutan) and in the Old World monkey, *Macaca mulata* (Grewal *et al.* 1999). As in humans, the great apes express multiple copies of their FRG1-related loci, whereas in *Macaca mulata* only two *FRG1* loci were detectable, one of which is presumed to be homologous to the human chromosome 4q35 *FRG1* gene. There is striking similarity between the distribution of *FRG1* and the dispersed 3.3 kb repeat family in primates.

The human *FRG1* gene is 22.4 kb in size, contains nine exons, and encodes a 1042 bp transcript that is predicted to yield a 258 amino acid protein. By utilizing two expressed single nucleotide polymorphisms (eSNPs), located in exons 1 and 5 of the *FRG1* gene respectively, muscle and lymphocyte cDNA isolated from both FSHD patients and normal individuals were examined. The demonstration in both tissues of similar levels of expression for each *FRG1* allele, in patients as well as controls, indicated there to be no evidence for allelic exclusion of the *FRG1* gene in FSHD patients (van Deutekom *et al.* 1996b). Although the *FRG1* gene, which is expressed in fetal and adult muscle, represents a good candidate gene for FSHD, no mutations of the *FRG1* gene have been found in FSHD patients. *FRG1*-like genes have been cloned and sequenced from both the pufferfish, *Fugu rubripes*, and from two nematode species, *Caenorhabditis elegans* and *Brugia mala* (Grewal *et al.* 1999). No functional role for the human FRG1 protein (FRG1P) has yet been determined, even though the protein is highly conserved in both vertebrates and non-vertebrates. Although polyclonal and monoclonal antibodies to FRG1P have been generated, immunohistochemical studies have failed to identify the subcellular location of the protein. Only after *in vitro* transfection studies, using an expression vector construct containing the FRG1P protein coupled to a FLAG epitope, could the expressed FRG1 protein be localized to the nucleolar region; it co-localized with ribosomal DNA (van der Maarel, personal communication). The question as to whether the *FRG1* gene has any functional role in the pathophysiology of FSHD still remains to be answered.

TUB4Q gene or pseudogene?

The *TUB4Q* gene, located 80 kb proximal to the D4Z4 repeats, contains 4 exons and encodes a putative 434 amino acid protein (van Geel *et al.* 1999). The nucleotide sequence of *TUB4Q* displays 88 per cent homology to the β2-tubulin protein domain. However, a high level of allelic sequence variability was observed, consistent with *TUB4Q* being a pseudogene. At least nine members of the *TUB4Q* multi-gene family have now been identified; these have been localized to the pericentromeric and telomeric regions of the genome and all appear to be derived from a large genomic duplication in the 4q35 region. It is possible that the inappropriate activation of this normally non-functional *TUB4Q* gene may have implications for the FSHD disease mechanism.

FRG2

The *FRG2* gene is a recently identified member of another multi-gene family that may be involved in muscle-specific gene expression. *FRG2*-related sequences are, as with many genes and pseudogenes from within the FSHD candidate region, dispersed across the genome. The *FRG2* gene contains 4 exons that encode a putative 277 amino acid protein that fails to exhibit homology to any known protein. Although *FRG2*-specific transcripts could not be identified in RNA isolated from skeletal muscle, lymphocytes, fibroblasts or brain, high-level expression of an *FRG2*-related transcript was detected in fibroblasts forced to undergo myogenic differentiation under the influence of an introduced MyoD expression vector (Silvere van der Maarel, personal communication). Whether the *FRG2* gene is involved in the pathophysiology of FSHD is yet unknown.

DUX4

A number of studies have consistently failed to identify a functional transcript associated with the D4Z4 repeat units, even though each repeat contained a large ORF encoding a putative homeobox-like protein. A genomic fragment, designated *HEFT1*, which is ~90 per cent identical to a single D4Z4 repeat was recently cloned, and an upstream potential promoter sequence identified (Ding *et al.* 1998). An homologous cDNA clone was then isolated and found to identify transcripts in both skeletal muscle- and cardiac muscle-derived mRNA, which, on sequencing, were found to encode a new transcription factor, DUX1, which possesses two potential homeodomains (Ding *et al.* 1998). Two additional related genes, DUX2 and DUX3, both with similar promoter sequences and ORFs, have subsequently been isolated (Beckers *et al.* 2001). However, all three DUX genes were found to map to the acrocentric chromosomes.

The same group has now identified a closely related *DUX4* gene present within each of the 3.3 kb D4Z4 elements (Ding *et al.* 1998)(Fig. 8.2). This *DUX4* gene is an intron-less gene, and lacks any polyadenylation signal (Gabriels *et al.* 1999). Computer-based promoter prediction analysis indicates that each D4Z4 repeat contains a number of potential regulatory sequences. A potential promoter-like sequence has been identified in the *DUX4* gene and is situated immediately upstream of a large homeobox-like ORF. This putative *DUX4* promoter is associated with a probable CpG island, and contains both a TACAA sequence that may represent a modified 'TATAA' box, and a consensus GC-box. This promoter is located immediately 5′ of an 'in-frame' translation initiation codon. To evaluate the functional activity of this potential promoter, a 191 bp genomic fragment encompassing the entire promoter region was cloned into a pGL-3 expression vector to yield a *DUX4*-luciferase fusion construct. Both wild-type and mutated constructs, containing sequence alterations in either the TACAA or the GC-box, were transfected into human rhabdomyosarcoma TE671 cells. Transient luciferase activities were then measured in cell extracts made 24 h following transfection. Mutations in either the TACAA or the GC-box were found to result in a significantly reduced expression of the luciferase reporter gene. *In vitro* transcription/translation studies using the *DUX4* ORF, in a rabbit reticulocyte system, yielded two labelled polypeptide products with apparent molecular weights of 38 kDa and 75 kDa which corresponded to the *DUX4* monomer and dimer, respectively. In a related experiment, a plasmid clone containing a 13.5 kb *Eco*RI fragment, comprising the two remaining D4Z4 repeats isolated from a FSHD patient, was injected into the leg muscle of a mouse. Rodents do not possess any D4Z4-like repeats, and so the rationale of the experiment was that if the ORF sequences in each repeat were functional and resulted in the production of at least some protein product, then this might be perceived by the recipient mouse as a foreign protein and might therefore invoke an immunological response against this protein. Indeed, all the six injected mice were found to produce antibodies to the ORF-encoded protein from the D4Z4 repeats (Coppee *et al.* 2000).

Expression studies in the FSHD candidate region

In a search for clues to help understand the possible underlying molecular mechanisms responsible for FSHD, a recent study directly compared mRNA expression patterns present in skeletal muscle from FSHD patients and normal controls (Tupler *et al.* 1999). Using an RNA subtraction hybridization technique to identify any differently expressed transcripts, FSHD dystrophic muscle was found to exhibit marked alterations in gene expression levels, showing evidence of significant underexpression or overexpression of a number of specific gene transcripts. Intriguingly, a number of the abnormally expressed genes are known to be transcriptional regulators; the deregulated expression of such factors may be reflected in the wide spectrum of genes that appear to be abnormally transcribed in FSHD muscle. Such deregulated gene expression muscle may also result in a breakdown of muscle molecular architecture. That these mRNA changes were absent in skeletal muscle samples from patients with Becker muscular dystrophy (BMD) patients and amyotrophic lateral sclerosis (ALS), indicates that the global misregulation of muscle-specific gene expression is specific to FSHD, and not a feature common to neuromuscular disease.

Various other studies have also revealed that several additional muscle-specific genes located within 4q35, the FSHD candidate region, are also upregulated; these include the *FRG1* gene, Lim protein genes, the actin-associated LIM protein gene (*ALP*), and the *SMT7* gene (Ehmsen *et al.* 1999; Forrester et al. 1999). However, whether such changes are the cause or consequence of FSHD pathophysiology is unknown. The application of the recently developed microarray-based technologies (Duggan *et al.* 1999) will allow us to investigate entire sets of muscle-specific genes in a single experiment. The current data indicating global misregulation of muscle gene expression in FSHD indicates that this disease may be particularly amenable to a microarray-based approach. Such a strategy may also help us to discriminate between primary causal mechanisms and the secondary effects of FSHD, as well as to monitor the effectiveness of any future therapeutic approaches when they are tested.

The D4Z4 repeats and chromatin structure

Some recent studies have assessed whether the D4Z4 repeats may be involved in determining the structure of the 4qter chromatin. Direct interactions between D4Z4 DNA sequences and nuclear proteins have been examined (Gabellini *et al.* 2000). Using mobility shift assays and *in vitro* DNase I footprinting, the presence of a 27 bp specific protein-binding site from D4Z4 was demonstrated. This site exhibited comparable binding activity in both human and mouse cultured muscle cells. A 27-kDa nuclear protein was identified that bound to the minimal binding site in D4Z4 with a high degree of specificity. Furthermore, this D4Z4 binding site was also able to activate an *in vitro* transcription test system. It is not known whether the specific binding of this protein to D4Z4 will result in the silencing of genes at 4q35.

DNA methylation

DNA methylation within the promoter region of a gene is usually associated with inactivation of expression of that gene, and is presumably the reason that most actively transcribed genes exhibit extremely low levels of promoter methylation. Methylation of DNA in most mammalian tissues occurs almost exclusively at CpG dinucleotides. Transcriptional inactivation of gene expression only seems to occur when at least 40 per cent of the CpG dinucleotides within the promoter region become methylated (Horan *et al.* 2000).

In the context of FSHD, it is pertinent to mention that vertebrate heterochromatin is preferentially methylated. The *DUX4* gene, a copy of which appears to be present in every D4Z4 repeat, is 'buried' in the strongly heterochromatic subtelomeric region and is, therefore, not normally expressed. In FSHD patients, however, the large deletion of the 3.3 kb repeats that contain the *DUX4* gene may lead to the opening up of the chromatin structures associated with the remaining few repeats. These structural changes could activate expression of the normally inactive *DUX4* gene, both in inappropriate tissues and or at abnormal times in tissue development. One way to monitor this inappropriate gene expression would be to determine whether methylation differences in the *DUX4* promoter region differed between skeletal muscles from FSHD patients as compared to normal control individuals. If FSHD-associated differences in the methylation pattern of the *DUX4* gene were detected, their specificity to the 4q35-located *D4Z4* repeats would need to be confirmed. Restriction of genomic DNA with *Bln*I should ensure that only 4q35-located D4Z4 repeats were being examined since the *Bln*I enzymatic step would have cleaved and removed the 10q26-derived D4Z4 repeats (Osborn *et al.* 1999; Upadhyaya and Osborn 2000). Interestingly, in patients with ICF syndrome (immunodeficiency centromeric instability and facial abnormalities), D4Z4 is hypomethylated whereas it is highly methylated in normal cells (Kondo *et al.* 2000).

Animal models

Mouse

The myodysgenesis (*myd*) mouse has been proposed to be a good model for FSHD (Mathews *et al.* 1995). The autosomal recessive mutation present in the *myd* mouse results in a diffuse and progressive skeletal myopathy, and is associated with reduced fertility. A degree of hearing impairment has been demonstrated in the homozygous *myd* mouse; this phenotypic feature is similar to that found in FSHD patients who may have some level of sensorineural hearing loss that appears to be localized to the cochlea (such hearing loss is often subclinical). The *myd* gene has been mapped to mouse chromosome 8 where it is located within the human 4q syntenic region (Lane *et al.* 1976). Comparative mapping has confirmed the general relationship between the most distal genes on human 4q and the most proximal genes in the mouse chromosome 8 syntenic region. Despite the chromosomal rearrangement of the syntenic groups within this region, conservation of gene order has been maintained between the group of genes in the human 4q35 region and on mouse chromosome 8. The *myd* gene is flanked distally by the mitochondrial uncoupling protein (*Ucp1*) gene, which has a human homologue located at 4q31, and proximally by the chloride channel 5 gene (*CLC5*) and the coagulation factor XI (*cf11*) gene, both of which have human homologues (*CLC5, F11*) located within 4q35. Grewal *et al.* (1998) localized the *frg1* gene, the mouse *FRG1* homologue, proximal to the *myd* gene, suggesting that *frg1* is not involved in the *myd* phenotype. An ongoing mapping project has been able to refine the map position of the *myd* gene, localizing it to a <1 Mb genomic region (K. Mathews, personal communication). Although the *myd* phenotype displays an autosomal recessive mode of inheritance, it is quite possible that it has a different mutational mechanism to FSHD. It may, nevertheless, still provide a good, albeit indirect, means of identifying the human *FSHD* gene.

Drosophila

A number of experimental fruit fly (*Drosophila*) cell lines have been generated in which a human D4Z4 (3.3 kb) repeat has been introduced into a 'white eye gene expression' system. Flies expressing these expression constructs exhibited variations in eye colour dependent upon how, if, or when the construct was expressed. Preliminary results indicate that the D4Z4 repeat has an effect on eye colour expression. In some flies, there was complete repression of normal eye colour, whereas in other lines an apparent developmental age effect was evident with normal eye colour present at birth that gradually changed with the age of the recipient fly. In a number of fly lines, no effect on eye colour was observed (Mathews 1999). These preliminary data indicate that some sequence element within the D4Z4 repeat is capable of suppressing gene expression in *Drosophila*, at least when placed in juxtaposition to that gene.

Possible FSHD disease mechanisms

A positional effect

The failure of extensive searches to identify a definitive *FSHD* gene within the 4q35 candidate region, coupled with the direct association between the level of D4Z4 repeat loss and the severity of FSHD disease expression, has resulted in investigators proposing a number of different pathognomic mechanisms. One of the major mutational mechanisms proposed is that the disease results from a positional effect, which is defined as a deleterious change in the level of gene expression brought about by a change in the position of the gene relative to its normal chromosomal environment but not associated with intragenic mutations or deletions (Bedell *et al.* 1996; Kleinjan and van Heyningen, 1998). Expression of a gene can be greatly influenced by its position in the genome. Euchromatin is decondensed during interphase, contains most of the genes and appears to replicate earlier in S phase. Heterochromatin is more condensed, replicates later in S phase and is associated with several repeat sequences. The chromosomal rearrangements can separate the promoter/transcription unit from an essential distant regulatory element thereby removing the effect of this regulator on the gene. It may also juxtapose the gene with an enhancer element from another gene, leading to inappropriate gene expression. The rearrangement could give rise to classical position effect variegation (PEV). PEV was first reported in *Drosophila* (Henikoff, 1990). PEV describes the variable, but heritably stable, inhibition of gene expression due to the juxtaposition of a euchromatic gene with a region of heterochromatin through chromosomal rearrangement. The degree of variegation is dependent on the distance of the gene from the breakpoint with shorter distances from the heterochromatic region, giving rise to more frequent suppression. In this model, the *FSHD* gene (or genes?) is (are) either being inappropriately activated or repressed as the direct result of some significant change in the surrounding structural or biochemical environment. One explanation is that it is the deletion of large numbers of 4q35-specific D4Z4 repeats that results in changes to the overall 3-D configuration of the chromosomal structure within the 4q terminal region, and it is this that exerts a positive or negative positional effect on a gene, or genes, that is (are) located more proximally in the 4q35 region. A related, and perhaps, complementary model proposes that it is an extension of the inactivating (?) influence of the telomeric heterochromatin into the normally protected more proximal genomic regions. The D4F104S1 repeat array is located only 25–30 kb from the 4q telomere and the large number of D4Z4 repeats normally present within the D4F104S1 locus ensures that there is usually at least a minimum of 38 kb, and often more than 300 kb, of D4Z4-related DNA that physically separates the 4q telomeric associated heterochromatin from the more proximally located euchromatic gene-rich regions of 4q35. Obviously, in the FSHD patient, the extensive loss of D4Z4 repeats will now place this gene-rich region immediately adjacent to the inactivating influence of the 4q telomeric heterochromatin, which is predicted to result in the spread of a wave of gene inactivation across this region. Thus, a position effect resulting in the inappropriate global regulatory influence of juxtaposed heterochromatic regions would fully explain the correlation between repeat size and the severity of the FSHD phenotype (Lunt *et al.* 1995b; Tawil *et al.* 1996; Zatz *et al.* 1995). It is perhaps interesting to speculate as to whether the larger deletions of D4Z4 repeats, which are postulated to result in the proximal euchromatic region being placed much closer to the telomere, also permit the heterochromatic influence to spread further into this euchromatic region, and hence, inactivate a larger number of genes. We certainly observe an extended clinical phenotype in those FSHD patients with the largest deletions and the most severe forms of the disease. Indeed, such severely affected patients may exhibit hearing loss, retinal vasculopathy, and even epilepsy and mental retardation.

The dynamic chromosomal interchanges between 4q35 and 10q26 may also represent some aspect of this position effect. It is now quite clear that it is the specific chromosomal environment of the D4Z4 deletions that is important in FSHD disease expression, with the disorder only developing when the large D4Z4-associated deletions are located on 4q35, regardless of whether the individual repeats originated from 4q35 or 10q26. The observation that large 10q26-associated D4Z4 repeat deletions are not apparently associated with any clinical phenotype suggests that there may be a lack of methylatable genes in the genomic region immediately adjacent to the 10q26 repeat array that are available to be affected by a similar positional effect. The region of sequence homology between 4q35 and 10q26 only extends some 35 kb proximal to the D4Z4 repeats and appears to lack any genes or gene-like sequences.

In humans, a position effect mechanism has been invoked to explain the presence of an aniridia phenotype in affected patients who do not have identifiable mutations within their *PAX6* genes, which underlie this disorder. The *PAX6* gene is located at 11p13, and no disruption of this gene was evident in two *de novo* aniridia patients. Careful cytogenetic and molecular analysis of these two patients revealed the presence of small genomic deletions, located ~11 kb from the 3′-UTR of the *PAX6* gene in both individuals (Lauderdale *et al.* 2000). Expression studies demonstrated that the *PAX6* genes of each patient were only transcribed from the normal allele, and not from the *PAX6* allele on the deleted chromosome. A number of experiments in *Drosophila* and yeast have clearly demonstrated that placing a gene in close physical proximity to either centromeric or telomeric sequences, or within or adjacent to any heterochromatic regions actively suppressed gene expression. An alteration of chromatin structure resulting from a spread of heterochromatic influence into the euchromatic domains is postulated. There is also clear evidence from these model systems of a gradient effect, with those genes located nearest to any heterochromatic region being more severely affected than those further away. Conversely, there are several examples in *Drosophila* of genes that absolutely require a heterochromatic environment to function normally, and hence these genes demonstrate a position effect when placed under a euchromatic influence. It is perhaps of interest that each D4Z4 repeat contains an internal *LSau* repeat, and this repeat family is normally found within heterochromatic regions. Position effects have been shown to exert their influence over large genomic distances (>500 kb) (Spofford 1976); hence we can imagine that the FSHD gene may also be located at some considerable distance from the D4F104S1 region. Thus, even though the disease demonstrates tight linkage to D4F10S1, and the severity of disease expression is increased with larger internal deletions of this locus, the location of the FSHD gene itself may be physically divorced from the mutational mechanism that causes the disorder. This would truly represent a positional effect! In order to test this hypothesis, one would have to examine the expression of the FSHD gene in the early embryo in an animal model.

Evidence for the FSHD gene within the D4Z4 repeat

The concept that one or more copies of the D4Z4 repeat encodes a functional protein is obviously supported by the recognition within each repeat of a potential homeodomain protein produced from a 405 bp ORF containing an 'in-frame' start codon.

Related homeodomain proteins are known to be involved in the regulation of development and morphogenesis. We can postulate that large D4Z4 tandem arrays induce and possibly stabilize heterochromatin formation, resulting in the inactivation of any repeat-associated genes in normal unaffected individuals. Then the extensive loss of these D4Z4 repeats in FSHD is associated with the destabilization of heterochromatic structures and the removal of its repressive influences, thereby permitting the inappropriate expression of genes that are normally inactive. Each D4Z4 repeat is known to contain the necessary coding sequence for the *DUX4* protein. However, whether this represents a functional gene or not is unknown. The apparent evolutionary conservation of *DUX4*-related genes, [this homeo-domain-like gene from both the rhesus monkey and humans is virtually identical (Winokur *et al.* 1996)] does indicate that this gene is likely to have some definite function, at least at some point during an animal's life. Thus, the *DUX4* gene product may function as a transcription factor that is normally not expressed in skeletal muscle, and that the aberrant production and potential interaction of this protein with the other factor(s) may be the basis of, (i) the observed upregulation of some of the 4q35-located genes, and (ii) the global disregulation of a number of muscle-specific genes (Ehmsen *et al.* 1999; Forrester *et al.* 1999; Tupler *et al.* 1999). According to this model (Gabriels *et al.* 1999), the destabilization of heterochromatin resulting from the loss of many D4Z4 repeats in FSHD patients, now permits expression of the *DUX4* gene in at least some of the repeats, and the resulting *DUX4* protein may be toxic to the muscle cells, perhaps as a result of strong dimerization potential of this protein. Such a model is consistent with a 'gain of function' mechanism that is likely to result from the dominant negative effect of such a mutation. This model is also supported by the finding that haplosufficiency for 4q, resulting in the complete loss of one set of the chromosome 4-located D4Z4 repeat arrays, does not cause FSHD (Tupler *et al.* 1996), and that clinical severity in FSHD is negatively correlated to the number of D4Z4 repeats that remain in the 4q35 located tandem array. The observations that FSHD patients often exhibit an assymetric progression of the disease, and that monozygotic twins with FSHD often exhibit discordant phenotypes, may be taken as evidence for the expression of the FSHD gene in a variable temporal and spatial manner in different tissues. Although we may have identified a definitive molecular mutational 'footprint' for FSHD disease expression, precisely which gene, or genes, are involved and the exact mechanism through which the mutation finds expression in the clinical phenotype, remain unknown.

Therapy

Currently, there is no specific treatment available for FSHD. Therapy may involve surgery such as scapular fixation, tendon transfers and blepharorrhaphy (Padberg 1998; Twyman *et al.* 1996). A pilot trial in which patients were treated with prednisone, showed no benefit to the patients, either in muscle strength, or in increased muscle mass (Tawil *et al.* 1997). In a preliminary three-month trial, albuterol, a β2-agonist that normally increases muscle mass and causes satellite cells to proliferate, has provided some encouraging evidence of improvements to both muscle strength and mass (Kissel *et al.* 1998; Kissel 1999).

The FSHD enigma

Does FSHD represent an inherited disease with a unique pathogenetic mechanism? Although there is some evidence for genetic heterogeneity in FSHD, the vast majority of cases involve a mutational mechanism located at 4q35. Unfortunately, the 4q35 genomic region containing the FSHD locus is still not fully defined, and any hypothesis that attempts to explain the underlying disease mechanism must take into account the high sequence complexity of this region, with its highly repetitive nature and its sequence homologies to loci on many other chromosomes.

A number of puzzling FSHD disease-associated features need to be considered when attempting to explain any proposed disease-causing mechanism:

- Monosomy of the 4q35 region does not produce disease.
- The lack of any discernible disease phenotype associated with large deletions of the 10q26-located D4Z4 repeat arrays, despite the almost identical sequence of the 4q35- and 10q26-located ORF.
- The dynamic nature of the interchromosomal exchanges between chromosome 4 and 10-located repeats, both in affected and normal individuals, and the overall plasticity of these two chromosomal regions.
- The significant levels of somatic mosaicism (ranging from normal to disease size range) observed in both asymptomatic parents and in affected individuals.
- The inverse correlation that is only demonstrated between the chromosome 4-located D4Z4 repeat copy number and clinical severity.
- Marked intra-familial variable clinical expression.
- The discordance in the clinical phenotype in monozygotic twins.
- The assymetrical involvement of this disease.
- Abnormalities of gene expression in FSHD muscle.

Some critical questions which remain unanswered:

Is there more than one disease gene involved in disease expression?

Is the *FSHD* gene only active in diseased muscle?

Is FSHD due to the up-regulation or down-regulation of gene expression?

The overall pathophysiology of FSHD is still not understood and the underlying molecular and biochemical defect is unknown. Despite the absence of any detectable genetic instability or molecular variation within families, it is evident that the D4Z4 repeats are directly related to the severity of disease expression, even though the underlying mutational mechanism remains to be elucidated. The identification of the *FSHD* gene and the characterization of the *FSHD* gene product should enable us not only to offer accurate molecular diagnosis for this disorder, and other related conditions, but may also help to resolve some of the apparent complexity of the 4q35 *FSHD* region. Finally, elucidation of the *FSHD* gene sequence and function should provide us with a much better insight into the underlying pathophysiology of the disease, and lead in the future to a possible effective treatment.

Acknowledgements

We are grateful to Dr Nick Thomas for his comments, Mr Neil Kent for his help with the illustrations and Dr Mark Rogers for Fig. 8.1.

References

Altherr, M.R., Bengtsson, C.M.T., Rachelle, P., Markovich, B.S., and Winokur, S.T. (1995). Efforts toward understanding the molecular basis of facioscapulohumeral muscular dystrophy. *Muscle & Nerve*, suppl. 2, S32–S38.

Altschul, S.F., Gish, W., Miller, W., Myers, E.W., and Lipman, D.J. (1990). Basic local alignment search tool. *Journal of Molecular Biology*, **215**, 403–10.

Bakker, E., Van der Weilen, M.J., Voorhoeve, E., Ippel, P.F., Padberg, G.W., and Frants, R.R. (1996). Diagnostic, predictive and prenatal testing for facioscapulohumeral muscular dystrophy: diagnostic approach for sporadic and familial cases. *Journal of Medical Genetics*, **33**, 29–35.

Beckers, M.C., Gabriels, J., van der Maarel, S., De Vniese, A., Frants, R.R, Collen, D, Belayew, A. (2001). Active genes in junk DNA? Characterization of *DUX* genes embedded within 3.3kb repeated elements. *Gene*, **264**, 51–7.

Bedell, M.A., Jenkins, N.A., and Copeland, N.G. (1996). Good genes in bad neighbourhoods. *Nature Genetics*, **12**, 229–32.

Brouwer, O.F., Ruys, C.J.M., Brand, R., De Laat, J.A.P.M., Grote, J.J., and Padberg, G.W. (1991). Hearing loss in facioscapuohumeral muscular dystrophy. *Neurology*, **41**, 1878–81.

Brouwer, O.F., Padberg, G.W., Bakker, E., Wijmenga, C., and Frants, R.R. (1995). Early onset facioscapuohumeral muscular dystrophy. *Muscle & Nerve*, suppl. 2, S67–S73.

Cacurri, S., Piazzo, N., Deidda, G., Vignetti, E., Galluzzi, G., and Colantoni, L. (1998). Sequence homology between 4qter and 10qter loci facilitates the instability of subtelomeric *Kpn*I repeat units implicated in facioscapuohumeral muscular dystrophy. *American Journal of Human Genetics*, **63**, 181–90.

Campbell, L., Potter, A., Ignatius, J., Dubowitz, V., and Davies, K. (1997). Genomic variation and gene conversion in spinal muscular atrophy, implications for disease process and clinical phenotype. *American Journal of Human Genetics*, **61**, 40–50.

Clark, L.N., Koehler, U., Ward, D.C., Wienberg, J., and Hewitt, J. (1996). Analysis of the organisation and localisation of the FSHD—associated tandem array in primates: implications for the origin and evolution of the 3.3 kb repeat family. *Chromosoma*, **105**, 180–189.

Coppee, P., Gabriels, J., Matteotti, C., Daneubourg, G., Zador, E., Wuytack, F., Dux, L., Collen, D., and Belayew, A. (2000). Study of *DUX4* gene present in the D4Z4 repeats of the 4q35 chromosome locus. Presented at FSHD Consortium meeting at American Society of Human Genetics, Philadelphia.

Deidda, G., Caccuri, S., Grisanti, P., Piazzo, N., and Felicetti, L. (1995). Physical mapping evidence for a duplicated region on chromosome 10qter showing high homology with the FSHD locus on chromosome 4qter. *European Journal of Human Genetics*, **3**, 155–67.

Deidda, G., Caccuri, S., Piazzo, N., and Felicetti, L. (1996). Direct detection of 4q35 rearrangements implicated in facioscapuohumeral muscular dystrophy (FSHD). *Journal of Medical Genetics*, **33**, 361–5.

Ding, H., Beckers, M.C., Plaisance, S., Marynen, P., Collen, D., and Belayew, A. (1998). Characterisation of a double homeodomain protein (DUX1) encoded by a cDNA homologous to 3.3 kb dispersed repeated elements. *Human Molecular Genetics*, **7**, 1681–94.

Duggan, D.J., Bittner, M., Chen, Y., Meltzer, P., and Trent, J.M. (1999). Expression profiling using cDNA microarrays. *Nature Genetics*, **21**, 10–4.

Ehmsen, J.T., Forrester, J.D., Figlewicz, D.A., Simon, M., Hewitt, J.E., and Winokur, S.T. (1999). Isolation and characterisation of a novel gene, SM7, in the facioscapulohumeral muscular dystrophy (FSHD) region. Presented at the FSHD Consortium Meeting at the American Society of Human Genetics, San Francisco.

Felice, K.J., North, W.A., Moore, S.A., and Mathews, K.D. (2000). FSH dystrophy 4q35 deletion in patients presenting with facial-sparing scapular myopathy. *Neurology*, **54**, 1927–30.

Fisher, J. and Upadhyaya, M. (1997). Molecular genetics of muscular dystrophy (FSHD) *Neuromuscular Disorders*, **7**, 55–62.

Fitzsimons, R.B. (1999). Facioscapulohumeral muscular dystrophy. *Current Opinion in Neurology*, **12**, 501–11.

Flint, J., Wilkie, A.O., Buckle, V.J., Winter, R.M., Holland, A.J., and McDermid, H.E. (1996). The detection of subtelomeric chromosomal rearrangements in idiopathic mental retardation. *Nature Genetics*, **9**, 132–40.

Forrester, J., Morsch, R., Sowden, J.E., Griggs, R.C., Tawil, R., and Figlewicz, D.A. (1999). Gene expression studies on chromosome 4q35. Presented at the FSHD consortium meeting at the American Society of Human Genetics, San Francisco.

Funakoshi, M., Goto, K., and Arahata, K. (1998). Epilepsy and mental retardation in a subset of early onset 4q35-facioscapulohumeral muscular dystrophy. *Neurology*, **50**, 1791–4.

Gabellini, D., Green, M.R., and Tupler, R.G. (2000). Analysis of protein-DNA interactions at the level of D4Z4, the DNA repetitive element causally related to facioscapulohumeral muscular dystrophy. FSHD Research Consortium at the American Society of Human Genetics, Philadelphia.

Gabriels, J., Beckers, M.C., Ding, H., DeVriese, A., Plaisance, S., van der Maarel, S. *et al.* (1999). Nucleotide sequence of the partially deleted D4Z4 locus in a patient with FSHD identifies a putative gene within each 3.3 kb element. *Gene*, **236**, 25–32.

Galluzzi, G., Deidda, G., Cacurri, S., Colantoni, L., Piazzo, N., Vigneti, E. *et al.* (1999). Molecular diagnosis of 4q35 rearrangements in facioscapulohumeral muscular dystrophy (FSHD): application to family studies for correct genetic advice and a reliable prenatal diagnosis of the disease. *Neuromuscular Disorders*, **9**, 190–8.

Gilbert, J.R., Speer, M.C., Stajich, J.M., Clancy, R., Lewis, K., Qiu, H. *et al.* (1995). Exclusion mapping of chromosomal regions which cross- hybridise to FSHD1A-associated markers in FSHD1B. *Journal of Medical Genetics*, **32**, 770–3.

Goto, K., Lee, O.H., Matsuda, C., Nakamura, A., Mitsunaga, Y., Furukawa, T., Sahashi, K., and Arahata, K. (1995). DNA rearrangements in Japanese facioscapulohumeral muscular dystrophy patients: clinical correlation. *Neuromuscular Disorders*, **5**, 201–8.

Grewal, P.K., van Geel, M., Frants, R.R., de Jong P., and Hewitt, J.E. (1999). Recent amplification of the human FRG1 gene during primate evolution. *Gene*, **227**, 79–88.

Griggs, R.C., Tawil, R., McDermott, M., Forrester, J., Figlewicz, D., and Weiffenbach, B. (1995) Monozygotic twins with facioscapulohumeral dystrophy (FSHD): implications for genotype/phenotype correlation. *Muscle & Nerve*, **2**, S50–S55.

Henikoff, S. (1990). Position effect variegation after 60 years. *Trends in Genetics*, **6**, 422–6.

Hewitt, J.E., Lyle, R., Clark, L.N., Valleley, E.M., Wright, T.J., Wijmenga, C. *et al.* (1994). Analysis of tandem repeat locus D4Z4 associated with facioscapulohumeral muscular dystrophy. *Human Molecular Genetics*, **3**, 1287–95.

Horan, M.P., Cooper, D.N., and Upadhyaya, M. (2000). Hypermethylation of the neurofibromatosis type 1 (NF1) gene promoter is not a common event in the inactivation of the NF1 gene in NF1-specific tumours. *Human Genetics*, **107**, 33–9.

Hsu, Y.D., Kao, M.C., Shyu, W.C., Lin, J.C., Huang, N.E., Sun, H.F. *et al.* (1997). Application of chromosome 4q35-qter marker (pFR-1) for DNA rearrangement of facioscapulohumeral muscular dystrophy patients in Taiwan. *Journal of Neurological Science*, **149**, 73–9.

Jardine, P., Koch, M.C., Lunt, P.W., Maynard, J., Bathke, K.D., Harper, P.S., and Upadhyaya, M. (1994). *De novo* facioscapulohumeral muscular dystrophy defined by DNA probe p13E11 (D4F104S1). *Archives of Diseases in Childhood*, **71**, 221–7.

Kissel, J.T., McDermott, M.P., and Natarajan, R. *et al.* (1998). Pilot trial of albuterol in facioscapulohumeral muscular dystrophy. *Neurology*, **50**, 1402–6.

Kissel, J.T. (1999). Facioscapulohumeral dystrophy. *Seminars in Neurology*, **19**, 35–43.

Kleinjan, D.J. and van Heyningen, V. (1998). Position effect in human genetic diseases. *Human Molecular Genetics*, **7**, 1611–8.

Kohler, J., Rupilius, B., Otto, M., Bathke, K., and Koch, M.C. (1996). Germline mosaicism in 4q35 facioscapulohumeral muscular dystrophy (FSHD1A) occurring predominantly in oogenesis. *Human Genetics*, **98**, 485–90.

Kondo, T., Bobek, M.P., Kuick, R., Lamb, B., Zhu, X., Narayan, A. *et al.* (2000). Whole-genome methylation scan in ICF syndrome: hypomethylation of non-satellite DNA repeats D4Z4 and NBL2. *Human Molecular Genetics*, **9**, 597–604.

Laforet, P., de Toma, C., Eyward, B., Becane, H. M., Jeanpierre, M., Fardeau, M., and Duboc, D. (1998). Cardiac involvement in genetically confirmed facioscapulohumeral muscular dystrophy (FSHD). *Neurology*, **51**, 1454–6.

Landouzy, L. and Dejerine, J. (1885). De la myopathie atrophique progressive. *Revues Medicales Francaises*, **5**, 81, 253.

Lane, P.W., Beamer, T.C., and Myers, D.D. (1976). Myodystrophy, a new myopathy on chromosome 8 of the mouse. *Journal of Heredity*, **67**, 135–8.

Lauderdale, J.D., Wilensky, J.S., Oliver, E.R., Walton, D.S., and Glaser, T. (2000). 3′ deletions cause aniridia by preventing *PAX6* gene expression. *Proceedings of the National Academy of Sciences of the USA*, **97**, 13755–9.

Lee, J.H., Goto, K., Matsuda, C., and Arahata, K. (1995). Characterisation of a tandemly repeated 3.3 kb *Kpn*I unit in the facioscapulohumeral muscular dystrophy (FSHD) gene region on chromosome 4q35. *Muscle & Nerve*, suppl. 2: S6–S13.

Lemmers, R.J., van der Maarel, S.M., van Deutekom, J.C., van der Wielen, M.J., Deidda, G., Dauwerse, H.G. *et al.* (1998). Inter- and intrachromosomal sub-telomeric rearrangements on 4q35: implications for facioscapulohumeral muscular dystrophy (FSHD) aetiology and diagnosis. *Human Molecular Genetics*, **7**, 1207–14.

Lemmers, R.J.L.F., de Kievit, P., van Geel, M., van der Wielen, M.J.R., Bakker, E., Padberg, G.W. *et al.* (2000). *Xap*I improves diagnosis of facioscapulohumeral muscular dystrophy (FSHD). Presented at the FSHD International Consortium Research Meeting, Philadelphia, USA.

Lunt, P.W. and Harper, P.S. (1991). Genetic counselling in facioscapulohumeral muscular dystrophy. *Journal of Medical Genetics*, **28**, 655–64.

Lunt, P., Jardine, P.E., Koch, M., Maynard, J., Osborn, M., Williams, M. *et al.* (1995a). Phenotypic-genotypic correlation will assist genetic counselling in 4q35-facioscapulohumeral muscular dystrophy. *Muscle & Nerve*, suppl. 2, S103–S109.

Lunt, P.W., Jardine, P.E., Koch, M.C., Maynard, J., Osborn, M., Williams, M., *et al.* (1995b). Correlation between fragment size at D4F104S1 and age at onset or at wheelchair use with a possible generational-effect, accounts for much phenotypic variation in 4q35-facioscapulo-humeral muscular dystrophy (FSHD). *Human Molecular Genetics*, **4**, 951–8.

Lyle, R., Wright, T.J., Clark, L.N., and Hewitt, J.E. (1995). The FSHD associated repeat, D4Z4, is a member of a dispersed family of homeobox-containing repeats, subsets of which are clustered on the short arms of the acrocentric chromosomes. *Genomics*, **28**, 389–97.

Mathews, K.D., Rapisarda, D., Bailey, H.L., Murray, J.C., Schleper, R.L., and Smith, R. (1995). Phenotypic and pathological evaluation of the *myd* mouse, a candidate model for facioscapulohumeral dystrophy. *Journal of Neuropathology and Experimental Neurology*, **54**, 601–6.

Mathews, K. (1999). D4Z4 represses gene transcription in *Drosophila*. Presented at the FSHD Consortium in San Franscisco at the American Society of Human Genetics.

Muira, K., Kumagai, T., Matsumoto, A., Iriyama, E., Watanabe, K., Goto, K., and Arahata, K. (1998). Two cases of chromosome 4q35-linked early onset facioscapulohumeral muscular dystrophy with mental retardation and epilepsy. *Neuropaediatrics*, **29**, 239–41.

Munsat, T.L. (1986). Facioscapulohumeral dystrophy and the scapuloperoneal syndrome. In Engel, A.G., Banker, B.O. eds. *Myology*, McGraw Hill, New York.

Osborn, M.J., Cooper, D.N., and Upadhyaya, M. (1999). Methylation studies in Facioscapulohumeral Muscular Dystrophy. *American Society of Human Genetics*, **65**, A2748.

Padberg, G.W. (1982). Facioscapulohumeral disease. MD Thesis, Leiden University.

Padberg, G.W. (1998). Facioscapulohumeral muscular dystrophy. In *Neuromuscular Disorders. Clinical and Molecular Genetics* (ed. A.E.H. Emery), pp. 105–21. Wiley, Chichester.

Padberg, G.W., Vogels, O.J.M., and van der Kooi, E.L. (1998). The clinical picture of FSHD. *Muscle & Nerve*, suppl. 7, S25.

Rogers, M.T., Zhao, F., Harper, P.S., and Stephen, S.D. (2000). Hearing impairment in FSHD. (submitted)

Sarfarazi, M., Upadhyaya, M., Padberg, G., Pericak-Vance, M., Siddique, T., Lucotte, G., Lunt, P. (1989). An exclusion map for facioscapulohumeral (Landouzy-Dejerine) disease. *Journal of Medical Genetics*, **26**, 481–4.

Sarfarazi, M., Wijmenga, C., Upadhyaya, M., Weiffenbach, B., Hyser, C., Mathews, K. *et al.* (1992). Regional mapping of facioscapulohumeral muscular dystrophy gene on 4q35-combined analysis of an international consortium. *American Journal of Human Genetics*, **51**, 396–403.

Spofford, J.B. (1976). Position-effect variegation in *Drosophila*. In *Genetics and Biology of Drosophila*, vol. 1c, (eds. M. Ashburner and E. Novitski), pp. 955–1019. Academic Press, London.

Tawil, R., Storvick, D., Feasby, T.E., Weiffenbach, B., and Griggs, R.C. (1993). Extreme variability of expression in monozygotic twins with FSH muscular dystrophy. *Neurology*, **43**, 345–8.

Tawil, R., Myers, G.J., Weiffenbach, B., and Griggs, R.C. (1995). Scapuloperoneal syndromes. Absence of linkage to the 4q35 FSHD locus. *Archives of Neurology*, **52**, 1069–72.

Tawil, R., Forrester, J., Griggs, R.C., Mendell, J., Kissel, J., McDermott, M. *et al.* (1996). Evidence for anticipation and association of deletion size with severity in facioscapulohumeral muscular dystrophy. *Annals of Neurology*, **39**, 744–8.

Tawil, R., McDermott, M.P., Pandya, S., King, W., Kissel, J., Mendell, J.R., and Griggs, R.C. (1997). A pilot trial of prednisone in facioscapulohumeral muscular dystrophy. *Neurology*, **48**, 46–9.

Tawil, R., Figlewicz, D.A., Griggs, R.C., Weiffenbach, B. and the FSH consortium (1998). Facioscapulohumeral dystrophy: a distinct regional myopathy with a novel pathogenesis. *Annals of Neurology*, **43**, 279–82.

Tupler, R., Bernardinelli, A., Barbierato, L., Frants, R., Hewitt, J.E., Lanzi, G. *et al.* (1996). Monosomy of distal 4q does not cause facioscapulohumeral muscular dystrophy. *Journal of Medical Genetics*, **33**, 366–70.

Tupler, R., Barbierato, L., Memmi, M., Sewry, C.A., De Grandis, D., Maraschio, P. *et al.* 1998). Identical *de novo* mutation at the D4F104S1 locus in monozygotic male twins affected by facioscapulohumeral muscular dystrophy (FSHD) with different clinical expression. *Journal of Medical Genetics*, **35**, 778–83.

Tupler, R., Perini, G., Pellegrino, M.A., and Green, M.R. (1999). Profound misregulation of muscle-specific gene expression in facioscapulohumeral muscular dystrophy. *Proceedings of National Academy of Sciences, USA*, **96**, 12650–4.

Twyman, R.S., Harper, G.D., and Elgar, M.A. (1996). Thoracoscapular fusion in facioscapulohumeral dystrophy: clinical view of a new surgical method. *Journal of Shoulder and Elbow Surgery*, **5**, 201–5.

Upadhyaya, M., Sarfarazi, M., Lunt, P.W., Broadhead, W., and Harper, P.S. (1989). A genetic linkage study of facioscapulohumeral disease with 24 polymorphic DNA probes. *Journal of Medical Genetics*, **26**, 490–3.

Upadhyaya, M., Lunt, P.W., Sarfarazi, M., Broadhead, W., Daniels, J., Owen, M., and Harper, P.S. (1990). DNA marker applicable to presymptomatic and prenatal diagnosis of facioscapulohumeral disease. *Lancet*, **336**, 1320–1.

Upadhyaya, M., Lunt, P.W., Sarfarazi, M., Broadhead, W., Daniels, J., Owen, M., and Harper, P.S. (1991). A closely linked DNA marker for facioscapulohumeral disease on chromosome 4q. *Journal of Medical Genetics*, **28**, 665–71.

Upadhyaya, M., Lunt, P., Sarfarazi, M., Broadhead, W., Farnham, J., Harper, P.S. (1992). The mapping of chromosome 4q markers in relation to facioscapulohumeral muscular dystrophy (FSHD). *Americal Journal of Human Genetics*, **51**, 404–10.

Upadhyaya, M., Jardine, P., Maynard, J., Farnham, J., Sarfarazi, M., Wijmenga, C. *et al.* (1993). Molecular analysis of British facioscapulohumeral dystrophy families for 4q DNA rearrangements. *Human Molecular Genetics*, **2**, 981–7.

Upadhyaya, M., Maynard, J., Osborn, M., Jardine, P., Harper, P.S., and Lunt, P.W. (1995a). Germinal mosaicism in facioscapulohumeral muscular dystrophy (FSHD). *Muscle & Nerve*, suppl. 2, S45–S49.

Upadhyaya, M., Osborn, M., Maynard, J., Altherr, M., Ikeda, J., and Harper, P.S. (1995b). Towards the finer mapping of facioscapulohumeral muscular dystrophy at 4q35: Construction of a laser microdissection library. *American Journal of Medical Genetics*, **60**, 244–51.

Upadhyaya, M., Maynard, J., Rogers, M.T., Lunt, P.W., Jardine, P., Ravine, D., and Harper, P.S. (1997). Improved molecular diagnosis of facioscapulohumeral muscular dystrophy (FSHD): validation of the differential double digestion for FSHD. *Journal of Medical Genetics*, **34**, 476–9.

Upadhyaya, M., MacDonald, M., and Ravine, D. (1999). Molecular prenatal diagnosis in 12 facioscapulohumeral muscular dystrophy (FSHD) families. *Prenatal Diagnosis*, **19**, 959–65.

Upadhyaya, M. and Osborn, M. (2000). Methylation studies in the FSHD candidate region. Presented at the The Third International Symposium on the Cause and Treatment of Facioscapulohumeral Muscular Dystrophy in Washington.

Van der Kooi, A.J., Visser, M.C., Rosenberg, N., van den Berg-vos, R., Wokke, J.H.J., Bakker, E., and de Visser, M. (2000). Extension of the clinical range of facioscapulohumeral dystrophy: report of six cases. *Journal of Neurology, Neurosurgery and Psychiatry*, **69**, 114–6.

Van der Maarel, S.M., Deidda, G., Lemmers, R.J., Bakker, B., van der Wielen M., Sandkuijl, L., Hewitt, J.E. *et al.* (1999). A new dosage test for subtelomeric 4; 10 translocations improves conventional diagnosis of facioscapulohumeral muscular dystrophy (FSHD). *Journal of Medical Genetics*, **36**, 823–8.

Van der Maarel, S., Deidda, G., Lemmers, R.J., van Overveld, P.G., van der Wielen, M., Hewitt, J.E. *et al.* (2000). *De novo* facioscapulohumeral muscular dystrophy: frequent somatic mosaicism, sex-dependent phenotype and the role of mitotic transchromosomal repeat interaction between chromosomes 4 and 10. *American Journal of Human Genetics*, **66**, 26–35.

van Deutekom, J.C.T., Wijmenga, C., van Tienhoven, E.A.E., Gruter, A.M., Hewitt, J.E., Padberg, G.W. *et al.* (1993). FSHD associated DNA rearrangements are due to deletions of integral copies of a 3.3 kb tandemly repeated unit. *Human Molecular Genetics*, **2**, 2037–42.

van Deutekom, J.C.T., Hofker, M.H., Romberg, S., van Geel, M., Rommens, J., Wright, T.J. *et al.* (1995). Search for the FSHD gene using cDNA selection in a region spanning 100 kb on chromosome 4q35. *Muscle & Nerve*, suppl. 2, S19–S26.

van Deutekom, J.C.T., Bakker, E., Lemmers, R.J.L.F., van der Wielen, M.J.R., Bik, E., Hofker, M.H. *et al.* (1996a). Evidence for subtelomeric exchange of 3.3 kb tandemly repeated units between chromosomes 4q35 and 10q26: implications for genetic counselling and etiology of FSHD1. *Human Molecular Genetics*, **5**, 1997–2003.

van Deutekom, J.C.T., Lemmers, R.J.L.F., Grewal, P.K., van Geel, M., Romberg, S., Dauwerse, H.G. *et al.* (1996b). Identification of the first gene (FRG1) from the FSHD region on human chromosome 4q35. *Human Molecular Genetics*, **5**, 581–90.

van Geel, M., Heather, L.J., Lyle, R., Hewitt, J.E., Frants, R.R., and de Jong, P. (1999). The FSHD region on human chromosome 4q35 contains potential coding regions among pseudogenes and a high density of repeat elements. *Genomics*, **61**, 55–65.

van Overveld, P.G.M., Lemmers, R.J.LF., Deidda, G., Sandkuijl, L., Padberg, G.W., Frants, R.R., and van der Maarel, S.M. (2000). Interchromosomal repeat array interactions between chromosomes 4 and 10: a model for subtelomeric plasticity. *Human Molecular Gßenetics*, **9**, 2879–84.

Wijmenga, C., Frants, R.R., Brouwer, O.F., Moerer, P., Weber, J.L., and Padberg, G.W., (1990). Location of facioscapulohumeral muscular dystrophy gene on chromosome 4. *Lancet*, **336**, 651–3.

Wijmenga, C., Hewitt, J.E., Sandkuijl, L.A., Clark, L.N., Wright, T.J., Dauwerse, H.G. *et al.* (1992). Chromosome 4q DNA rearrangements associated with facioscapulohumeral muscular dystrophy. *Nature Genetics*, **2**, 26–30.

Wijmenga, C., van Deutekom, J.C.T., Hewitt, J.E., Padberg, G.W., van Ommen, G.B., Hofker, M.H., and Frants, R.R. (1994) Pulsed-field gel electrophoresis of the D4F104S1 locus reveals the size and the parental origin of the facioscapulohumeral muscular dystrophy (FSHD)-associated deletions. *Genomics*, **19**, 21–6.

Wilhelmsen, K.C., Blake, D.M., Lynch, T., Mabutas, J., De Vera, M., Neystat, M. *et al.* (1996). Chromosome 12 linked autosomal dominant scapuloperoneal muscular dystrophy. *Annals of Neurology*, **39**, 507–20.

Winokur, S.T., Bengtsson, U., Feddersen, J., Mathews, K.D., Weiffenbach, B., Bailey, H. *et al.* (1996). The evolutionary distribution and structural organisation of the homeobox–containing repeat D4Z4 indicates a functional role for the ancestral copy in the FSHD region. *Human Molecular Genetics*, **5**, 1567–75.

Wright, T.J., Wijmenga, C., Clark, L.N., Frants, R.R., Williamson, R., and Hewitt, J.E. (1993) Fine mapping of the FSHD region orientates the rearranged fragment detected by the probe p13E–11. *Human Molecular Genetics*, **2**, 1673–8.

Zatz, M., Marie, S.K., Passos-Bueno, M.R., Vainzof, M., Campiotto, S., Cerqueira, A., *et al.* (1995). High proportion of new mutations and possible anticipation in Brazilian facioscapulohumeral muscular dystrophy families. *American Journal of Human Genetics*, **56**, 99–105.

Zatz, M., Marie, S.K., Cerquiera, A., Vainzof, M., Pavanello, R.C.M., Passos-Bueno, M.R. (1998). The facioscapulohumeral muscular dystrophy (FSHD) gene affects males more severely and more frequently than females. *American Journal of Medical Genetics*, **77**, 155–61.

Chapter 9

Distal muscular dystrophy

Bjarne Udd and Hannu Somer

Distal myopathy—distal dystrophies

Distal myopathies are considered rare disorders, and this is probably true, although, there are no genetic epidemiological studies available. Developments during the past decade with a number of reports on new phenotypes suggest that distal myopathies may be less rare than previously considered and maybe not always well understood. Many of the disorders are relatively benign diseases and, therefore, may have escaped diagnostic procedures. Many patients with distal myopathy have earlier been considered to be cases of type 2 Charcot–Marie-Tooth disease. This is still a major differential diagnostic challenge.

Distal myopathy has prevailed as the main general term used for this group of primary myopathies. Since they are progressive and genetic disorders, the use of distal dystrophies as the collective term is also correct. In fact, much of the pathology in affected muscles shows findings compatible with dystrophic changes, including fibre necrosis, regeneration, splitting and replacement by fat and connective tissue. During the past decade distal myopathies have entered the new field of molecular genetic clarification. All major entities previously defined on clinical grounds have proved to be distinct categories also by molecular genetic resolution.

Clinical phenotypes of distal myopathy

Welander distal myopathy (WDM)

In 1951 the Swedish neurologist published a series of 249 patients with distal muscle weakness entitled 'Myopathia distalis tarda hereditaria' (Welander 1951). Her patients were all from a limited geographic area to the north of Stockholm. The disease appeared around the age of 40–50 years with progressive clumsiness and weakness of hand muscles. Finger extensors were more affected than flexors. Muscle atrophy was slowly progressive involving both posterior and anterior compartments of the lower leg resulting in stumbling gait. Deep tendon reflexes were preserved at an early stage of the disease. Many patients complained of increased cold sensation in their hands.

Histopathological findings show rimmed vacuoles and general myopathic-dystrophic features including increase of connective tissue and fat (Borg et al. 1989; 1993).

Electromyography (EMG) is usually myopathic at an early stage, and by MRI or CT fatty degeneration in anterior and posterior lower leg muscles develop along with clinical weakness. Serum CK is slightly elevated or normal (Åhlberg *et al.* 1994).

The disease may cause functional disability, because of severe hand muscle involvement in elderly patients. WDM is known to exist in neighbouring countries, but reports from more distant countries are few. Inheritance of WDM is autosomal dominant and linkage was recently established on chromosome 2p (Åhlberg *et al.* 1999).

Tibial muscular dystrophy (TMD)—late onset distal myopathy (LODM)

TMD was first described in 66 Finnish patients by Udd *et al.* (1993). Symptoms with gradually reduced dorsiflexion of ankles appear after the age of 35 years, and in mild cases the onset may be delayed well into the seventh decade (Fig. 9.1). Patients can no longer stand and walk on their heels and mild to moderate foot drop will develop. Progression is slow and patients usually maintain their walking ability, although they may need a cane in later years. Upper extremities are clinically not involved and extensor digitorum brevis muscles are normal. Deep tendon reflexes are preserved. Muscle biopsy shows a spectrum of changes depending on the stage of the disease process and the involvement of the particular muscle. In a large series of biopsies from tibial anterior muscle, rimmed vacuoles were detected in the majority of patients (Udd *et al.* 1998).

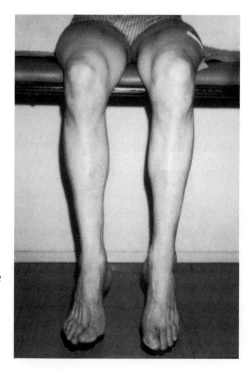

Fig. 9.1 Atrophy of tibialis anterior on both sides with mild foot drop in a male patient with TMD at the age of 52 years. Note prominence of the anterior edge of the tibial bone. Symptoms of ankle dorsiflexion weakness had been slowly progressive over 15 years.

EMG shows myopathic changes with reduced amount of low amplitude motor unit potentials, frequent fibrillations and occasional complex repetitive discharges in the anterior tibial muscle. Imaging with CT/MRI enforce the clinical impression of selective muscle involvement with fatty degenerative changes in the anterior compartment of lower legs (Fig. 9.2). Patchy lesions in the hamstrings, minor gluteus and calf muscles may occur (Udd *et al.* 1991). Serum CK is slightly elevated or normal.

TMD is inherited as an autosomal dominant trait and the gene has been mapped to chromosome 2q (Haravuori *et al.* 1998a). TMD is not rare in Finland with a prevalence above 6/100 000. Descendants of Finnish immigrants with TMD have been diagnosed in Sweden, Germany and Canada. One completely unrelated family with TMD and confirmed linkage to the TMD locus on 2q has been reported from northern France (deSeze *et al.* 1998).

In 1974 Markesbery and Griggs described an American family of French–English ancestry with LODM. Symptoms were largely similar to the later described TMD. Weakness started with mild drop foot after the age of 40 years. At variance with TMD, progression to the proximal muscles was more evident in the LODM family and patients developed atrophy in the upper limb and intrinsic muscles. Cardiomyopathy was confirmed on autopsy in one patient. LODM has been linked to the TMD locus on 2q suggesting that the two disorders may be allelic (Haravuori *et al.* 1998b).

Distal myopathy with rimmed vacuoles (DMRV)

In 1981 Nonaka *et al.* described a few patients from two families who developed weakness of the anterior compartment muscles of the lower legs in early adulthood. In contrast to the previous categories of WDM and TMD this disorder showed an autosomal recessive mode of inheritance. Sunohara *et al.* (1989) reviewed 37 Japanese patients and further described the phenotype. Gait disturbances were the first symptoms and besides the lower leg muscle weakness, neck flexor muscles and iliopsoas muscles were also affected. In the upper limbs distal muscles were more severely involved than the proximal ones. Patients display a combination of waddling and steppage gait. The disease

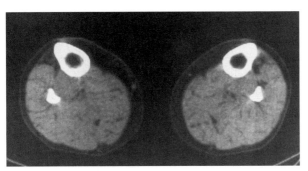

Fig. 9.2 CT-scan with transverse section of the thickest part of the lower legs in a 69 years old female patient with TMD: highly selective fatty degeneration of tibialis anterior bilaterally and compensatory bulging of the long toe extensor muscle into the degenerated anterior tibial compartment.

is fairly progressive causing patients to become non-ambulant within a time interval of 12 years (Nonaka *et al.* 1998).

Needle EMG shows myopathic changes either alone or in combination with mild neurogenic findings. Serum CK is slightly elevated or normal. Sporadic cases have been diagnosed outside the Japanese population in various neuromuscular centres. The disease was mapped to chromosome 9p1-q1 (Ikeuchi *et al.* 1997). This locus shows large overlap with the locus assigned for recessive hereditary inclusion body myopathy (AR h-IBM) (Mitrani-Rosenbaum *et al.* 1996)

Miyoshi myopathy (MM)

The Japanese neurologist Miyoshi has described an early adult onset distal myopathy with initial weakness and atrophy of the calf muscles (Miyoshi *et al.* 1986). The primary study was based on clinical material of 17 patients and autosomal recessive inheritance was shown. Onset is around the age of 20 years (15–30) with difficulty in climbing stairs and hopping due to reduced push off caused by pronounced muscle weakness and atrophy in the calfs. In the upper extremities the forearm muscles become involved and grip strength is reduced, although, small hand muscles are relatively spared. The disease is moderately progressive. After 10–15 years of disease duration, patients usually needed the help of a cane. After 20–25 years some of the patients were confined to the wheelchair.

Typical with MM is the very high CK activity; the values exceeding the upper normal limit by 10–100 times. The early and severe involvement of calf muscles is usually evident on inspection and easily established by CT or MRI. Gastrocnemius muscle biopsy shows necrotic fibres and dystrophic changes whereas a biopsy from other muscles may show mild changes of nonspecific myopathy. Rimmed vacuoles were not observed.

Originally, MM was thought to be relatively rare and occur mainly in the Japanese population. This has turned out not to be the case. There are several reports on MM patients from various European, American and African countries (Argov *et al.* 2000; Eymard *et al.* 2000; Barohn *et al.* 1991). In 1995 Bejaoui *et al.* mapped MM to a locus on chromosome 2p, overlapping the locus already defined for limb-girdle muscular dystrophy type 2B (LGMD2B). Later studies soon showed that both disorders are caused by mutations in the novel muscle gene *dysferlin*, which is associated with membranes of the muscle cell and organelles.

Early onset dominant distal myopathy (MPD1)

In 1995 Laing *et al.* published linkage assignment to chromosome 14q for a dominant distal myopathy occurring in one Australian family. Onset of symptoms varied from infancy to early adulthood with mild foot drop as the leading sign. On examination there was involvement of distal upper limb, sternocleidomastoid muscles and slight weakness of face and tongue. The disease was very slowly progressive. Muscle biopsy findings in proximal muscles revealed nonspecific myopathic changes. Rimmed vacuolar fibres were not observed.

Clinical findings and evolution of the disease is similar to the disorder published in an almost 100-year-old description of a single patient reported to have had distal myopathy (Gowers 1902). Scoppetta *et al.* (1995) described an Italian family with onset of mild foot drop in childhood and later involvement of neck flexor, proximal and facial muscles. Indications for linkage to chromosome 14q were found in this Italian and in another German family presenting a similar early onset distal myopathy (Voit *et al.* 2001).

Other phenotypes in single families

Distal myopathy with sarcoplasmic bodies

Edström *et al.* (1980) described one family with autosomal dominant distal myopathy in three generations. Weakness and atrophy started in hand muscles, thenar and finger flexors around the age of 40 years. The disease progressed to involve proximal muscles and 15 years later patients lost their walking ability. Some had cardiomyopathy and specific features were found on muscle biopsy showing sarcoplasmic bodies with abundant intermediate sized filaments and myofibrillar degeneration. Molecular genetic investigations are in progress.

Distal myopathy with pes cavus and areflexia

A large Italian family with an autosomal dominant distal myopathy presenting unusual pes cavus and early loss of deep tendon reflexes has been described (Servidei *et al.* 1999). Symptoms and signs varied within the family; as with the age of onset between 10 and 50 years. Both anterior and posterior compartments in the lower legs were involved and patients had vocal cord weakness and dysphagia. Serum CK was mildly elevated and the course of the disease mild to moderate. Some patients were nonambulant in their 60s. Muscle biopsy showed rimmed vacuolar myopathic-dystrophic features. Molecular genetic linkage studies disclosed linkage to a new locus for distal myopathies on chromosome 19p.

Distal myopathy with vocal cord and pharyngeal weakness (MPD2)

Recently a large American family was reported with late onset dominant distal myopathy and with involvement of vocal cord and pharyngeal muscles (Feit *et al.* 1998). Symptoms varied among the family members and the progression regarding walking ability was mild. CK was slightly elevated and histopathology showed rimmed vacuolar myopathic changes. The size of the family allowed genetic linkage of the disorder to a locus on 5q, that overlaps the locus previously assigned for autosomal dominant LGMD1A (Speer *et al.* 1992).

Dominant adult onset distal myopathy

In 1999 Felice *et al.* described an American family with autosomal dominant distal myopathy. Patients developed weakness of anterior compartment lower leg muscles in adulthood. Distal upper limb muscles and proximal muscles were involved later. The overall progression of the disease was moderate to slow. Inclusions or rimmed vacuoles were not observed on muscle biopsy showing nonspecific myopathy. Molecular genetic linkage studies excluded all five distal myopathy loci, indicating yet another gene responsible for this disorder.

Very late onset dominant distal myopathy

In one French family described by Penisson-Besnier *et al.* (1998) patients developed weakness and atrophy of lower leg muscles, predominantly in the posterior compartment, in their 60s and 70s. Progression was moderate and walking difficulties occurred 10 years after onset of weakness. Remarkable findings on deltoid muscle biopsy were rimmed and nonrimmed vacuoles and sarcoplasmic masses immunoreactive for desmin and dystrophin. Filaments of 15–20 nm were encountered on electron microscopy and serum CK was slightly elevated.

Juvenile onset dominant distal myopathy

Three members of an Austrian family had onset of lower leg anterior compartment weakness in their teens (Zimprich *et al.* 2000). The course of the disease was mild. Facial or sternocleidomastoid muscle weakness did not develop over 20 years of disease duration. The mode of inheritance appeared to be autosomal dominant and CK values were slightly or moderately increased up to eight-fold the upper normal limit. Myopathic changes and rimmed vacuolar fibres were encountered on muscle biopsy.

Juvenile–adult variable onset distal myopathy

In 1971 Sumner *et al.* described a British family having autosomal dominant distal myopathy with variable presentation. The age of onset varied from 15 to 50 years. Three patients had initial weakness in their hands, more evident in finger extensors than in the flexor muscles, whereas two patients had weakness and atrophy starting in the anterior compartment muscles of lower legs. Progression was slow and patients remained ambulant. EMG and muscle biopsy findings were considered purely myopathic although the methodology did not entirely correspond to the currently used methods.

New adult onset dominant distal myopathy in a Finnish family (MPD3)

Recently a new type of distal myopathy was detected in a Finnish family. (Mahjneh *et al.* 2000). Onset of weakness and atrophy occurred after age 30 and varied within the family; some had onset in the intrinsic hand muscles and others in the anterior lower leg muscles asymmetrically. In the single individual a distinction between WDM or TMD was very difficult. Atrophy of the extensor digitorum brevis muscles makes a difference to TMD and the initial symptom of index finger extensor weakness was not as marked as in WDM. Rimmed vacuolar fibres on muscle biopsy were regularly observed, occasionally with eosinophilic inclusions. Patients in this family lack the founder haplotype for WDM and the TMD locus 2q was excluded by linkage.

Distal phenotypes in other myopathies

Desmin related disorders—myofibrillar myopathies (MFM)

One of the first well described families reported as a distal myopathy was a large American-European family of Jewish ethnicity (Milhorat *et al.* 1943). This family was studied later with new methodology and histopathological findings of desmin accumulation were reported in 1994 (Horowitz and Schmalbruch 1994). Recently molecular genetic studies have disclosed a mutation in the desmin gene as the cause of the disease (Sjöberg *et al.* 1999). Patients had onset of weakness in the anterior compartment of their lower legs between 25 and 45 years and later of hands and fingers both extensors and flexors. Some patients developed cardiac conduction disturbances very early in the course of the disease, requiring a pace-maker. Walking ability was lost after 6–10 years from onset.

In families with desmin related disease caused by mutations in the αB-crystallin gene (Vicart *et al.* 1998), distal weakness may dominate the involvement of skeletal muscles, although patients have cardiomyopathy as the leading clinical problem (Fardeau *et al.* 1978). The same was true in a Swedish family with MFM without defect in desmin or αB-crystallin, but linked to a new locus on chromosome 10q (Melberg *et al.* 1999)

Oculopharyngodistal myopathy (OPDM)

So far reported in a few Japanese patients only is a very late onset distal myopathy with prominent weakness of extraocular and pharyngeal muscles causing ptosis and dysphagia. Distal atrophies without specific predilection occurred in both upper and lower limbs. The autosomal dominant disorder was slowly progressive with preserved walking ability. Rimmed vacuolar histopathological findings were shown on muscle biopsy (Satoyoshi *et al.* 1977). One sibpair in a consanguineous family has been reported, suggesting also recessive inheritance (Uyama *et al.* 1998).

Distal presentation in LGMD2G

LGMD2G is a recessive dystrophy usually presenting with a conventional LGMD pattern of severe proximal weakness in adolescence. In some patients, however, at onset, weakness and atrophy may be seen predominantly in the anterior distal leg muscles. This variable presentation may occur even within the same family. Muscle biopsy findings show rimmed vacuolar pathology, which is unusual in the LGMD2 group of disorders (Moreira *et al.* 1997).

Classification of distal myopathies—Table 9.1(a–c)

Until 1995 all classification of the different disorders relied on well documented clinical and genetic characteristics. Four major entities were previously defined on these grounds: WDM, TMD/LODM, DMRV and MM (Somer 1995). During the past few years advances in molecular genetic research have shown that these entities now also can be determined by molecular genetic linkage data, and in the case of MM by mutations in

Table 9.1 Classification of distal myopathies (AD, autosomal dominant; AR, autosomal recessive)

	Code	Trait	Locus gene	Onset age	CK	Initial muscle weakness
(a) Definite entities						
Welander distal myopathy	WDM	AD	2p	>30–40	1–4x	Finger, hand extensors
Tibial muscular dystrophy	TMD	AD	2p	>35	1–4x	Anterior lower legs
Late onset distal myopathy	LODM	AD	2p	>40	1–3x	
Nonaka early adult distal myopathy	DMRV	AR	9p-q	15–30	1–5x	Anterior lower legs
Miyoshi early adult distal myopathy	MM	AR	2p dysferlin	15–25	10–100x	Posterior lower legs
Early onset distal myopathy	MPD1	AD	14q	2–25	1–3x	Anterior lower legs
(b) Single families						
Distal myopathy with sarcoplasmic bodies		AD		>40	1–3x	Thenar, finger flexors
Distal myopathy with pes Cavus and areflexia		AD	19p	15–50	1–3x	Lower legs, dysphonia and dysphagia
Distal myopathy with vocal cord and pharyngeal signs	MPD2	AD	5q	35–60	1–8x	Asymmetric legs and hands
Adult onset distal myopathy		AD		20–40	2–6x	Foot drop + proximal
Very late distal myopathy		AD		50–60	1–2x	Posterior lower legs
Juvenile onset distal myopathy		AD		14	1–8x	Anterior lower legs
Variable onset distal myopathy		AD		15–50		Forearm or lower legs extensors > flexors
New Finnish distal myopathy	MPD3	AD		>30	1–3x	Hands or anterior lower legs
(c) Distal phenotypes in other myopathies						
Myofibrillar myopathy – desmin related myopathies	MFM	AD	Desmin, αB-crystallin	20–40	1–4x	Lower legs, hands + cardiomyopathy
Oculopharyngeal distal muscular dystrophy	OPDM	AD		>40	1–4x 1–3x	Lower legs and hands + ptosis
Distal myopathy in telethoninopathy		AR	Telethonin 17q	10–15	3–17x	Anterior lower legs

Table 9.2 Differential diagnosis in distal myopathies

Charcot-marie-tooth disease (neuronal), CMT2
Distal spinal muscular atrophy
Hereditary motor neuropathy, HMN
FSH dystrophy
Inclusion body myositis, IBM
Myotonic dystrophy, DM1
Scapuloperoneal syndromes
Central core disease
Nemaline myopathy
Debranching enzyme deficiency
Phosphorylase b kinase deficiency
Lipid storage myopathy

the responsible gene, dysferlin. In addition, chromosome 14 linked early onset dominant distal myopathy MPD1 can be considered an established definite entity.

There are many distal myopathies so far described in single families only. Clinical and molecular data suggest that these may be separate entities. Many muscle diseases may in some patients have an apparently distal clinical presentation, although another clinical or histopathological feature makes them to be classified on other grounds. These disorders will probably never be defined as distal myopathies and are listed here as: distal phenotypes in other myopathies.

Histopathology

The main findings on muscle biopsy in WDM were described already by Welander (1951), and were subsequently updated by using new methods (Edström *et al.* 1975; Borg *et al.* 1989; 1991; 1993; Lindberg *et al.* 1991) Tibialis anterior is the suggested muscle for biopsy. Taken at an early stage, before drop foot has evolved (usually between 25 and 45 years), muscle biopsy does not show significant structural abnormality although changes may be present on EMG. Later the muscle will show nonspecific myopathy: increased amount of internal nuclei and variation of fibre size, and rimmed vacuolar fibres. On electron microscopy the rimmed vacuoles appear as autophagic vacuoles with myeloid figures, small vesicles, debris material and filamentous inclusions (15–18 nm) similar to those in inclusion body myositis. Intranuclear inclusions have been observed (Borg *et al.* 1991; 1993; Lindberg *et al.* 1991). At the late stage there is a marked increase of fat and connective tissue. Specific findings to allow diagnosis on histopathological grounds are not known.

Muscle biopsy findings in TMD are fairly similar to those in WDM. Anterior tibial muscle shows early changes at least 10 years before clinical symptoms appear: scattered few necrotic fibres and increased amount of internal nuclei. With early weakness (usually between 35 and 45 years) dystrophic features are present (Fig. 9.3): large variation of fibre size, round and thin atrophic fibres without grouping, increased fat and connective tissue, fibre splits, rare necrotic fibres and regeneration, and, in the majority of patients

Fig. 9.3 Biopsy taken from tibialis anterior muscle in a 36 years old TMD male patient with early symptoms of ankle dorsiflexion weakness and inability to walk on his heels. General dystrophic features with increased variation in fibre size, fibre splitting, increased amount internalized nuclei, endomysial connective tissue, fat cells, and fibres with rimmed vacuoles (H&E 150×).

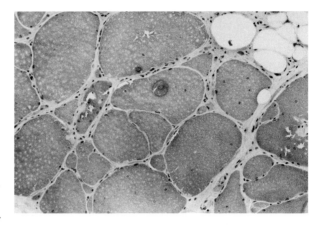

rimmed vacuolar degeneration (Partanen *et al.* 1994; Udd *et al.* 1998). After some 20 years from onset, the anterior tibial muscle shows endstage pathology with fat and connective tissue replacement. Ultrastructural findings consist of autophagic vacuoles not bound by any membrane, and occasional cytoplasmic filamentous (15–20 nm) inclusions (Udd *et al.* 1993). Proximal muscles and gastrocnemius muscle show normal or minimal myopathic findings. Interestingly, in the first described large consanguineous family, rimmed vacuoles were not observed on muscle biopsy, not even in some rare homozygotes with LGMD phenotype (Udd *et al.* 1991).

In the LODM family histopathological changes in proximal muscles were much more pronounced with both nonrimmed and rimmed vacuoles and dark cytoplasmic masses corresponding to granulofilamentous material on electron microscopy (Markesbery and Griggs 1974).

Frequent rimmed vacuoles on muscle biopsy is the main histopathological characteristic of DMRV (Nonaka *et al.* 1999). However, inflammatory infiltrates are not present. On electron microscopy the rimmed vacuoles in DMRV conform to the general aspects of autophagic vacuoles. By specific immunohistochemistry they are shown to contain both lysosomal constituents and also increased amounts of material needed for nonlysosomal degradation (Kumamoto *et al.* 1994; 2000).

In MM muscle biopsy shows nonspecific dystrophy. Rimmed vacuoles are not present, whereas necrotic and regenerating fibres are more common than in the other distal myopathies. Nonsense mutations in the dysferlin gene are responsible for pathogenesis, which is reflected by absent labelling of dysferlin on immunohistochemical stains with dysferlin antibodies (Matsuda *et al.* 1999). In sporadic patients with MM phenotype this will be the method of choice for differential diagnosis.

Finding excessive accumulation of desmin and bodies in muscle fibres is yet another direct clue for differential diagnosis in patients with sporadic or unknown familial distal myopathy phenotype, indicating MFM disorder. Fibre type specific changes have not been reported in distal myopathies.

Genetics and molecular biology

Although rimmed vacuoles are not a specific finding, they are much more frequently encountered in distal myopathies compared to the LGMDs. In those disorders which so far have been associated with specific gene loci, most of the corresponding gene products are sarcomeric-cytoplasmic proteins, and none of them is part of the dystrophin associated protein-complex. Dysferlin is associated with membranes of the sarcolemma and other organelles. Desmin, myotilin and telethonin are parts of the sarcomeric structure, and αB-crystallin is a cytoplasmic chaperone belonging to the family of heat-shock proteins.

Welander distal myopathy (WDM)

In WDM there is a unique core haplotype on 2p in all Swedish patients indicating one single founder mutation in the population. WDM patients in Finland also carry the identical haplotype (Åhlberg *et al.* 1999). In her thesis Welander described some rare patients as 'grossly atypical', and in one of these families both their parents were typical WDM patients. On clinical grounds these patients were considered probable homozygotes for the dominant gene (Welander 1957). This particular family is no longer available for molecular genetic studies. However, in one large family included in the primary linkage studies of WDM, one patient proved to be homozygote for the founder haplotype. Clinically this particular patient had a more severe phenotype and earlier involvement of proximal muscles. A number of genes at the 2p13 locus have been studied, so far without mutations (Åhlberg *et al.* 1999).

Tibial muscular dystrophy (TMD)

In TMD there is also one common haplotype for the linked 2q region among Finnish TMD patients (Haravuori *et al.* 1998b). In one large and consanguineous TMD family there were two different phenotypes: the common TMD distal myopathy and, in eight patients, a severe childhood onset LGMD type of disease. In accordance with the clinical genetic evaluation three of those available proved to be homozygous for the TMD founder haplotype (Udd *et al.* 1998). Thus, homozygosity for gene defects at the 2q locus is capable of causing yet another recessive limb-girdle dystrophy, LGMD2J (Haravuori *et al.* 2000). Patients in the LODM family have a different haplotype on 2q segregating with the disease, suggesting that TMD and the slightly different LODM might be allelic disorders. In the French TMD family patients had a different 2q haplotype.

Within the narrowed critical region only one muscle gene has been identified; the gene encoding the giant sarcomeric protein titin. Molecular studies in TMD have so far not been able to show mutations in titin, even though positional and functional molecular findings are suggestive. By Western blotting calpain3 was shown to be defect in the TMD haplotype homozygous patient with LGMD phenotype (Haravuori *et al.* 2001). Primary defects in the calpain3 gene cause LGMD2A. Since titin is known to bind calpain3, preventing it from rapid autodegradation, this secondary calpain3 defect in the homozygous patient further supports titin as the candidate gene in TMD. Apoptotic myonuclei and aberrations in the location of the signalling molecules nuclear factor kappaB (NF-κB) and its inhibitor kappaB (IκB), in congruence with previous studies in LGMD2A were also shown in TMD (Haravuori *et al.* 2001). Similar calpain3 defect and apoptic myonuclei were disclosed in the mdm-mouse, which is a natural mutant linked to chromosome 2 and thought to be a titin mutant, yet without known mutation (Haravuori *et al.* 2001). The linked chromosomal region of mdm-mouse is syntenic with the linked human TMD-region. Mdm-mouse could, therefore, be an animal model for TMD.

Dysferlinopathy—Miyoshi myopathy

Mutations in dysferlin have been shown to be responsible for both MM and LGMD2B. Details of the gene structure and detected mutations are reported in Chapter 7 in context with LGMD2B. Families have been published where these two phenotypes existed in different individuals within the same family (Iliaroshkin *et al.* 1996; Weiler *et al.* 1996). Why the same homozygous mutation is able to cause these different phenotypes is not understood. Interacting modifiers have been discussed (Weiler *et al.* 1999). In some patients with primary dysferlin mutation and absent dysferlin protein a secondary decrease of calpain3 has been observed (Anderson *et al.* 2000).

Recently, Illa *et al.* (2001) described a family with homozygous mutation in the dysferlin gene and a slightly different third phenotype. At onset patients had mild foot drop followed by rapid progression to the proximal muscles and disability. On imaging, however, severe fatty degenerative changes were shown in all lower leg muscles, both in the posterior and the anterior and lateral compartments. In some families with a slightly later onset of the disease linkage to a locus on chromosome 10 has been suggested (Linssen *et al.* 1998), indicating genetic heterogeneity.

Dysferlin is associated with membranes and regulated membrane fusion, and is not a component of the dystrophin associated protein complex at the sarcolemma. Partial reduction of sarcolemmal labelling and simultaneous increase of cytoplasmic reactivity of dysferlin has been observed in variable dystrophies (Piccolo *et al.* 2000). Whether these are significant regarding pathophysiology or are nonspecific secondary epiphenomenon is not clear.

LGMD1A

Independently of the linkage studies in LGMD1A and MPD2, Salmikangas *et al.* (1999) described a new sarcomeric protein, myotilin, and found that its genomic location also overlapped the 5q loci for LGMD1A and MPD2. Subsequently, a mutation in myotilin has been reported in one LGMD1A family (Hauser *et al.* 2000), while the situation in the MPD2 family has not been published.

LGMD2G

LGMD2G has been mapped to chromosome 17 and mutations in the sarcomeric protein telethonin (titin-cap, Tcap protein) were reported (Moreira *et al.* 1997). Telethonin is a ligand of the giant sarcomeric protein titin at the Z-disc end. The exact role of telethonin is not known. Interestingly, this is another gene to cause distal presentation coexisting with a proximal LGMD phenotype.

Therapy and management

There is no cure for any of the distal myopathies available. Distal myopathies are often relatively mild disorders with fairly late onset and slow progression. In WDM and TMD orthoses are commonly used for wrist and ankle stabilization. In DMRV and MM walking aids are needed, and in later adulthood corresponding equipment when ambulation is lost. Respiratory problems are hardly ever part of the disease evolution. Cardiomyopathy is more often seen in the MFMs than in the 'pure' distal myopathies. As a pilot intervention in TMD, tibial posterior tendon transposition to replace lost function of the anterior tibial and long toe extensor muscles has been performed with good functional outcome.

References

Åhlberg, G., Jakobsson, F. *et al.* (1994). Distributioin of muscle degeneration in Welander distal myopathy – a magnetic resonance imaging and muscle biopsy study. *Neuromuscular Disorder,* **4**, 55–62.

Åhlberg, G., von Tell, D. *et al.* (1999). Genetic linkage of Welander distal myopathy to chromosome 2p13. *Annals of Neurology,* **46**(3), 399–404.

Anderson, L. and Harrison, R. (2000). Secondary reduction in calpain3 expression in patients with limb girdle muscular dystrophy type 2B and Miyoshi myopathy (primary dysferlinopathies). *Neuromuscular Disorder,* **10**, 553–9.

Argov, Z., Sadeh, M. *et al.* (2000). Muscular dystrophy due to dysferlin deficiency in Libyan Jews. Clinical and genetic features. *Brain* 2000, **123**, 1229–37.

Barohn, R., Miller, R. *et al.* (1991). Autosomal recessive distal dystrophy. *Neurology,* **41**, 1365–9.

Bejaoui, K., Hirabayashi, K. *et al* (1995). Linkage of Miyoshi myopathy (distal autosomal recessive muscular dystrophy) to chromosome 2p12–14. *Neurology,* **45**, 494–8.

Borg, K., Solders, G. *et al.* (1989). Neurogenic involvement in distal myopathy (Welander). *Journal of Neurological Sciences,* **91**, 53–70.

Borg, K., Åhlberg, G. *et al.* (1991). Welander's distal myopathy: clinical, electrophysiological and muscle biopsy observations in young and middle aged adults with early symptoms. *Journal of Neurological Neurosurgical Psychiatry,* **54**, 494–8.

Borg, K., Åhlberg, G. *et al.* (1993). Muscle fibre degeneration in distal myopathy (Welander) – ultrastructure related to immunohistochemical observations on cytoskeletal proteins and leu-19antigen. *Neuromuscular Disorder,* **2**, 149–55.

de Seze, J., Udd, B. *et al.* (1998). The first European tibial muscular dystrophy family outside the Finnish population. *Neurology,* **51**, 1746–8.

Edström, L. (1975). Histochemical and histopathological changes in skeletal muscle in late-onset hereditary distal myopathy (Welander). *Journal of Neurological Sciences*, **26**, 147–57.

Edström, L., Thornell, L. *et al.* (1980). A new type of hereditary distal myopathy with characteristic sarcoplasmic bodies and intermediate (skeletin) filaments. *Journal of Neurological Sciences*, **47**, 171–89.

Eymard, B., Laforet, P. *et al.* (2000). Miyoshi distal myopathy: specific signs and incidence (in French). *Revue Neurologique*, **156**(2), 161–8.

Fardeau, M., Godet-Guilain, J. *et al.* (1978). Une novelle affection musculaire familiale, definie par l'accumulation intra-sarcoplasmic d'un materiel granulo-filamentaire dense en microscopie electronique. *Revue Neurologique (Paris)*, **134**, 411–25.

Feit, H., Silbergleit, A., *et al.* (1998). Vocal cord and pharyngeal weakness with autosomal distal myopathy: clinical description and gene localization to chromosome 5q31. *American Journal of Human Genetics*, **63**, 1732–44.

Felice, K., Meredith, C. *et al.* (1999). Autosomal dominant distal myopathy not linked to the known distal myopathy loci. *Neuromuscular Disorders*, **9**(2), 59–65.

Gowers, W., (1902). Myopathy and a distal form. *British Medical Journal*, **2**, 89–92.

Haravuori, H., Mäkelä-Bengs, P. *et al.* (1998a). Assignment of the tibial muscular dystrophy (TMD) locus on chromosome 2q31. *American Journal of Human Genetics*, **62**, 620–6.

Haravuori, H., Mäkelä-Bengs, P. *et al.* (1988b). Tibial muscular dystrophy and late onset distal myopathy are linked to the same locus on chromosome 2q. *Neurology*, **50**(suppl. 4), A186 (abstract).

Haravuori, H., Vihola, A. *et al.* (2000). LGMD2J in patients homozygous for 2q31 linked distal myopathy (TMD) - caused by secondary calpainopathy? *Neurology*, **54**(suppl. 3) A435 (abstract).

Haravuori, H., Vihola, A. *et al.* (2001). Secondary calpain3 deficiency in 2q linked muscular dystrophy – *titin is the candidate gene*. *Neurology*, **56**, 869–77.

Hauser, s., Horrigan, M. *et al.* (2000). Myotilin is mutated in limb girdle muscular dystrophy 1A. *Human Molecular Genetics*, **9**, 2147–7.

Horowitz, S. and Schmalbruch, H. (1994). Autosomal dominant distal myopathy with desmin storage: a clinicopathologic and electrophysiologic study of a large kinship. *Muscle Nerve* **17**, 151–60.

Ikeuchi, T., Asaka, T. *et al.* (1997). Gene locus for autosomal recessive distal myopathy with rimmed vacuoles maps to chromosome 9. *Annals of Neurology*, **41**, 432–7.

Laing, N., Laing, B. *et al.* (1995). Autosomal dominant distal myopathy: linkage to chromosome 14. *American Journal of Human Genetics*, **56**, 422–7.

Iliaroshkin, S., Ivanova-Smolenskaja, I. *et al.* (1996). Clinical and molecular analysis of large family with three distinct phenotypes of progressive muscular dystrophy. *Brain*, **119**, 1895–909.

Illa, I., Serrano-Munuera, C. *et al.* (2001). Distal anterior compartment myopathy: a dysferlin mutation causing a new muscular dystrophy phenotype. *Annals of Neurology*, **49**, 130–4.

Kumamoto, T., Ueyama, H. *et al.* (1994). Muscle fiber degredation in distal myopathy with rimmed vacuoles. *Acta Neuropathologica*, **87**, 143–8.

Kumamto, T., Ito, T. *et al.* (2000). Increased lysosome-related proteins in the skeletal muscles of distal myopathy with rimmed vacuoles. *Muscle Nerve*, **23**, 1686–93.

Laing, N., Laing, B. *et al.* (1995). Autosomal dominant distal myopathy: linkage to chromosome 14. *American Journal of Human Genetics*, **56**, 422–7.

Lindberg, C., Borg, K. *et al.* (1991). Inclusion body myositis and Welander distal myopathy: a clinical, neurophysiological and morphological comparison. *Journal of Neurological Sciences*, **103**, 76–81.

Linssen, W., de Visser, M. *et al.* (1988). Genetic heterogeneity in Miyoshi type distal muscular dystrophy. *Neuromuscular Disorders*, **8**, 317–20.

Mahjneh, I., Udd, B. *et al.* (2000). A distinct phenotype of distal myopathy in a large Finnish family. *Journal of Neurology*, **3**, 247 (abstr).

Markesbery, W., Griggs, R. *et al.* (1974). Late onset hereditary distal myopathy. *Neurology*, **23**, 127–34.

Matsuda, C., Aoki, M. *et al.* (1999). Dysferlin is a surface membrane-associated protein that is absent in Miyoshi myopathy. *Neurology*, **53**, 1119–22.

Melberg, A. Oldfors, A. *et al.* (1999). Autosomal dominant myofibrillar myopathy with arrhythmogenic right ventricular cardiomyopathy linked to chromosome 10q. *Annals of Neurology*, **46**, 684–92.

Milhorat, A. and Wolff, H. (1943). Studies in diseases of muscle: XIII. Progressive muscular dystrophy of atrophic distal type: report on a family: report of autopsy. *Archives of Neurological Psychiatry*, **49**, 655–64.

Mitrani-Rosenbaum, S., Argov, Z. *et al.* (1996). Hereditary inclusion body myopathy maps to chromosome 9p1-q1. *Human Molecular Genetics*, **5**, 159–63.

Miyoshi, K., Kawai, H. *et al.* (1986). Autosomal recessive distal muscular dystrophy as a new type of progressive muscular dystrophy: seventeen cases in eight families, including an autopsied case. *Brain*, **109**, 31–54.

Moreira, E., Vanizof, M. *et al.* (1997). The seventh form of autosomal recessive limb-girdle muscular dystrophy is mapped to 17q11–12. *American Journal of Human Genetics*, **61**, 151–9.

Nonaka, I. (1999). Distal myopathies. *Current Opinion in Neurology*, **12**, 493–9.

Nonaka, I., Sunohara, N. *et al.* (1981). Familial distal myopathy with rimmed vacuole and lamellar (myeloid) body formation. *Journal of Neurological Science*, **51**, 141–55.

Partanen, J., Laulumaa, V. *et al.* (1994). Late onset foot-drop muscular dystrophy with rimmed vacuoles. *Journal of Neurological Science*, **125**, 158–67.

Penisson-Besnier, I., Dumez, C. *et al.* (1998). Autosomal dominant late adult onset distal leg myopathy. *Neuromuscular Disorder* **8**, 459–466.

Piccolo, S., More, S. *et al.* (2000). Intracellular accumulation and reduced sarcolemmal expression in limb-girdle muscular dystrophies. *Annals of Neurology*, **48**, 902–12.

Salmikangas, P., Mykkänen, O. *et al.* (1999). Myotilin, a novel sarcomeric protein with two IgG-like domains, is encoded by a candidate gene for limb-girdle muscular dystrophy. *Human Molecular Genetics*, **8**, 13229–36.

Satoyoshi, E. and Kinoshita, M. (1977). Oculopharyngodistal myopathy: report of four families. *Archives of Neurology*, **34**, 89–92.

Scoppetta, C., Casali, C. *et al.* (1995). Infantile aurosomal dominant distal myopathy. *Acta Neurologica Scandinavia*, **92**, 122–6.

Servidei, S., Capon, F. *et al.* (1999). A distinctive autosomal dominant vacuolar neuromyopathy linked to 19p13. *Neurology*, **53**(4), 830–7.

Sjöberg, G., Sasvedra-Matiz, C. *et al.* (1999). A missense mutation in the desmin rod domain is associated with autosomal dominant distal myopathy, and exerts a dominant negative effect on filament formation. *Human Molecular Genetics*, **8**, 2191–98.

Somer, H. (1995). Workshop report: distal myopathies. *Neuromuscular Disorders*, **5**, 249–52.

Speer, M., Yamaoka, L. *et al.* (1992). Identification of a new autosomal dominant limb-girdle muscular dystrophy locus on chromosome 5q. *American Journal of Human Genetics*, **50**, 1211–7.

Sumner, D., Crawfurd, M. *et al.* (1971). Distal muscular dystrophy in an English family. *Brain*, **94**, 51–59.

Sunohara, N., Nonaka, I. *et al.* (1989). Distal myopathy with rimmed vacuole formation. A follow up study. *Brain*, **112**, 65–83.

Udd, B., Haravuori, H. *et al.* (1998). Tibial muscular dystrophy—from clinical description to linkage on chromosome 2q31. *Neuromuscular Disorders*, **8**, 327–32.

Udd, B., Kääriäinen, H. *et al.* (1991). Muscular dystrophy with separate phenotypes in a large family. *Muscle Nerve*, **14**, 1050–8.

Udd, B., Partanen, J. *et al.* (1993). Tibial muscular dystrophy. Late adult-onset distal myopathy in 66 Finnish patients. *Archives of Neurology*, **50**, 604–608.

Uyama, E., Uchino, M. *et al.* (1998). Autosomal recessive oculopharyngodistal myopathy in light of distal myopathy with rimmed vacuoles and oculopharyngeal muscular dystrophy. *Neuromuscular Disorder*, **8**, 119–25.

Vicart, P., Caron, A. *et al.* (1998). A missense mutation in the alpha B-crystallin chaperone gene causes a desmin-related myopathy. *Nature Genetics*, **20**, 92–95.

Voit, T., Kutz, P. *et al.* (2001). Autosomal dominant distal myopathy: further evidence of a chromosme 14 locus. *Neuromuscular Disorders*, **11**, 11–19.

Weiler, T., Greenberg, C. *et al.* (1996). Limb-girdle muscular dystrophy and Miyoshi myopathy in an aboriginal Canadian kindred map to LGMD2B and segregate with the same hapotype. *American Journal of Human Genetics*, **59**, 872–8.

Weiler, T., Bashir, R. *et al.* (1999). Identical mutation in patients with limb girdle muscular dystrophy type 2B or Miyoshi myopathy suggests a role for modifier gene(s). *Human Molecular Genetics*, **8**(5), 871–7.

Welander, L. (1951) Myopathia distalis tarda hereditaria. *Acta Medica Scandinavia* **141** (suppl. 265), 1.

Welander, L. (1957). Homozygous appearance of distal myopathy. *Acta Genetica*, **7**, 321–5.

Zimprich, F., Djamshidian, A. *et al.* (2000). An autosomal dominant early adult-onset distal muscular dystrophy. *Muscle Nerve*, **23**, 1876–9.

Chapter 10

Oculopharyngeal muscular dystrophy: the muscular dystrophies

Bernard Brais and Fernando M.S. Tomé

History

In 1915, Taylor of Boston reported the familial association of eyelid ptosis and dysphagia in a family of French–Canadian descent (Taylor 1915). The more common autosomal dominant (MIM 164300) form of Oculopharyngeal muscular dystrophy (OPMD) became a distinct muscular dystrophy in 1962 (Victor *et al.* 1962). It was described as causing, usually after the age of 50, a selective progressive ptosis and dysphagia. Pathological changes were considered suggestive of a muscular dystrophy. André Barbeau established the existence of a large French–Canadian cluster of OPMD (Barbeau 1965; 1966; 1969; Letendre *et al.* 1966). Barbeau also demonstrated that proximal limb weakness was also part of the clinical presentation. In 1980, Tomé and Fardeau identified on electron microscopy unique filamentous intranuclear inclusions (INI) in the deltoid muscles of three unrelated OPMD patients (Tomé and Fardeau 1980). Since, these INI have been considered a specific histological marker of OPMD (Tomé *et al.* 1997). OPMD has a worldwide distribution. Cases have been described in 33 countries: Armenia, Australia, Brazil, Belgium, Canada, Denmark, France, Germany, Holland, Hungary, Israel, Ireland, Italy, Japan, Lebanon, Malaysia, Mexico, New Zealand, Norway, Poland, Portugal (also in the Azores), Romania, Russia, Spain (also in the Canaries), Sweden, Switzerland, Czech Republic, Taiwan, United Kingdom, United States, Uzbekistan, Uruguay and Yugoslavia. However, OPMD is particularly prevalent in the French–Canadian population (1 : 1000) and in Bukhara Jews living in Israel (1 : 600) (Blumen *et al.* 1997; Brais *et al.* 1995). Most North American cases of OPMD descend from three French sisters who arrived in Québec in 1648 (Brais *et al.* 1998a,c). Numerous other historically distinct OPMD mutations have also been introduced in North America by Louisiana Cajuns, Hispanic Americans from the Southwestern United States, Jews of Eastern European extraction, Italians, Mennonites, and descendants of British immigrants (Brais *et al.* 1998c; Grewal *et al.* 1998; 1999; Scacheri *et al.* 1999; Stajich *et al.* 1997a,b). A large OPMD cluster described also in Bukhara Jews living in Israel (Blumen *et al.* 1993; 1996; 1997; 1999; 2000). The OPMD locus was mapped to chromosome 14q11.1 (Brais *et al.* 1995). In 1998, short $(GCG)_n$

repeat mutations in the poly(A) binding protein nuclear 1 (*PABPN1*) gene were found to cause OPMD (Brais *et al.* 1998c).

Clinical features

Dominant OPMD usually presents with both dysphagia and eyelid ptosis in the late 40s or early 50s (Fig. 10.1). Brais *et al.* have proposed the following diagnostic criteria for dominant OPMD: (1) a positive family history of two or more generations of OPMD, (2) at least one palpebral fissures at rest smaller than 8 mm (or previous corrective surgery), and (3) a swallowing time greater than 7 s when asked to drink 80 ml of ice-cold water (Brais *et al.* 1995). The decade-specific penetrances for carriers of a dominant $(GCG)_9$ mutation are: 1 per cent (<40), 6 per cent (40–49), 31 per cent (50–59), 63 per cent (60–69), 99 per cent (>69) (Brais *et al.* 1997). Therefore, dominant $(GCG)_9$ OPMD is fully penetrant past 70. Other signs observed in affected individuals carrying a $(GCG)_9$ mutation are: proximal upper extremity weakness (38 per cent), facial muscle weakness (43 per cent), limitation of upper gaze (61 per cent), dysphonia

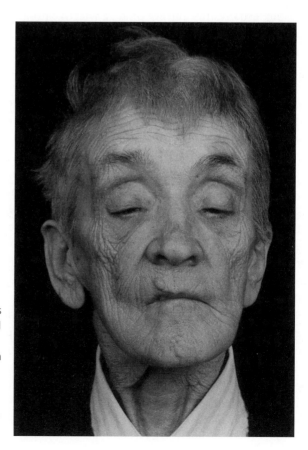

Fig. 10.1 A 76-year-old OPMD patient with severe blepharoptosis despite previous surgery. Forehead wrinkling caused by constant frontalis muscle contraction is evident. Atrophy of facial and anterior neck muscles is prominent. (Reproduced from *Neuromuscular Disorders: Clinical and Molecular Genetics*, edited by Emery 1998. Courtesy of John Wiley and Sons.)

(67 per cent), proximal lower extremity weakness (71 per cent) and tongue atrophy and weakness (82 per cent) (Bouchard *et al.* 1997).

Severity of the dominant OPMD phenotype is variable (Bouchard *et al.* 1997a). Severe cases have an earlier onset, before the age of 45, of ptosis and dysphagia, and will develop an incapacitating proximal leg weakness. OPMD cases are considered severe if they have symptomatic proximal leg weakness before age 60. They represent 5–10 per cent of cases. These cases will eventually need a wheelchair. The most severe OPMD phenotype was observed in individuals homozygotes for dominant OPMD mutations (Blumen *et al.* 1996; 1999; Brais *et al.* 1998c). The study of four French–Canadian and three Bukhara Jewish OPMD homozygotes documented that on average the onset was 18 years earlier than in $(GCG)_9$ heterozygotes. The severity of the OPMD phenotype may well be proportional to the size of the mutation, but this important issue has not yet been adequately addressed.

The much rarer recessive OPMD (MIM 257950) appears to have a similar clinical phenotype as the dominant form with an older age of onset. The recessive OPMD family members previously described have since been found to be cases of mitochondrial neurogastrointestinal encephalomyopathy syndrome (MNGIE, MIM 550900) caused by mutations in the thymidine phosphorylase *ECGF1* gene (M. Sadeh personal communication) (Fried *et al.* 1975). Only one case to date of recessive OPMD has been confirmed molecularly and pathologically (Brais *et al.* 1998c). This patient had a very late onset of ptosis at 67 while her dysphagia started at the more usual age of 50 (Pouget and Pellissier, personal communication). Recessive cases may be under-diagnosed because of a milder phenotype and the absence of clear family history. The predicted prevalence of the recessive form is in the order of 1 : 10 000 in Québec, France and Japan (Brais *et al.* 1998c).

Serum CK levels have been reported to be elevated, two to five times the normal value, in OPMD cases with severe leg weakness (Barbeau 1966). In most cases, however, they are normal or only slightly elevated. Electromyography (EMG) of weak muscles usually reveals discrete signs of a myopathic process (Bouchard *et al.* 1997). Very mild neuropathic findings have been reported, but are felt to be related in most cases to old age or concomitant disease (Bouchard *et al.* 1997; Hardiman *et al.* 1993). However, there has been no correlation study to establish if patients with the larger mutations are more at risk to develop a peripheral neuropathy. The ice-cold swallowing test developed by J.-P. Bouchard has an 87 per cent sensitivity and an 88.7 per cent specificity for the dysphagia in OPMD (Bouchard *et al.* 1997). This test consists in timing the swallowing of 80 ml of ice-cold water. The dysphagia is considered to be confirmed if the individuals take more than 7 s to swallow the small volume. Genetic testing and muscle biopsy are the most valuable means of establishing the diagnosis of OPMD.

Pathology

Biopsies from different muscles have been studied in OPMD. It is, however, the study of deltoid muscle that has most often been reported. All biopsies show variation in fibre diameter with the presence of some atrophic angulated muscle fibres (Tomé *et al.* 1997). Hypertrophic and segmented fibres are seen in several biopsies. Necrotic fibres are rarely seen. Ragged red fibres are occasionally observed. Predominance of type 1 fibres is often observed, but fibre type grouping does not occur. Rimmed vacuoles (RV) and intranuclear inclusions (INI) are both characteristic of OPMD.

Rimmed vacuoles are non-membrane bound and have irregular outlines. Their rimmed borders consist of dark staining material which extends to the neighbouring cytoplasm. The content of RV is variable. They may contain cytoplasmic debris and myelin bodies. Collection of filaments, 15–18 nm in diameter, is occasionally observed within the vacuoles and in the neighbouring cytoplasm. They are similar to the filaments observed in inclusion-body myositis (IBM) (Askanas *et al.* 1991; Askanas and Engel 1995; Leclerc *et al.* 1993). Acid phosphatase activity is found in many vacuoles. RV are observed in all biopsies but are usually not numerous. RV mean frequency in muscle fibres is in the order of 0.6 per cent of fibres (range: 0.1–3.5 per cent) (Tomé *et al.* 1997).

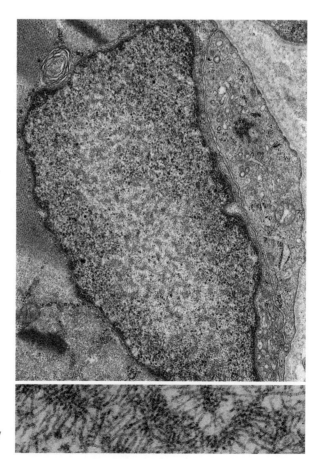

Fig. 10.2 Ultrastructural features of a skeletal muscle intranuclear filamentous OPMD inclusion. The upper panel demonstrates the tubular nature of the filaments and their organization in palisades (upper panel, ×100 000; lower panel ×23 000). (Reproduced from *Neuromuscular Disorders: Clinical and Molecular Genetics*, edited by Emery 1998. Courtesy of John wilsey and Sons.)

OPMD intranuclear inclusions are formed by tubular filaments (Fig. 10. 2). The INI are about 8.5 nm in outer diameter, 3 nm in inner diameter and up to 0.25 μm in length. They are often arranged in tangles or palisades. They are found exclusively within the nuclei of muscle fibres, never in the cytoplasm. They are not seen in the nuclei either of satellite cells or other cell types present in the biopsies (fibroblasts, endothelial cells, pericytes, adipocytes, Schwann and perineurial cells of intramuscular nerves). The INI replace the normal nuclear structure. They do not contain DNA. Their size is very variable. In a given ultrathin section the frequency of nuclei in which filamentous inclusions are seen varied from 2 to 5 per cent (mean: 4 per cent) in heterozygote patients. In homozygote OPMD cases, on average twice as many muscle nuclei containing INI are observed than in heterozygotes (9.4 vs 4.9 per cent, $p < 0.02$) (Blumen et al. 1999). Percentage of nuclei containing INIs appears to be variable between muscles. They are more frequent in most affected muscles. For example, Coquet et al. reported that 8 per cent of nuclei contained INIs in the more affected cricothyroid pharyngeal compared to 4 per cent in the deltoid of the same patient (Coquet et al. 1990). The areas containing the intranuclear inclusions may be detected on semi-thin sections of material prepared for electron microscopy and embedded in acrylic resins. The INI correspond to clearer zones surrounded by nucleoplasm. Studies of serial semi-thin sections show the presence of clear zones at different levels of most nuclei of the muscle fibres suggesting that all nuclei have inclusions.

Following the identification of the mutated gene in OPMD, much work centered on the identification of the proteins present in the INI. Mutated Poly(A)binding protein nuclear (PABPN1) was shown to be integral part of the muscle OPMD inclusions (Becher et al. 2000; Calado et al. 2000b; Uyama et al. 2000) Using both immuno-electron microscopy and fluorescence confocal microscopy, the OPMD-specific nuclear inclusions are decorated by anti-PABPN1 antibodies (Calado et al. 2000b). In addition, the inclusions were shown to be decorated by antibodies directed against ubiquitin and proteasomal subunits. This suggests that the polyalanine expansions in PABPN1 induce misfolding and aggregation of ubiquitin-tagged proteins that cells are not able to breakdown through the proteosome machinery. Interestingly, the nuclear inclusions were found to sequester poly(A) mRNA (Calado et al. 2000b).

Genetics

The OPMD locus maps to chromosome 14q11.1 (Brais et al. 1995; 1997; 1998c; Grewal et al. 1998; Porschke et al. 1997; Stajich et al. 1997a; Teh et al. 1997). Linkage studies suggested that dominant OPMD was a genetically homogeneous condition. A positional cloning strategy led to the identification of short $(GCG)_{8-13}$ expansions in the poly(A) binding protein nuclear 1 (PABPN1, previously abbreviated *PABP2*) gene in all dominant OPMD cases (Fig. 10.3) (Brais et al. 1998c). They consist of mitotically and meiotically stable insertions of GCG-triplets in the first exon of the gene. The secondary mutation of an existent mutation is in the order of 1 : 500 meioses (Brais et al. 1998c). Dominant mutations consist in the addition of two to seven (GCG) repeats to

Fig. 10.3 Genomic *PABPN1* sequence of OPMD dominant mutations and the corresponding protein expansions of the homopolymeric polyalanine domain.

Genomic sequence of *PABPN1* OPMD (GCG)$_n$ dominant mutations

ATG GCG GCG GCG GCG GCG GCG **(GCG)$_{2-7}$** GCA GCA GCA GCG

Expansions in the PABPN1 N-terminus polyalanine domain

M A A A A A A A A A A **(A)$_{2-7}$** G A A G G R G S

the usual (GCG)$_6$ stretch. The study of 81 non-French–Canadian families originating from 17 countries documented the existence of 6 different mutation sizes. The percentage of these families sharing the different mutations are: 5 per cent (GCG)$_8$, 40 per cent (GCG)$_9$, 26 per cent (GCG)$_{10}$, 21 per cent (GCG)$_{11}$, 7 per cent (GCG)$_{12}$ and 1 per cent (GCG)$_{13}$. In French Canadians and Bukhara Jews, OPMD is caused by two distinct (GCG)$_9$ founder mutations (Blumen *et al.* 2000). The molecular basis of autosomal recessive OPMD appears to be at least in some cases the double inheritance of the (GCG)$_7$ polymorphism (Brais *et al.* 1998c). The observed inter-familial phenotype variability may depend on the differences in sizes of the (GCG)$_n$ mutations, but this important issue still needs to be addressed fully.

In the case of severe dominant OPMD cases, approximately 20 per cent carry both a dominant mutation and a (GCG)$_7$ polymorphism in their other copy of the *PABPN1* gene (Brais *et al.* 1998c). This polymorphism has a 1–2 per cent prevalence in Japan, North America and Europe. OPMD compound heterozygotes have been diagnosed in many different countries (Brais *et al.* 1998c; Mirabella *et al.* 2000). The (GCG)$_7$ allele is, therefore, an example of a polymorphism which can act either as a modifier of a dominant phenotype or as a recessive mutation. Nevertheless, the cause of the increased severity in 80 per cent of severe cases is still unknown. Strikingly, severe cases cluster in families, suggesting that other genetic factors modulate severity (Brais *et al.* 1998b). Patients with severe OPMD are not more likely to transmit the severe phenotype to their children than patients affected with the classical form. The more severe phenotypes observed in homozygotes and compound heterozygotes for a dominant and a recessive mutation suggest a clear gene dosage effect (Blumen *et al.* 1999; Brais *et al.* 1998c; 1999).

Molecular basis and pathogenesis

At the protein level, the OPMD mutations cause the lengthening of a predicted N-terminus polyalanine domain (Fig. 10. 3). PABPN1 is an abundant mostly nuclear protein involved in the polyadenylation of all messenger RNAs (Bienroth *et al.* 1993; Krause *et al.* 1994; Nemeth *et al.* 1995; Wahle 1991; Wahle *et al.* 1993). The biphasic polyadenylation process depends, for its first step on polyadenine polymerase (PAP), the cleavage and polyadenylation specificity factor (CPSF), cleavage factors I$_m$ and II$_m$ (CFI$_m$ and CFII$_m$) and the cleavage stimulation factor (CstF) (Wahle and Ruegsegger 1999). The final rapid elongation of the poly(A) tails is dependent on the adjoining of PABPN1 to the polyadenylation complex (Wahle and Ruegsegger 1999). PABPN1 travels with the mRNA to the cytoplasm. The protein falls off when the mRNA is taken over by the translation machinery. PABPN1 is then actively transported back into the nuclei (Calado *et al.* 2000a; Chen *et al.* 1999).

Different lines of evidence suggest that polyalanine oligomers form resistant macro-molecules *in vivo* and *in vitro*. Polyalanine oligomers are known to be very resistant to protease digestion or chemical degradation (Forood *et al.* 1995). They form β-sheet structure *in vitro* (Forood *et al.* 1995). Polyalanine oligomers containing more than 8 alanines in a row form fibrils spontaneously (Billingsley *et al.* 1994). Furthermore, PABPN1 molecules in OPMD muscle INI are more resistant to salt extraction than the other proteins of the nucleoplasm (Calado *et al.* 2000b). Various fusion proteins with long polyalanine domains accumulate as INI (Gaspar *et al.* 2000; Rankin *et al.* 2000). In one transfection experiment, a long 37 Ala-GFP fusion protein caused nuclear inclusion formation and cell death (Rankin *et al.* 2000). Lastly, the observation that proteins in the INIs are tagged with ubiquitin without being degraded strongly suggests that indeed the mutated PABPN1 has acquired new pathogenic physical characteristics (Calado *et al.* 2000b).

Different versions of a polyalanine toxicity gain-of-function pathogenetic hypothesis have been proposed for OPMD (Brais *et al.* 1998c; 1999). They are all based on the presumed altered physical properties of the expanded polyalanine PABPN1 domain. The abnormal physical characteristics are suggested to cause both PABPN1 accumulation and interference with normal cellular processes. It is proposed that beyond 10 alanines, the normal number of alanines in PABPN1, the polyalanine domains polymerize to form stable β-sheets that are resistant to nuclear proteosomal degradation. The polyalanine

Table 10.1 Possible altered mechanisms leading to cell death in OPMD

I- Intranuclear Inclusion-dependent:

1- Physical rupture of the nuclear membrane
2- Disruption of transcriptional domains
3- Disruption of chromosomal domains
4- Sequestering of mRNAs coding for proteins vital for cell survival
5- Sequestering of PABPN1 in sufficient quantity to interfere with normal mRNA processing
6- Sequestering of other proteins:
6.1) Proteins interacting normally with PABPN1
6.2) Proteins involved in protein folding (e.g. chaperones such as HSP70, HDJ2)
6.3) Proteins of the ubiquitin/proteasome pathway
6.4) Other proteins with polyalanine domains

II- Intranuclear Inclusion-independent:

1- Interfere with normal function of PABPN1 in mRNA polyadenylation
2- Interfere with the mRNA processing machinery
3- Interfere with PABPN1 shuttling between nucleus and cytoplasm
4- Interfere with mRNA nuclear export
5- Interfere with initiation of translation
6- Interaction of PABPN1 with other soluble polyalanine containing proteins

macromolecules grow with time to form the OPMD PABPN1-containing intranuclear filaments that are seen on electron microscopy (Calado *et al.* 2000b; Tomé *et al.* 1997; Tomé and Fardeau 1980) When a significant portion of a nucleus is occupied by the inclusions, they may sufficiently alter normal cellular processes to lead to fatal nuclear dysfunction. On the other hand, cytoplasmic functions could also be pathologically altered, considering that PABPN1 shuttles between the nuclei and the cytoplasm (Calado and Carmo-Fonseca 2000; Calado *et al.* 2000a; Chen *et al.* 1999). The possible pathophysiological mechanisms that could lead to cellular demise can be classified as either intranuclear inclusion-dependent or -independent (Table 10.1). Though there is an apparent accumulation of mRNA in the INI, there does not appear to be any alteration in the PABPN1-dependent final elongation of the poly(A) tails. (Calado *et al.* 2000b) This mRNA accumulation, however, raises the possibility that the polyalanine expansions in PABPN1 may interfere with the normal cellular traffic of poly(A) mRNA by trapping mRNA in the INI (Calado *et al.* 2000b). The demonstration that INI can readily be produced by transfection will allow the study of how mutated PABPN1 plays a part in late-onset diseases with intranuclear inclusions (Shanmugam *et al.* 2000).

Genetic counseling

In the dominant form of OPMD, one of the biological parents should have developed OPMD provided they live long enough. Parents of recessive cases are unlikely to be alive at the time their children are diagnosed and should not have been affected. For the dominant form each child and sib has a 50 per cent risk of having inherited this fully penetrant mutation. For cases of recessive OPMD the risk for sibs is 25 per cent and less than 1 per cent for their children. Patients with more severe phenotypes are not more likely to transmit the severe phenotype to their children than patients affected with the more usual form. Individuals inheriting a dominant mutation from the affected parent and a recessive mutation from the other will develop a severe form of OPMD (Brais *et al.* 1998c). Much care should be taken before requesting the predictive testing of an asymptomatic individual. It is unclear if these individuals will benefit from the test, considering that there is no medical therapy or prevention for this disease. Presymptomatic testing should, therefore, be performed in the context where genetic counselling and psychological support can be offered.

Prenatal diagnosis

Prenatal testing is usually not offered, considering the late-onset and the nature of the physical limitations caused by this disease.

Management

The clinical diagnosis of dominant OPMD can readily be made based on the three previously described diagnostic criteria. The following other diagnoses can also be entertained: myotonic muscular dystrophy (MIM 160900), autosomal dominant distal myopathy (MIM 158580), mitochondrial myopathies with or without PEO including mitochondrial neurogastrointestinal encephalomyopathy syndrome (MNGIE, MIM 550900) and myasthenia gravis. The absence of fluctuation of symptoms and a positive history usually distinguish it from myasthenia gravis. If in doubt, an EMG, neostigmine testing and OPMD genetic testing should be performed. Polymyositis and progressive bulbar palsy can usually be excluded because of the absence of ptosis in these conditions. Late-onset, usually in their 60s, of isolated familial ptosis without dysphagia can be distinguished from OPMD by genetic testing and lack of dysphagia. The clinical diagnosis of recessive OPMD is more problematic. Late onset ptosis and dysphagia without a clear family history should raise this diagnostic possibility and lead to genetic testing.

Until the identification of the OPMD *PABPN1* mutations, definitive diagnosis relied on electron microscopy for OPMD INI (Tomé and Fardeau 1994). This approach has now been replaced by DNA testing (Brais *et al.* 1998c). Autosomal dominant and recessive OPMD being allelic, the molecular diagnosis of both conditions is quite straight forward. A single polymerase chain reaction (PCR) is required to establish the carrier status of an individual (Brais *et al.* 1998c). The test has a >99 per cent sensitivity and specificity. This test is offered commercially and in numerous academic laboratories worldwide. The major indications for DNA testing of a symptomatic individuals are: (1) confirmation of the diagnosis in a family never previously tested, (2) the clinical picture presents a diagnostic dilemma, (3) the patient has a severe earlier onset form of the disease, and (4) the patient may suffer from recessive OPMD.

There is no medical treatment for OPMD. The surgical treatments presently available are used to correct the ptosis and improve swallowing in moderately to severely affected individuals. Two types of operations are used to correct the ptosis: resection of the levator palpebral aponeurosis and frontal suspension of the eyelids (Codère 1993). Resection of aponeurosis is easily done but usually needs to be repeated within five years (Rodrigue and Molgat 1997). Frontal suspension of the eyelids consist in using a thread of skeletal muscle fascia as a sling that is inserted in the tarsal plate of the upper eyelid and attached at its ends in the frontalis muscle, which is relatively preserved in OPMD (Codère 1993). Its major advantage is that it is permanent, however, it requires general anaesthesia. Surgery is recommended when the ptosis interferes with vision or cervical pain appears secondary to the constant dorsiflexion of the neck. Contraindications to blepharoplasty are marked ophthalmoplegia, a dry-eye syndrome or poor orbicularis oculi function.

Surgical evaluation for symptomatic dysphagia should be prompted by marked weight loss, near-fatal choking, which is extremely rare, or recurrent pneumonia (Duranceau *et al.* 1983). Cricopharyngeal myotomy will alleviate symptoms in most cases. Usually, this surgery requires an over-night hospitalization and a one-week convalescence. Dysphagia will reappear slowly over years in most cases. Severe dysphonia and lower esophageal sphincter incompetence are contraindications to surgery (Duranceau 1997).

Repetitive dilatations of the upper-esophageal sphincter with bougies does alleviate some of the symptoms in many patients, but need to be repeated more than twice a year (Mathieu *et al.* 1997).

References

Askanas, V. and Engel, W.K. (1995). New advances in the understanding of sporadic inclusion-body myositis and hereditary inclusion-body myositis. *Current Opinion in Rheumatology*, 7, 486–96.

Askanas, V., Serdaroglu, P., Engel, W.K., and Alvarez, R.B. (1991). Immunolocalization of ubiquitin in muscle biopsies of patients with inclusion body myositis and oculopharyngeal muscular dystrophy. *Neuroscience Letters*, 130, 73–6.

Barbeau, A. (1965). La myopathie oculaire au Canada Français. *L'Union Médical du Canada*, 94, 1186–7.

Barbeau, A. (1966). In *Symposium über progressive Muskeldystrophie* (ed. Kuhn, E.). Springer-Verlag, Berlin, pp. 102–9.

Barbeau, A. (1969). In *Progress in neuro-ophthalmology.* (ed. Brunette, J.-R. and Barbeau, A.) Vol. 2. Excerpta Medica, Amsterdam, p. 3.

Becher, M.W., Kotzuk, J.A., Davis, L.E., and Bear, D.G. (2000). Intranuclear inclusions in oculopharyngeal muscular dystrophy contain poly(A) binding protein 2. *Annals of Neurology*, 48, 812–5.

Bienroth, S., Keller, W., and Wahle, E. (1993). Assembly of a processive messenger RNA polyadenylation complex. *The EMBO Journal*, 12, 585–94.

Billingsley, G.D., Cox, D.W., Duncan, A.M.V., Googfellow, P.J., and Grzeschil, K.-H. (1994). Regional localization of loci on chromosome 14 using somatic cell hybrids. *Cytogenetics & Cell Genetics*, 66, 33–8.

Blumen, S.C., Brais, B., Korczyn, A.D., Medynsky, S., Chapman, J., Asherov, A. *et al.* (1999). Homozygotes for oculopharyngeal muscular dystrophy have a severe form of the disease. *Annals of Neurology*, 46, 115–8.

Blumen, S.C., Korczyn, A.D., Lavoie, H., Medynski, S., Chapman, J., Asherov, A. *et al.* (2000). Oculopharyngeal MD among Bukhara Jews is due to a founder (GCG)9 mutation in the PABP2 gene. *Neurology*, 55, 1267–70.

Blumen, S.C., Nisipeanu, P., Sadeh, M., Asherov, A., Blumen, N., Wirguin, Y., *et al.* (1997). Epidemiology and inheritance of oculopharyngeal muscular dystrophy in Israel. *Neuromuscular Disorders*, 7, S38–S40.

Blumen, S.C., Nisipeanu, P., Sadeh, M., Asherov, A., Tomé, F.M.S., and Korczyn, A.D. (1993). Clinical features of oculopharyngeal muscular dystrophy among Bukhara Jews. *Neuromuscular Disorders*, 3, 575–7.

Blumen, S.C., Sadeh, M., Korczyn, A.D., Rouche, A., Nisipeanu, P., Asherov, A. *et al.* (1996). Intranuclear inclusions in oculopharyngeal muscular dystrophy among Bukhara Jews. *Neurology*, 46, 1324–8.

Bouchard, J.-P., Brais, B., Brunet, D., Gould, P.V., and Rouleau, G.A. (1997). Recent studies on oculopharyngeal muscular dystrophy in Quebec. *Neuromuscular Disorders*, 7, S22–S9.

Brais, B., Bouchard, J.-P., Jomphe, M., Desjardins, B., Dubé, M.-P., Gosselin, F. *et al.* (1998a). When genetics and history converge: the fine-mapping and North American introduction and diffusion of the French Canadian oculopharyngeal muscular dystrophy mutation. *American Journal of Human Genetics*, 63, 229.

Brais, B., Bouchard, J.P., Tomé, F.M.S., Fardeau, M., Codère, F., Duranceau, A. *et al.* (1998b). Genetic evidence for the involvement of other genes in modulating the severity of oculopharyngeal muscular dystrophy (OPMD). *Annals of Neurology*, 44, 455–6.

Brais, B., Bouchard, J.-P., Xie, Y.-G., Rochefort, D.L., Chrétien, N., Tomé, F.M.S. *et al.* (1998c). Short GCG expansions in the PABP2 gene cause oculopharyngeal muscular dystrophy. *Nature Genetics*, 18, 164–7.

Brais, B., Bouchard, J.-P., Ya-Gang, X., Gosselin, F., Fardeau, M., Tomé, F.M.S. *et al.* (1997). Using the full power of linkage analysis in 11 French Canadian families to fine map the oculopharyngeal muscular dystrophy gene. *Neuromuscular Disorders*, 7, S70–S5.

Brais, B., Rouleau, G.A., Bouchard, J.-P., Fardeau, M., and Tomé, F.M.S. (1999). Oculopharyngeal muscular dystrophy. *Seminars in Neurology*, 19, 59–66.

Brais, B., Xie, Y.-G., Sanson, M., Morgan, K., Weissenbach, J., Korczyn, A.D. *et al.* (1995). The oculopharyngeal muscular dystrophy locus maps to the region of the cardiac α and β myosin heavy chain genes on chromosome 14q11.2-q13. *Human Molecular Genetics*, 4, 429–34.

Calado, A. and Carmo-Fonseca, M. (2000). Localization of poly(A)-binding protein 2 (PABP2) in nuclear speckles is independent of import into the nucleus and requires binding to poly(A) RNA. *Journal of Cell Science*, 113, 2309–18.

Calado, A., Kutay, U., Kuhn, U., Wahle, E., and Carmo-Fonseca, M. (2000a). Deciphering the cellular pathway for transport of poly(A)-binding protein II. *RNA*, 6, 245–56.

Calado, A., Tome, F.M.S., Brais, B., Rouleau, G.A., Kuhn, U., Wahle, E. *et al.* (2000b). Nuclear inclusions in oculopharyngeal muscular dystrophy consist of poly(A) binding protein 2 aggregates which sequester poly(A) RNA. *Human Molecular Genetics*, 9, 2321–8.

Chen, Z., Li, Y., and Krug, R.M. (1999). Influenza A virus NS1 protein targets poly(A)-binding protein II of the cellular 3'-end processing machinery. *The EMBO Journal*, 18, 2273–83.

Codère, F. (1993). Oculopharyngeal muscular dystrophy. *Canadian Journal of Ophthalmology*, 28, 1–2.

Coquet, M., Vital, C., and Julien, J. (1990). Presence of inclusion body myositis-like filaments in oculopharyngeal muscular dystrophy: ultrastructural study of 10 cases. *Neuropathology and Applied Neurobiology*, 16, 393.

Duranceau, A. (1997). Cricopharyngeal myotomy in the management of neurogenic and muscular dysphagia. *Neuromuscular Disorders*, 7, S85–S9.

Duranceau, A.C., Beauchamp, G., Jamieson, G.G. and Barbeau, A. (1983). Oropharyngeal dysphagia and oculopharyngeal muscular dystrophy. *Surgical Clinics of North America*, 63, 825–32.

Forood, B., Pérez-Payá, E., Houghten, R.A., and Blondelle, S.E. (1995). Formation of an extremely stable polyalanine B-sheet macromolecule. *Biochemical and Biophysical Research Communications*, 211, 7–13.

Fried, K., Arlozorov, A., and Spira, R. (1975). Autosomal recessive oculopharyngeal muscular dystrophy, *Journal of Medical Genetics*, 12, 416–8.

Gaspar, C., Jannatipour, M., Dion, P., Laganiere, J., Sequeiros, J., Brais, B. *et al.* (2000). CAG tract of MJD-1 may be prone to frameshifts causing polyalanine accumulation. *Human Molecular Genetics*, 9, 1957–66.

Grewal, R.P., Cantor, R., Turner, G., Grewal, R.K., and Detera-Wadleigh, S.D. (1998). Genetic mapping and haplotype analysis of oculopharyngeal muscular dystrophy. *Neuroreport*, 9, 961–5.

Grewal, R.P., Karkera, J.D., Grewal, R.K., and Detera-Wadleigh, S.D. (1999). Mutation analysis of oculopharyngeal muscular dystrophy in Hispanic American families. *Archives of Neurology*, 56, 1378–81.

Hardiman, O., Halperin, J.J., Farrell, M.A., Shapiro, B.E., Wray, S.H., and Brown, R.H.J. (1993). Neuropathic findings in oculopharyngeal muscular dystrophy. A report of seven cases and a review of the literature. *Archives of Neurology*, 50, 481–8.

Krause, S., Fakan, S., Weis, K., and Wahle, E. (1994). Immunodetection of poly(A) binding protein II in cell nucleus. *Experimental Cell Research*, 214, 75–82.

Leclerc, A., Tomé, F.M.S., and Fardeau, M. (1993). Ubiquitin and beta-amyloid-protein in inclusion body myositis (IBM), familial IBM-like disorder and oculopharyngeal muscular dystrophy: an immunocytochemical study. *Neuromuscular Disorders*, 3, 283–91.

Letendre, J., Tétreault, C., and Barbeau, A. (1966). Dystrophie musculaire oculo-pharyngienne, *Montréal Médical*, 17, 11–3.

Mathieu, J., Lapointe, G., Brassard, A., Tremblay, C., Brais, B., Rouleau, G.A. *et al.* (1997). A pilot study on upper oesophageal sphincter dilatation for the treatment of dysphagia in patients with oculopharyngeal muscular dystrophy. *Neuromuscular Disorders*, 7, S100–S4.

Mirabella, M., Silvestri, G., de Rosa, G., Di Giovanni, S., Di Muzio, A., Uncini, A. *et al.* (2000). GCG genetic expansions in Italian patients with oculopharyngeal muscular dystrophy. *Neurology*, 54, 608–14.

Nemeth, A., Krause, S., Blank, D., Jenny, A., Jenö, P., Lustig, A., *et al.* (1995). Isolation of genomic and cDNA clones encoding bovine poly(A) binding protein II. *Nucleic Acids Research*, 23, 4034–41.

Porschke, H., Kress, W., Reichmann, H., Goebel, H.H., and Grimm, T. (1997). Oculopharyngeal muscular dystrophy and carnitine deficiency in a Nothern German family. *Neuromuscular Disorders*.

Rankin, J., Wyttenbach, A., and Rubinsztein, D.C. (2000). Intracellular green fluorescent protein-polyalanine aggregates are associated with cell death. *Biochemical Journal*, 348, 15–9.

Rodrigue, D. and Molgat, Y.M. (1997). Surgical correction of blepharoptosis in oculopharyngeal muscular dystrophy. *Neuromuscular Disorders*, 7, S82–S4.

Scacheri, P.C., Garcia, C., Hébert, R., and Hoffman, E.P. (1999). Unique *PABP2* mutation in 'Cajuns' suggest multiple founders of oculopharyngeal muscular dystrophy in populations with French ancestry. *American Journal of Medical Genetics*, 86, 477–81.

Shanmugam, V., Dion, P., Rochefort, D., Laganiere, J., Brais, B. and Rouleau, G. A. (2000). PABP2 polyalanine tract expansion causes intranuclear inclusions in oculopharyngeal muscular dystrophy, *Annales of Neurology*, 48, 798–802.

Stajich, J.M., Gilchrist, J.M., Lennon, F., Lee, A., Yamaoka, L., Rosi, B. *et al.* (1997a). Confirmation of linkage of oculopharyngeal muscular dystrophy to chromosome 14q11.2-q13. *Annals of Neurology*, 40, 801–4.

Stajich, J.M., Gilchrist, J.M., Lennon, F., Lee, A., Yamaoka, L., Rosi, B. *et al.* (1997b). Confirmation of linkage of oculopharyngeal muscular dystrophy to chromosome 14q11.2-q13 in American families suggests the existence of a second causal mutation. *Neuromuscular Disorders*, 7, S75–S81.

Taylor, E.W. (1915). Progressive vagus-glossopharyngeal paralysis with ptosis: a contribution to the group of family diseases. *The Journal of Nervous and Mental Diseases*, 42, 129–39.

Teh, B.T., Sullivan, A.A., Farnebo, F., Zander, C., Li, F.Y., Strachan, N. *et al.* (1997). Oculopharyngeal muscular dystrophy; report and genetic studies of an Australian kindred. *Clinical Genetics*, 51, 52–5.

Tomé, F.M.S., Chateau, D., Helbling-Leclerc, A., and Fardeau, M. (1997). Morphological changes in muscle fibres in oculopharyngeal muscular dystrophy. *Neuromuscular Disorders*, 7, S63–S9.

Tomé, F.M.S. and Fardeau, M. (1980). Nuclear inclusions in oculopharyngeal muscular dystrophy. *Acta Neuropathologica*, 49, 85–7.

Tomé, F.M.S. and Fardeau, M. (1994). In *Myology*. (ed. Engel, A.G. and Franzini-Armstrong, C.) Vol. 2. McGraw-Hill, New York, pp. 1233–45.

Uyama, E., Tsukahara, T., Goto, K., Kurano, Y., Ogawa, M., Kim, Y.J. *et al.* (2000). Nuclear accumulation of expanded PABP2 gene product in oculopharyngeal muscular dystrophy. *Muscle Nerve*, 23, 1549–54.

Victor, M., Hayes, R., and Adams, R.D. (1962). Oculopharyngeal muscular dystrophy: a familial disease of late life characterized by dysphagia and progressive ptosis of the eyelids. *New England Journal of Medicine*, 267, 1267–72.

Wahle, E. (1991). A novel poly(A)-binding protein acts as a specificity factor in the second phase of messenger RNA polyadenylation. *Cell*, 66, 759–68.

Wahle, E., Lustig, A., Jenö, P., and Maurer, P. (1993). Mammalian Poly(A)-binding protein II: physical properties and binding to polynucleotides. *Journal of Biological Chemistry*, 268, 2937–45.

Wahle, E. and Ruegsegger, U. (1999). 3'-End processing of pre-mRNA in eukaryotes. *FEMS Microbiol Rev*, 23, 277–95.

Chapter 11

Dilated cardiomyopathy and related cardiac disorders in muscular dystrophy

J. Andoni Urtizberea, Denis Duboc,
Ketty Schwartz, and Gisèle Bonne

Introduction

Heart dysfunction in muscular dystrophy has been noted a long time ago but did not draw much attention until recently. As Duchenne patients live longer and better nowadays, this complication has become, over the years, a major concern as well as a growing cause of death. The spectrum of cardiac abnormalities turned out to be much broader than originally thought: congestive heart failure, secondary to left ventricular dysfunction, is the commonest risk in many muscular dystrophies but rhythm disturbances and/or conduction defects can also be complications of their own, sometimes indicative of a given neuromuscular disease. In parallel, substantial advances have been made over the last ten years concerning the molecular origins of many other hereditary cardiomyopathies, irrespective of muscular dystrophy. Cardiogeneticists have thus been very successful in identifying the majority of genes responsible for hypertrophic cardiomyopathies, a distinct group of cardiac muscle diseases. They are currently focusing on dilated cardiomyopathy (DCM) with the same momentum. In the meantime, the spectrum of genetic diversity in muscular dystrophies has expanded formidably and generated new insights into muscle physiology.

For historic reasons, and despite obvious similarities between skeletal and cardiac muscles, cardiologists and neurologists have lived in two different worlds. Times are changing, for the benefit of all. There is an urgent need to join efforts for a better understanding of disease mechanisms and figuring out therapeutic solutions. We have a great deal to learn from each other. Additionally, these newcomers in our field now play a crucial role in the multidisciplinary integrated approach of patients with muscular dystrophy by shedding a more therapy-oriented light on pathogenesis and management. They bring with them new concepts, new technologies and greater hopes for a cure.

Definitions

Dilated cardiomyopathy (DCM)   Is a primary or secondary myocardial disorder characterized by dilatation of the cardiac chambers and faulty systolic contraction. It is a major cause of congestive heart failure and therefore a great provider of morbidity and mortality in the general population. The vast majority of DCM cases result from secondary aetiologies such as coronary artery disease, drug toxicity (adriamycin), hypertension, myocarditis, or systemic diseases but many others remain idiopathic.

Out of these primary disorders, approximately one-third are of hereditary origin with autosomal dominant inheritance being the most common. X-linked, autosomal recessive, and mitochondrial transmission have also been reported. Thus far, DCM was clinically categorized according to the presence or absence of associated conduction defects. Among all cases of DCM, the proportion of patients with muscular dystrophy, even if proportionally minimal, is of great interest from a scientific/fundamental viewpoint. The molecular determinants of DCM were poorly understood until very recently as opposed to the fast-moving field of hypertrophic cardiomyopathies, a distinct clinical and pathological entity, in which gene harvesting has been more swift and fruitful. Six loci have now been assigned to DCM group of diseases four of which have been cloned and mutations identified (cardiac actin, lamin A/C, delta-sarcoglycan, desmin).

Related cardiac disorders   There is a wide spectrum of conduction defects (incomplete or complete heart blocks, at the atrioventricular level or below, in the bundle branches) and rhythm disturbances (premature beats or atrial or ventricular origin, ventricular arrhythmias, sinus tachy- or bradycardia; etc.) They usually reflect that something is wrong in the nodal tissue, a specialized cardiac tissue comprising the sinus and the His–Purkinje system. They represent a major cause of sudden death especially in Emery–Dreifuss muscular dystrophies and myotonic dystrophy. They can be the key feature or, a secondary event following advanced myocardial degeneration. Coronary disease is exceptionally seen in muscular dystrophy except in cases where patients may be exposed to other risks (diabetes, hypercholesterolaemia).

Muscular dystrophy   Muscular dystrophy is basically defined by histological changes (necrotic and regenerative processes, fibre size variability, and fatty replacement) and encompasses a great variety of clinical conditions characterized by progressive proximal muscle weakness. As opposed to other neuromuscular disorders in which cardiac involvement also exists and which will be addressed in the differential diagnosis, our attention will be focused exclusively on DCM and related disorders with muscular dystrophy.

Investigations of cardiac involvement

Until recently, the cardiac evaluation of a myopathic patient was hampered by the non-specificity of symptoms and the lack of reliable tools to assess them. With the advent of advanced technologies and better follow-up in many patients, this is no longer the case.

Clinical evaluation

With the exception of rare instances of sudden death, cardiac disease is rarely symptomatic in muscular dystrophy. On the other hand, ancillary examinations clearly demonstrate that cardiac involvement is much more frequent than clinical signs indicate. Two situations should be distinguished: Firstly, when a patient already diagnosed with muscular dystrophy undergoes regular cardiac evaluation and where left ventricular dysfunction, for instance, is expected to occur at some point in time. Secondly, when the cardiac abnormality is a presenting symptom or complication and where muscular dystrophy will be diagnosed subsequently on biological and/or clinical grounds.

Detection of heart failure

Early symptoms are usually insidious: fatigue, loss of appetite, insomnia, cough, abdominal pain, palpitations, or mild ankle swelling are non-specific and often misleading signs. Later, dyspnea can occur but must be distinguished from ventilatory insufficiency. Dyspnea that persists despite adequate ventilatory support suggests cardiac etiology. The significance of palpitations is unclear in these patients. They can reflect either sinusal tachycardia—which is almost constant in DMD—or simple anxiety.

In a wheelchair bound patient, clinical assessment is generally more difficult (weight measurement is often problematic, for instance) and subject to misinterpretation (the commonest source of lower leg oedema in a Duchenne patient is of veinous, and not necessarily cardiac, origin).

Given the total absence of correlation between the severity of heart involvement and the clinical manifestations—even at the skeletal muscle level—it has been suggested to consider systematically every DMD boy above age 9 as being at risk for cardiac involvement, at least in theory. The same applies to Becker muscular dystrophy (BMD) patients irrespective of their ambulatory status.

At a later, sometimes terminal, stage of cardiac failure, symptoms can be overt and comparable to those seen in other causes of congestive heart failure (CHF): weight gain, gross oedema, enlarged liver, congestive veins, and sustained tachycardia.

Sudden death/near miss episodes

Sudden death is by definition unpredictable and thus being inaugural especially in myotonic dystrophy and nucleopathies where skeletal muscle weakness can be minimal if not absent. Syncopes, episodes of fainting or simple irregular heart beats may precede such an event and should therefore be worked up extensively.

Recognition of muscular dystrophy in a cardiac patient

Most non-specialized cardiologists are not very familiar with muscular dystrophy. The only exception perhaps relates to myotonic dystrophy which is a well known cause of cardiac arrhythmia or heart block. Other muscular dystrophies are more difficult to suspect in patients presenting with overt CHF or isolated conduction defects but with very little apparent skeletal muscle involvement. Careful neurological evaluation can detect subtle signs suggesting a primary muscle involvement but it is usually not that easy. In cases of advanced CHF, for instance, generalized weakness is trivial and attributed sometimes wrongly, to chronic hypoxia. Hence, CK levels may be helpful in that context but normal values do not preclude muscular dystrophy. Eventually, the best clue is provided by a muscle biopsy, a procedure which should be more widely indicated / performed in patients with apparently isolated severe CHF.

Ancillary examinations

Chest radiography

With the advent of sophisticated ultrasound echocardiography, chest X-ray is now of less value. At a typical advanced stage of CHF, it shows a globular heart, congested pulmonary vasculature, and sometimes pleural effusion. It can also remain close to normal for a long time. Hence, the cardiothoracic ratio is not often correlated to the severity heart dysfunction. Furthermore, spine deformities, which are commonplace in these patients, make the interpretation of such radiological findings more difficult. Conversely, the existence of major thoracic deformities and abnormal ventilatory distribution in the lungs (atelectasia) may indicate the patient is at risk for cor pulmonale (cf. differential diagnosis).

Electrocardiogram

ECG is generally useful for both detecting and monitoring cardiac disease in a patient with a neuromuscular condition. This relatively cheap, widely accessible tool is also part of the long-term follow-up in every patient with muscular dystrophy especially in myotonic dystrophy. Abnormal findings on ECG are commonplace even in very young DMD boys and occasionally in female carriers. ECG classically shows tall R waves and an R/S ratio greater than 1 in the right precordium leads. As myocardial fibrosis progresses, deep Q waves can be noted in the anterior left ventricular region (Chenard 1988). Axis deviation is more rarely seen. Unfortunately, and despite many attempts to establish correlations with the clinical progression of the disease, these abnormalities are of poor prognostic value.

Isolated presenting conduction defects are in principle more suggestive of myotonic dystrophy or Emery–Dreifuss muscular dystrophy rather than DMD or BMD. Nevertheless, such abnormalities can occur in association with advanced stages of CHF in dystrophinopathies. Even for a non-specialist, the duration of the PR interval is an excellent clue to conduction defects and can easily be measured. Interpretation of other findings, blocks, premature beats, conduction delays are left to the cardiologist but are too often non-specific.

24-hour Holter monitoring

Holter monitoring is a non-invasive technique quite helpful in detecting permanent or non-permanent hyperexcitability or paroxysmal conduction defects. Sinus tachycardia is almost consistent in all DMD patients after age 10. One can note atrioventricular blocks, atrial flutter, premature atrial contractions or sinus pauses, depending on the aetiology. Premature ventricular beats and ventricular tachycardia are less common. Some authors advocate the importance of late potentials on the signal-average ECG as predictive of malignant arrhythmia (Kubo 1993).

Electrophysiological studies

Whenever conduction defects or rhythm disturbances are present, notably in myotonic dystrophy and nucleopathies, it is essential to document them thoroughly. Electrophysiological studies are therefore recommended and consist in monitoring invasively the His–Purkinje system and in potentiating this search by pharmacological agents if necessary. This can only be done in specialized centres where resuscitation measures can be taken instantly. This can be coupled with cardiac catheterization only when pulmonary arterial hypertension is anticipated.

Echocardiography

Echocardiography is a very valuable tool and has become a routine test over the years. In parallel, technological advances have made it more accurate and more user friendly in its approach. However, four circumstances hamper the validity of such a test: severe chest or spinal deformities, poor myocardial echogenicity, improper ventricular positioning and marked hypovolaemia. It is therefore recommended to examine the patient on a lateral position. Several parameters can be measured accurately even though inter-observers discrepancies may persist. M-mode echocardiography can evaluate the presence of mitral valve prolapse, posterior wall systolic and diastolic maximum velocities, and left ventricular wall thickness, mass, fractional shortening, and ejection fraction. The 2D (and soon 3D) mode in combination with Doppler and colour flow mapping helps visualize the cardiac anatomy (chambers, valves), possible regurgitation, and more importantly, regional and global left ventricular contraction patterns. Intracardiac thrombi can also be detected in the same way. In routine practice, LVEF (left ventricular ejection fraction, normal value above 40 per cent) coupled with FS (fractional shortening, normal value above 20 per cent) are the two most critical measurements in a follow-up perspective (de Kermadec et al. 1994). Some argue however that wall motion indexes may be of more predictive value of left ventricular dysfunction than LVEF.

Radioisotope monitoring

Myocardial isotope scanning is to date the most accurate and objective method to evaluate ejection fraction and myocardial perfusion, even in a patient with substantial chest deformities or advanced fibrosis. In that context, myocardial perfusion imaging using thallium-201 single-photon emission computed tomography (SPECT) is less relevant to the assessment of left ventricular dysfunction than radionuclide ventriculography (Tamura 1993). The latter provides a good idea of LVEF at rest and after a pharmacologically induced exercise. Positon emission tomography (PET) imaging is more recent, less accessible but also of great scientific value notably in myotonic dystrophy and to a lesser extent in DMD (Annane 1998; Quinlinvan *et al.* 1996). These sophisticated methods are of rather good prognostic value but cannot be repeated routinely.

Neuroendocrine evaluation

It is well established that CHF triggers neuroendocrine activation. Plasma ANP (atrial natriuretic peptide) and norepinephrine (PNE) levels are therefore useful indicators of DCM and CHF (Ishikawa *et al.* 1995; 1999). Nevertheless, their predictive value in the context of muscular dystrophy is still debated and to our knowledge, they are not widely used.

Endomyocardial biopsy

Such an invasive and potentially hazardous procedure is exceptionally recommended for diagnostic purposes in proven muscular dystrophy with suspected cardiac involvement. It is ethically questionable and only performed routinely in very few centres (Maeda *et al.* 1995). So far, histological findings have been shown to be non-specific except for the lack of dystrophin in BMD/DMD patients. This may change in future, especially in pure and severe cases of DCM, as a growing number of defective proteins are now being discovered (cardiac actin, δ-sarcoglycan, etc.) and for which immunocytochemistry, at least in recessive disorders, will be available in a diagnostic perspective. At this point, it is too early to say whether or not a systematic screening of mutations in the corresponding candidate genes would be a better approach, but it is likely.

Strategies and timing

It is essential to differentiate two types of cardiac disturbances. When the myocardium is altered, structural or functional changes occur in the ventricles and may lead to cardiomyopathy and CHF. When the specialized cardiac tissue is involved, decreased automaticity of the impulse-generating centres may result in bradycardia and extrasystoles, while conduction defects can generate heart blocks, malignant arrhythmias, and sudden death. The consequences and therapeutic strategies are therefore different.

Cardiac investigations are better conducted within a multidisciplinary framework. However, very few expert muscle centres have a specifically dedicated cardiomyologist and/or the adequate sophisticated diagnostic equipment. In our experience, the interaction with cardiologists proves essential, fruitful and requires much attention and consideration from both sides.

The timing of cardiac investigations is not yet clearly defined. In DMD, the tendency is to schedule them earlier, from age 9 onwards. Later, yearly ECG and echocardiography monitoring are generally satisfactory. When the patient is close to spine surgery time, in general, around age 13–14, a thorough evaluation of the left ventricular dysfunction is necessary almost every six months, in order to detect a fast progressing cardiomyopathy that may impede general anesthesia.

In myotonic dystrophy and nucleopathies, and apart from cases of overt and symptomatic bradycardia, a yearly ECG is a minimum. Holter monitoring is needed every two years whereas electrophysiological studies for both diagnostic purposes and follow-up should be discussed on a case-by-case basis.

Etiologies

The muscular dystrophies are a clinically and genetically heterogeneous group of myopathies that differ widely in their frequency and pattern of cardiac involvement. Myocardial disease manifesting predominantly as cardiomyopathy and congestive heart failure is characteristic of dystrophinopathies (including DMD, BMD and XLDCM) sarcoglycanopathies and LGMD 1D, whereas conduction system abnormalities that cause heart block, arrhythmias, and sudden death are more commonly seen in limb-girdle type 1B, myotonic dystrophy, and Emery–Dreifuss muscular dystrophies (Cox and Kunkel 1997). A distinction should be made between muscular dystrophies in which cardiac disease is a cardinal feature and those in which cardiac abnormalities are occasionally reported.

Disorders with cardiac disease as a cardinal feature

Dystrophinopathies

Duchenne muscular dystrophy   Duchenne muscular dystrophy is the very first instance of muscular dystrophy in which cardiac involvement was reported. It was even mentioned in the early Conte's reports back in 1836. Later, the first cardiac histological studies confirmed their original clinical impression (Ross 1883). Since 1987, we have known that dystrophin is the defective protein, both in skeletal muscle and myocardium, two tissues where it is normally highly expressed. Interestingly, it has never been possible to establish a link between the type or the location of mutations and the clinical cardiac severity of the disease. No correlation either has ever been described between the severity of cardiomyopathy and other clinical parameters (including the age of onset, vital capacity, and the severity of skeletal muscle involvement). For some time, an angiotensin-converting enzyme (ACE) polymorphism was thought to be a risk factor but it has never been confirmed in larger series (Reynolds *et al.* 1993).

Cardiac disease is so much associated with dystrophinopathies that some experts often question the diagnosis of DMD in the absence of cardiomyopathy after age 18. As mentioned earlier, the development of cardiac involvement is very insidious and rarely symptomatic (Boland *et al.* 1996; Nigro *et al.* 1994). This means that the cardiomyopathy is likely to be quite advanced and therefore beyond any therapeutic action. Sinus tachycardia is present in most patients after age 5 and persists throughout life and precedes the left ventricular dysfunction.

At the other end of the spectrum, a growing number of young ambulant DMD boys below 10 years of age are now being diagnosed with early, and sometimes substantial, left ventricular dysfunction. This is due to the sophistication of cardiac evaluation and to a better follow-up in general. Once again, there is currently no way to extract/isolate this subgroup at risk from mainstream DMD patients. For unknown reasons, the cardiomyopathy in DMD can progress very rapidly at any stage of the disease. We have followed a couple of young children, around 11–12 years of age, in whom heart function deteriorated dramatically within three months without any associated clinical symptoms whatsoever.

The natural history of cardiac disturbances is partly known: as myocardium is gradually replaced by fibrous tissue, the left ventricular walls become thin and show decreased systolic contraction and diastolic relaxation. A mitral valve prolapse is frequent but its significance is yet debated as it can be observed in severe thoracic deformities. At a later stage, conduction and arrhythmias may occur with an increased exposure to sudden death. Very few studies have documented the causes of death in these patients but one can imagine that with better and customized respiratory care, cardiac insufficiency may well be or become the most common source of mortality in this population in future.

Becker muscular dystrophy Becker muscular dystrophy is an allelic variant of DMD characterised by a slower disease course at the skeletal muscle level and a great clinical variability ranging from mild DMD phenotype to simple myalgias and elevated CK. It occurs at one tenth the frequency of DMD. In some instances of BMD, dilated cardiomyopathy is the predominating symptom and may require heart transplantation. It is likely that a couple of patients in the overall population of transplanted individuals are in fact undiagnosed BMD cases.

Skeletal involvement and cardiomyopathy are not correlated even though involvement of heart muscle seems more prominent in BMD patients with mildly affected skeletal muscles (Visser 1992). One explanation might be that ambulant BMD patients do exercise their heart more than those who are wheelchair dependent and that this may be deleterious in the long run. The diagnosis of BMD is firmly established on muscle biopsy (reduction of dystrophin staining) and/or by screening the dystrophin gene by multiplex-PCR. Cardiac involvement is not associated with specific mutations. Ambulant BMD patients with terminal CHF can be considered positively for heart transplantation with a generally good outcome.

X-linked dilated cardiomyopathy (XLDCM) A significant proportion of X-linked cases of dilated cardiomyopathy with subclinical skeletal muscle involvement are caused by dystrophin-gene defects resulting from mutations similar to those found in DMD and BMD, and others most notably at the 5′ end of the gene (Ferlini *et al.* 1998; 1999; Muntoni *et al.* 1993; 1995; 1997; Towbin *et al.* 1993). The nosological boundary with mild forms of Becker muscular dystrophy is very narrow. In our experience, CK elevation and/or minimal changes on the muscle CT-scan, and/or asymptomatic pseudohypertrophic calves are the best clues to possible XLDCM. The most likely pathophysiological explanation is the difference in the dystrophin expression pattern: in XLCMD, cardiac dystrophin is usually absent in the myocardium while its expression in skeletal muscle is preserved. However, it has recently been shown that dystrophin could also be quantitatively normal in the heart of some XLCMD patients. This finding would suggest the existence of a conformational change in the molecule itself that could in turn lead to the disruption of the sarcoglycan complex (Franz *et al.* 2000).

Nucleopathies

This term is used here to encompass the newly recognized group of muscular dystrophies in which, emerine and lamin A/C, two proteins of the nuclear envelope, are defective.

X-Linked Emery–Dreifuss muscular dystrophy (XLEDMD)   Cardiac involvement is often the key and presenting feature in XLEDMD, a condition otherwise characterized by a slowly progressive muscular dystrophy with multiple early contractures (in the elbows, cervical spine and Achilles tendons) and mutations in the STA gene which codes for the protein emerin. Cardiac arrhythmias are mostly atrial in origin—atrial fibrillation, atrial paralysis, and atrioventricular heart block—and may be progressive. In addition, some degree of dilated cardiomyopathy may be observed as disease progresses. Very few patients are severely physically disabled and therefore, the prognosis depends almost exclusively on the risk of sudden death. Cardiac pacing is highly recommended as it can be life saving. As lethal cardiac involvement may also occur in female carriers, careful cardiological follow-up examinations are recommended.

Autosomal dominant Emery–Dreifuss muscular dystrophy (ADEDMD)   The ADEDMD phenotype differs a little clinically from XLEDMD. Of note is the broader spectrum of clinical severity within the same kindred as is often the case in autosomal dominant traits. Mutations in the lamin A/C gene have been identified recently and these findings outline the importance of proteins of the nuclear envelope (emerin, lamin A/C) in the genesis of Emery–Dreifuss muscular dystrophies (Bonne *et al.* 2000). The cardiac phenotype and skeletal involvement may differ in severity (Brodsky *et al.* 2000). More importantly, the clinical spectrum of nucleopathies has now extended to non-skeletal muscle disorders (DCM associated with conduction defects—(Fatkin *et al.* 1999), hereditary forms of lipodystrophy (Dunnigan syndrome) and other related muscular syndromes (limb girdle muscular dystrophy type 1B). Interestingly, it has been shown within one extended French pedigree that some patients harbouring the same mutation in the lamin A/C gene may exhibit cardiac symptoms with or without skeletal muscle involvement, thus suggesting the existence of modifying factors.

Limb girde muscular dystrophy type 1B   LGMD 1B is an autosomal dominantly inherited, slowly progressive limb girdle muscular dystrophy, characterized by severe age-related atrioventricular cardiac conduction disturbances and absence of early contractures. Fifty per cent of the patients over 35 years had had a pacemaker implanted.

It has been shown that ADEDMD and LGMD 1B were actually allelic disorders to the same locus on chromosome 1q. Mutations in the lamin A/C have subsequently been identified and this finding suggests that the associated skeletal muscle phenotype is much broader than in the classical Emery–Dreifuss muscular dystrophy (Muchir 2000).

Myotonic Dystrophy

Myotonic dystrophy and related conditions are alternatively classified in the muscular dystrophies or in the myotonic disorders. The degree of necrosis/regeneration of muscle fibres is usually very mild as proven by the inconsistent and slight elevation of CK levels. Nevertheless, heart involvement can be dramatic, life threatening and, sometimes, a presenting symptom preceding neurologic signs. Clinically, myotonic dystrophy is characterized by conduction disturbances and tachyarrhythmias whereas myocardial degeneration is rarely present (Philips and Harper 1997). Patients are particularly at risk during general anaesthesia. In that respect, prophylactic measures can be taken even in presymptomatic individuals. The pathogenesis of such problems is little known as many genes at the same 19q locus seem to be influenced by the adjacent and pathologic triplet (CTG) expansion located in the myotonin-protein kinase (Mt-PK) gene. The transgenic mouse for human Mt-PK develops cardiomyopathy but not the knockout mice. The diagnosis of myotonic dystrophy is easily achieved by DNA analysis on lymphocytes. Some correlation has been established between cardiac disease and the length of triplet expansion. (Tokgozoglu et al. 1995; Lazarus et al. 1999). The same kind of cardiac disturbances have also been reported in proximal myotonic myopathy (DM2), a condition that can mimic myotonic dystrophy but which is far less prevalent.

Disorders with occasional cardiac involvement

DMD female carriers   According to separate surveys carried out across Europe, a significant number of female carriers for the DMD/BMD defective are at risk for cardiac disease (Hoogerwaard et al. 1999; Politano et al. 1996). On average, less than one-third of examined carriers have a completely normal cardiac examination after ECG and echocardiographic screening. The risk seems slightly higher in DMD carriers than in BMD carriers and increases with time. Cardiac muscle biopsies normally show a mosaic pattern of absent (DMD) or reduced (BMD) dystrophin.

There is no correlation between the cardiomyopathy and manifestations of skeletal muscle involvement (cramps, muscle weakness) (Mirabella et al. 1993; Ogata et al. 2000). Such individuals should be notified of this potential risk when seeking genetic advice. However, no consensus exists as to which age should the first cardiac evaluation be performed. In the most extreme situations, cardiomyopathy with intractable CHF has been documented and occasionally leads to heart transplantation (Melacini et al. 1998; Quinlinvan and Dubowitz 1992). Interestingly, in one of these cases, the explanted heart did not show a skewed pattern of X-chromosome inactivation as in skeletal muscle suggesting a possible faulty regeneration in cardiomyocytes.

Sarcoglycanopathies   When severe childhood autosomal recessive muscular dystrophy (SCARMD) was first described in Tunisia in the earlier 1980s, heart disease had already been mentioned in order to stress the similarities with DMD (Ben Hamida *et al.* 1983). Unfortunately, the report was poorly documented from a cardiological perspective, and the prevalence of respiratory insufficiency in many of these patients made the evaluation of intrinsic ventricular dysfunction more difficult. Since then, most autosomal recessive muscular dystrophies have genetically been elucidated: among these, the four sarcoglycanopathies (LGMD 2C, 2D, 2E and 2F) correspond to molecular defects of the α, γ, β and δ-SG genes respectively (Bönnemann *et al.* 1995; Duggan *et al.* 1997; Nigro *et al.* 1996; Roberds *et al.* 1994). All four sarcoglycans belong to the dystrophin-glycoprotein complex and are expressed in skeletal and heart muscle, β-SG being more ubiquitous. Sarcoglycans are tightly bound to each other so that mutation in one normally results in partial or total absence of all of them. Similar patterns are found in cardiomyocytes. The role of the sarcoglycan subcomplex is still unclear. A role in signal transduction is most likely.

Cardiac involvement in sarcoglycanopathies is supported by the existence of a natural model of δ-sarcoglycan deficiency, the Syrian hamster, which exhibits a marked and lethal cardiomyopathy (Nigro *et al.* 1997). In human disease however, the situation is more complex and contrasted. The prevalence of the association between sarcoglycanopathy and cardiomyopathy is still debated. The first clinical evidence derives from a report on a 13-year-old patient with dilated cardiomyopathy with a loss of staining in α-SG and γ-SG in cardiac and skeletal muscle (Fadic *et al.* 1996). However, the molecular defect has never been documented in detail in this patient.

Heart involvement has been occasionally reported in all sub-types but one may wonder whether this feature is not underestimated due to the paucity of cases for each of them, and to the lack of rigorous cardiac assessment in the reported cases (Fadic *et al.* 1996; Melacini *et al.* 1999; Merlini *et al.* 2000; Piccolo *et al.* 1995; Towbin 1998; van der Kooi *et al.* 1998). We actually know very little about the natural history of each clinical entity and that is the reason why establishing a long-term prognosis in these patients is not easy.

γ-sarcoglycan deficient patients (LGMD 2C) seem to be the most at risk for cardiac disease (Ben Hamida *et al.* 1996). In a recent paper, and on a homogeneous genetic background (10 Gypsy patients with the same C283Y mutation in the γ-sarcoglycan gene) it has been shown that cardiac abnormalities were frequent (close to 50 per cent) and particularly affected the right ventricule (Calvo 2000). In α-sarcoglycan deficiency (LGMD 2D), this complication is fairly rare, involving less than 20 per cent of cases (Eymard *et al.* 1997).

In β-sarcoglycan deficiency (LGMD 2E), the risk was originally thought to be minimal until recently when two early deaths (around age 20) due to severe cardiomyopathy were reported in two cousins harbouring the same mutation in β-sarcoglycan gene (Bönnemann *et al.* 1996).

The situation is more complex regarding δ-sarcoglycan deficiency (LGMD 2F). On the one hand, the very few patients reported so far in the literature present with severe DMD phenotype but do not demonstrate overt cardiac disease. On the other hand, there is now some strong evidence to think that mutations in the δ-sarcoglycan gene can cause DCM without skeletal muscle involvement (Tsubata *et al.* 2000), a finding more in accordance with what occurs in the δ-sarcoglycan deficient Syrian hamster. Molecular diagnosis of sarcoglycanopathies is available in specialized centres. Dystrophinopathy should be ruled out first by immunostaining and blotting before embarking on a tedious and sometimes unfruitful mutation search in the sarcoglycan genes. As a matter of fact, the four sarcoglycanopathies are clinically indistinguishable whereas immunocytochemistry might be helpful in some instances to target one specific gene (α, β, γ, or δ).

The general conclusion is therefore to rigorously monitor patients with sarcoglycan deficiencies in order to detect asymptomatic cardiac disease. That will provide new insights into the natural history of these conditions.

FSHD   Cardiac disturbances are not a common feature in facioscapulohumeral muscular dystrophy (Padberg 1982). In recent studies however, significant conduction defects or rhythm anomalies have been reported in a couple of patients with molecularly confirmed FSHD (Ohno *et al.* 1991; Laforêt *et al.* 1998). The authors suggest that these complications are probably overlooked and that closer cardiac monitoring should be planned.

Limb girdle muscular dystrophies   Apart from the four sarcoglycanopathies (LGMD 2C to 2F) and one allelic variant of nucleopathies (LGDM 1B), only one other form of LGMD is reported to be associated with cardiac disease. In *LGMD 1D*, an autosomal dominant subtype described in a Northern American kindred, the phenotype resembles that of LGMD 1B with unspecific adult-onset limb girdle muscular dystrophy, dilated cardiomyopathy, and cardiac conduction defects. A locus has been assigned to the long arm of the chromosome 6q with a maximum lod-score of 4.99, in a region distinct from the LAMA2 locus which normally encodes merosin, a protein defective in congenital muscular dystrophy (Messina *et al.* 1997). In other types of recessive (LGMD 2A, 2B, 2G, 2H and 2I) or dominant (LGMD 1A, 1C, 1E) limb girdle muscular dystrophies, heart involvement has never been regarded as a core feature. Some authors nevertheless reported cases with marked heart involvement but at a time when molecular diagnosis was insecure (Hoshio *et al.* 1987; Kawashima *et al.* 1990).

Congenital muscular dystrophies

Congenital muscular dystrophies (CMD) represent a very heterogeneous group of autosomal recessive myopathies with an early onset and a variable clinical progression. Classically, cardiac involvement is more an exclusion than an inclusion criteria for CMD but it has occasionally been reported in a few merosin-deficient cases when children were carefully assessed from a cardiological point of view (Reed *et al.* 1996; Cil *et al.* 1994; Dubowitz 1995).

Differential diagnosis

Cor pulmonale

In the past, when most patients would not benefit from assisted ventilation, one major cause of cardiac disturbances in Duchenne patients was the insidious development of cor pulmonale due to chronic respiratory failure with resulting hypoxemia. The correction of hypoxia is therefore a prerequisite for the evaluation of any intrinsic cardiomyopathy in this type of patients. This is discussed in detail in Chapter 11.

Other neuromuscular conditions

Cardiac involvement is not specific to some forms of muscular dystrophy. It has also been documented in other neuromuscular conditions such as infantile acid maltase deficiency (Pompe's disease), carnitine deficiency, mitochondrial disease (Kearns-Sayre syndrome), periodic paralysis, polymyositis, and desmin-storage myopathies. In most cases, the clinical features and/or the histological findings on the skeletal muscle biopsy provide the best clue to the diagnosis. Subsequent genetic studies generally confirm this impression.

Random association

Minor cardiac abnormalities are frequent in the general population: extrasystoles, tachyarrythmias, incomplete blocks, etc. No overall surveys are available but one can estimate they occur in 1–2 per cent of the population. With more sophisticated tests, and advanced preventive screening programs, this figure is likely to increase in future. Therefore, the most relevant question when such anomalies are found in a patient with muscular dystrophy is: could it simply be a random association? This is particularly true in subtypes of muscular dystrophy in which cardiac disease is very rarely reported or seems quite intriguing. In our experience, random association can be ruled out when cardiac disturbances clearly co-segregate with the skeletal muscle disorder or when the proportion of involved cases within a given clinical subgroup is above 30 per cent. The other question would be: where is the threshold to state that a patient with a neuromuscular disorder has cardiac involvement? The sensitivity ratio differs from one cardiac test to the other, and probably from one centre to another. On the other hand, it is hardly conceivable to perform sophisticated investigations (radionuclide ventriculography, PET, or His–Purkinje system measurements, for instance) on every patient with neuromuscular disease. Standardization of procedures and attitudes is therefore necessary.

Therapeutic interventions

Therapeutic interventions are based on the fact that myopathic patients with heart involvement are basically at risk for sudden death and congestive heart failure. In addition, thrombo-embolic complications are also possible even if rarely reported. Even though we cannot tackle the degenerative process yet, taking place in the myocardium or in the specialized cardiac tissue, much else can be done to alleviate deleterious symptoms and help the patient live longer. More drastic improvement is expected from the development of innovative therapies based on cell/gene engineering but it will probably take time before they materialize at bedside.

Symptomatic treatment of congestive heart failure

There is no real consensus on the pharmacological treatment of CHF but this is not specific to DCM associated with muscular dystrophy. For the subcategory of patients with DMD, very few controlled studies are available. A prerequisite is to normalize ventilatory parameters before instituting any cardiac drug therapy. Digitalis and diuretics have long been used but are subject to many side effects including overdosage. The current trend is to prescribe angiotensin-converting enzyme inhibitors (ACEI) a commonly used and generally safe drug. Dry cough and slight hypotension are the two main side effects that can be tackled by adjusting the dosage. β-blockers, despite their negative inotropic effects have paradoxically been found to alleviate neurohormonal activation and sustain haemodynamic and clinical improvement in chronic CHF. The use of catecholamines is possible in theory (Mastumura *et al.* 1999), but less convenient in routine practice. Routine antiarrhythmic therapy does not appear to be indicated as arrhythmias are usually secondary to DCM itself.

Diverse regimens and combinations have been proposed, including tritherapy (digitalis, diuretics, ACEI) none of which appears to be the panacea (Ishikawa *et al.* 1995; 1999). In any case, echocardiographic monitoring should be instituted every six months to evaluate the therapeutic impact. Isotopic ventriculography would provide more objective measurements but cannot be repeated too often at that stage.

When LVEF declines to below 10 per cent and does not respond to any drug therapy, the outcome is generally fatal within a few months. At that point, heart transplantation could be the only solution. The rule, however, is not to propose non-ambulatory patients for transplantation for ethical reasons and shortage of donors. The patients who reportedly benefited from this life-saving technique are mostly patients either with BMD or Emery-Dreifuss muscular dystrophies, or DMD/BMD female carriers (Bittner *et al.* 1995; Casazza *et al.* 1988; Donofrio *et al.* 1989; Quinlivan *et al.* 1992; Rees *et al.* 1993). The outcome is generally good even though the follow-up period is still short.

Symptomatic treatment of conduction defects

There is little doubt about the crucial impact of pacemaker in conduction defects. It is a common, straightforward procedure that can be life saving. All sorts of devices exist, mono or dual chamber pacemakers, with or without defibrillating capacities, as well as a wide range of prices. In case of isolated but life-threatening heart block, a simple basic pacemaker is recommended, especially in myotonic dystrophy. When associated to potential ventricular arrhythmias, a more complex device should be considered.

Prophylactic measures

Whatever the type of muscular dystrophy, early detection of cardiac troubles is essential. The best example is given by cardiac management before spinal surgery, a commonplace procedure in Duchenne boys now. In the early days, anaesthetists were very reluctant to let such fragile patients undergo such a major, and stressful operation. Hence, a significant number of young patients died in the preoperative period due to unmasked cardiac failure. Ever since, patients have been more carefully monitored beforehand and orthopaedic surgeons are often asked to operate on them earlier, around 13 or 14 years of age, irrespective of the completion of spine growth. Thanks to this integrated approach, mortality of spine surgery in DMD teenagers has dramatically decreased over the past 10 years and a majority of them (85 to 90 per cent, at least in the French experience) can benefit from this functional surgery. A recent, but yet unpublished, French protocol has evaluated the possibility of preventing or delaying the occurrence of cardiomyopathy in DMD by administrating ACEI before any detectable left ventricular malfunction that is, in general, from age 10 onwards. Preliminary results after a 3-year follow-up did not, however, demonstrate any benefit in the pace of cardiac deterioration. Interestingly, the pre-inclusion studies showed, as mentioned earlier, the existence of a small subgroup of DMD patients characterized by a very early cardiomyopathy manifesting before age 9. The project is now to design the same kind of trial for younger patients, between age 6 and 8.

The other obvious example of useful prophylactic measures is the possibility of inserting a life-saving pacemaker in case of severe conduction defects (in patients with nucleopathies or myotonic dystrophy). The main issue now is as to which type of pacemaker should be implanted. Regular ones prevent sudden death caused by permanent or paroxystic heart block whereas the new generation of sophisticated pacemakers permits defibrillation in case of associated acute rhythm disturbances. An ongoing French study attempts to evaluate the possibility of preventing sudden death in myotonic dystrophic by implanting a pacemaker at an early stage when cardiac symptoms are minimal (widened PR interval).

More generally, it might be interesting to screen the general population of patients with conduction defects for genetic abnormalities such as mutations in the lamin A/C, emerin or the Mt-PK genes and subsequently identify within their relatives presymptomatic individuals at risk.

The prevention of thromboemboli in DMD patients is more controversial as the risk is more difficult to evaluate. Some prescribe low-dose aspirin or anti-aggregants daily while others do not.

Curative treatments

Several experimental therapeutic avenues are being explored but none of them have as yet reached the clinical level in man except myoblast transfer. Gene therapy was successfully experimented in the *mdx* mouse but the validity of the model for heart disease is questionable. Upregulation of utrophin, a protein sharing many similarities with dystrophin is potentially of interest. Developing pharmalogic agents that will increase endogenous utrophin expession in DMD and BMD is under way. However, clinical reports of explanted DMD heart suggest that utrophin is already upregulated in the myocardium. Results achieved in gene therapy applied to the δ-sarcoglycan deficient mouse look more promising. Nucleopathies could also be considered positively for gene therapy protocols as both genes, *STA* gene (emerin) and *LMNA* gene (lamin A/C) are of limited size and easy to target inside the cardiac conducting tissue. Stem cell therapy may also prove a possibility and is discussed further in Chapter 13.

Pathogenesis/Future prospects

The existence of two distinct patterns of cardiac disease (dilated cardiomyopathy on the one hand, conductions defects and rhythm disturbances on the other) suggests that two different cellular processes are involved: defects in mechanical stabilization of the plasma membrane and signal transduction impairments. In that context, many scientists speculate that the dystrophin–glycoprotein complex (DGC) could be one core element of the final common pathway leading to muscular dystrophy and dilated cardiomyopathy. This attractive hypothesis is also supported by evidence of dystrophin cleavage and disruption of sarcoglycans in non-hereditary models of DCM like the enterovirus-induced cardiomyopathy. (Badorff *et al.* 2000; Lee *et al.* 2000). On the other hand, defective nuclear proteins such as lamin A/C and emerin, and possibly Mt-PK could generate conduction defects and rhythm disturbances because of their potential impact on signal transduction. This dichotomy is partly confirmed in clinical experience but does not account for the wide spectrum of symptoms that sometimes occurs within the same kindred, notably in nucleopathies.

Spontaneous or genetically engineered animal models are relevant to the pathogenesis of DCM and muscular dystrophy (Ikeda and Ross 2000). Interestingly, the dystrophin-deficient *mdx* mouse does not exhibit any cardiac symptoms whereas the double knockouts for dystrophin and utrophin on the one hand, and for dystrophin and MyoD, on the other, do. The knockout mouse lacking γ-sarcoglycan, as well as the above mentioned δ-sarcoglycan deficient Syrian hamster also have marked heart involvement and subsequent lethal CHF. Apoptosis could play a role in this process (Hack *et al.* 1998). Knockout mice are in progress for lamin A/C and emerin, whereas knockout mice in myotonic dystrophic show contradictory findings.

The potential implication of the vascular smooth muscle has recently been hypothesized in the δ-sarcoglycan deficient mouse where microvascular abnormalities and inducible myocardial ischaemia have been noted. This, however, has not yet been reported in other models.

There is also a great deal to learn from disease mechanisms that have been unravelled in other cardiomyopathies without muscular dystrophy. The general and somewhat attractive idea is that dilated cardiomyopathy would stem from molecular defects in force transmitting proteins as opposed to hypertrophic cardiomyopathy that might be caused by defects in force generating proteins like the various components of the sarcomere. There is, however, growing evidence for some degree of overlap (Sakamoto *et al.* 1997). Cardiac α-actin, for instance, has recently been shown to cause both HCM or DCM. The pathophysiologic role of other proteins implicated in DCM (for example, tafazzin, desmin) is as yet poorly understood.

From a broader perspective, one may speculate that the discovery of new genes and new biochemical pathways will contribute to identifying the missing links in future. Modifying factors, of genetic and non-genetic nature, also have to be considered in order to explain the wide range of phenotypic variability and the intriguing absence of correlations between cardiac and skeletal muscle phenotypes.

Conclusion

Incorporating fundamental or clinical cardiologists into the field of myology is something very valuable that should be promoted in every centre. The Institute of Myology in Paris pioneered this new approach and clearly benefits, for the sake of its scientists and patients alike, from this mutual cross-fertilization. Cardiac and skeletal muscle tissues share many proteins. Their interaction and specific role in each tissue are probably very complex but their molecular structure remains comparable. Reaching the stage of curative therapies still represents a long-term goal but what has occurred in the past five years is very encouraging.

References

Annane, D., Fiorelli, M., Mazoyer, B., Pappata, S., Eymard, B., Radvanyi, H. *et al.* (1988). Impaired cerebral glucose metabolism in myotonic dystrophy: a triplet-size dependent phenomenon. *Neuromuscular Disorders*, 8, 39–45.

Badorff, C., Lee, G.H., and Knowlton, K.U. (2000). Enteroviral cardiomyopathy: bad news for the dystrophin-glycoprotein complex. *Herz*, 25, 227–32.

Barresi, R., Di Blasi, C., Negri, T., Brugnoni Vitali, A., Felisari, G., Salandi, A. *et al.* (2000). Disruption of heart sarcoglycan complex and severe cardiomyopathy caused by beta sarcoglycan mutations. *Journal of Medical Genetics*, 37, 102–7.

Ben Hamida, M., Fardeau, M., and Attia, N. (1983). Severe childhood muscular dystrophy affecting both sexes and frequent in Tunisia. *Muscle and Nerve*, 6, 469–80.

Ben Hamida, M., Ben Hamida, C., Zouari, M., Belal, S., and Hentati, F. (1996). Limb-girdle muscular dystrophy 2C: clinical aspects. *Neuromuscular Disorders*, 6, 493–4.

Bittner, R.E., Shorny, S., Streubel, B., Hubner, C., Voit, T., and Kress, W. (1995). Serum antibodies to the deleted dystrophin sequence after cardiac transplantation in a patient with Becker's muscular dystrophy. *New England Journal of Medicine*, 333, 732–3.

Boland, B.J., Silbert, P.L., Groover, R.V., Wollan, P.C., and Silverstein, M.D. (1996). Skeletal, cardiac, and smooth muscle failure in Duchenne muscular dystrophy. *Pediatric Neurology*, 14, 7–12.

Bonne, G.B., Di Barletta, M.R., Varnous, S., Bécane, H.M., Hammouda, E.H., Merlini, L. *et al.* (1999). Mutations in the gene encoding lamin A/C cause autosomal dominant Emery-Dreifuss muscular dystrophy. *Nature Genetics*, 21, 285–8.

Bönnemann, C.G., Modi, R., Noguchi, S., Mizuno, Y., Yoshida, M., Gussoni, E. *et al.* (1995). Beta-sarcoglycan (A3b) mutations cause autosomal recessive muscular dystrophy with loss of the sarcoglycan complex. *Nature Genetics*, **11**, 266–73.

Bönnemann, C.G., Passos-Bueno, M.R., McNally, E.M., Vainzof, M., de Sa Moreira, E., Marie. *et al.* (1996). Genomic screening for beta-sarcoglycan gene mutations: missense mutations may cause severe limb-girdle muscular dystrophy type 2E (LGMD 2E). *Human Molecular Genetics*, **5**, 1953–61.

Brodsky, G.L., Muntoni, F., Miocic, S., Sinagra, G., Sewry, C., Mestroni, L. (2000). Lamin A/C gene mutation associated with dilated cardiomyopathy with variable skeletal muscle involvement. *Circulation*, **101**(5), 473–6.

Calvo, F., Teijeira, S., Fernandez, J.M., Teijeiro, A., Fernandez-Hojas, R., Fernandez-Lopez, X.A. *et al.* (2000). Evaluation of heart involvement in gamma-sarcoglycanopathy (LGMD 2C). A study of ten patients. *Neuromuscular Disorders*, **10**, 560–6.

Casazza, F., Brambilla, G., Salvato, A., Morandi, L., Grande, E., and Bonacina, E. (1988). Dilated cardiomyopathy and successful cardiac transplantation in Becker's muscular dystrophy: follow-up after two years. *G Ital Cardiol*, **18**, 753–7.

Chenard, A.A., Becane, H.M., Tertrain, F., and Weiss, Y.A. (1988). Systolic time intervals in Duchenne muscular dystrophy: evaluation of left ventricular performance. *Clinical Cardiology*, **11**, 407–11.

Cil, E., Topaloglu, H., Caglar, M., and Osme, S. (1994). Left ventricular structure and function by echocardiography in congenital muscular dystrophy. *Brain Development*, **16**, 301–3.

Cox, G.F. and Kunkel, L.M. (1997). Dystrophies and heart disease. *Current Opinion in Cardiology*, **12**, 329–43.

de Kermadec, J.M., Becane, H.M., Chenard, A., Tertrain, F., and Weiss, Y. (1994). Prevalence of left ventricular systolic dysfunction in Duchenne muscular dystrophy: an echocardiographic study. *American Heart Journal*, **127**(3), 618–23.

De Visser, M. (1992). The heart in Becker muscular dystrophy, facioscapulohumeral dystrophy, and Bethlem myopathy. *Muscle nerve*, **15**, 591–6.

Donofrio, P.D., Challa, V.R., Hackshaw, B.T., Mills, S.A., and Cordell, R. (1989). Cardiac transplant in a patient with muscular dystrophy and cardiomyopathy. *Archives of Neurology*, **46**, 705–7.

Dubowitz, V. (1995). 41st ENMC international workshop on congenital muscular dystrophy. *Neuromuscular Disorders*, **6**, 295–305.

Duggan, D., Manchester, D., Stears, K., Mathews, D., Hart, C., and Hoffmann, E. (1997). Mutations in the delta sarcoglycan gene are a rare cause of autosomal recessive limb-girdle muscular dystrophy (LGMD2F). *Neurogenetics*, **1**, 49–58.

Eymard, B., Romero, N.B., Leturcq, F., Piccolo, F., Carrié, A., Jeanpierre, M. *et al.* (1997). Primary adhalinopathy (alpha-sarcoglycanopathy), clinical, pathological and genetic correlation in twenty patients with autosomal recessive muscular dystrophy. *Neurology*, **48**, 1227–34.

Fadic, R., Sunada, Y., Walclawik, A.J., Buck, S., Lewandoski, P.J., Campbell, K.P., and Lodz, B.P. (1996). Brief report: deficiency of a dystrophin-associated glycprotein (adhalin) in a patient with muscular dystrophy and cardiomyopathy. *New England Journal of Medicine*, **334**, 362–6.

Fanin, M., Melacini, P., Angelini, C., and Danieli, G.A. (1999). Could utrophin rescue the myocardium of patients with dystrophin gene mutations? *Journal of Molecular and Cellular Cardiology*, **31**, 1501–8.

Fatkin, D., MacRae, C., Sasaki, T., Wolff, M.R., Porcu, M., Frenneaux, M. *et al.* (1999). Missense mutations in the rod domain of the lamin A/C gene as causes of dilated cardiomyopathy and conduction-system disease. *New England Journal of Medicine*, **341**, 1715–24.

Ferlini, A., Nazzareno, G., Merlini, L., Sewry, C., Branzi, A., and Muntoni, F. (1998). A novel Alu-like element rearrangement in the dystrophin gene causes a splicing mutation in a family with X-linked dilated cardiomyopathy. *American Journal of Human Genetics*, **63**, 436–46.

Ferlini, A., Sewry, C., Melis, M.A., Mateddu, A., and Muntoni, F. (1999). X-linked dilated cardiomyopathy and the dystrophin gene. *Neuromuscular Disorders*, **9**, 339–46.

Franz, W.M., Müller, M., Müller, O.J., Hermann, R., Rothmann, T., Cremer, M. *et al.* (2000). Association of nonsense mutation of dystrophin gene with disruption of sarcoglycan complex in X-linked dilated cardiomyopathy. *Lancet*, **355**, 1781–5.

Hack, A.A., Ly, C.T., Jiang, F., Clendenin, C.J., Sigrist, K.S., Wollmann, R.L., and McNally, E.M. (1998). Gamma-sarcoglycan deficiency leads to muscle membrane defects and apoptosis independent of dystrophin. *Journal of Cell Biology*, **142**, 1279–87.

Hoogerwaard, E.M., van der Wouw, P.A., Wilde, A.A., Bakker, E., Ippel, P.F., Oosterwijk, J.C. *et al.* (1999). Cardiac involvement in carriers of Duchenne and Becker muscular dystrophy. *Neuromuscular Disorders*, **9**, 347–51.

Hoshio, A., Kotake, H., Saito, M., Ogino, K., Fujimoto, Y., Hasegawa, J. *et al.* (1987). Cardiac involvement in a patient with limb-girdle muscular dystrophy. *Heart Lung*, **16**, 439–41.

Ikeda, Y. and Ross, J. (2000). Models of dilated cardiomyopathy in the mouse and the hamster. *Current Opinion in Cardiology*, **15**, 197–201.

Ishikawa, Y., Bach, J.R., Sarma, R.J., Tamura, T., Song, J., Marra, S.W. *et al.* (1995). Cardiovascular considerations in the management of neuromuscular disease. *Seminars in Neurology*, **15**, 93–108.

Ishikawa, Y., Bach, J.R., and Minami, R. (1999). Cardioprotection for Duchenne's muscular dystrophy. *American Heart Journal*, **X**, 895–902.

Kawashima, S., Ueno, M., Kondo, T., Yamamoto, J., and Iwasaki, T. (1990). Marked cardiac involvement in limb-girdle muscular dystrophy. *American Journal of Medical Science*, **299**, 411–4.

Kubo, M., Matsuoka, S., Taguchi, Y., Akita, H., and Kuroda, Y. (1993). Clinical significance of late potential in patients with Duchenne muscular dystrophy. *Pediatric Cardiology*, **14**, 214–9.

Laforet, P., de Toma, C., Eymard, B., Becane, H.M., Jeanpierre, M., Fardeau, M., and Duboc, D. (1998). Cardiac involvement in genetically confirmed facioscapulohumeral muscular dystrophy. *Neurology*, **51**(5), 1454–6.

Lazarus, A., Varin, J., Ounnoughene, Z., Radvanyi, H., Junien, C., Coste, J. *et al.* (1999). Relationships among electrophysiological findings and clinical status, heart function, and extent of DNA mutation in myotonic dystrophy. *Circulation*, **99**, 1041–6.

Lee, G.H., Badorff, C., and Knowlton, K.U. (2000). Dissociation of sarcoglycans and the dystrophin carboxyl terminus from the sarcolemma in enteroviral cardiomyopathy. *Circulation Research*, **87**, 489–5.

Maeda, M., Nakao, S., Miyazato, H., Setoguchi, M., Arima, S., Higuchi, I. *et al.* (1995). Cardiac dystrophin abnormalities in Becker muscular dystrophy assessed by endomyocardial biopsy. *American Heart Journal*, **129**(4), 702–7.

Matsumura, T., Saito, T., Miyai, I., Nozaki, S., and Kang, J. (1999). Effective milrinone therapy to a Duchenne muscular dystrophy patient with advanced congestive heart failure. *Rinsho Shinkeigaku*, **39**, 643–8.

Melacini, P., Fanin, M., Angelini, A., Pegoraro, E., Livi, U., Danieli, G.A. *et al.* (1998). Cardiac transplantation in a Duchenne muscular dystrophy carrier. *Neuromuscular Disorders*, **8**, 585–90.

Melacini, P., Fanin, M., Duggan, D., Freda, M., Berardinelli, A., Danieli, G. *et al.* (1999). Heart involvement in muscular dystrophies due to sacoglycan gene mutations. *Muscle & Nerve*, **22**, 473–9.

Merlini, L., Kaplan, J.-C., Navarro, C., Barois, A., Bonneau, D., and Brasa, J. (2000). Homogeneous phenotype of the gypsy limb-girdle muscular dystrophy with the gamma-sarcoglycan C283Y mutation. *Neurology*, **54**, 1075–9.

Messina, D.N., Speer, M.C., Pericak-Vance, M.A., and McNally, E.M. (1997). Linkage of familial dilated cardiomyopathy with conduction defect and muscular dystrophy to chromosome 6q23. *American Journal of Human Genetics*, **61**, 909–17.

Mirabella, M., Servidei, S., Manfredi, G., Ricci, E., Frustaci, A., Bertini, E., (1993). Cardiomyopathy may be the only clinical manifestation in female carriers of Duchenne muscular dystrophy. *Neurology*, **43**, 2342–5.

Muchir, A., Bonne, G., van der Kooi, A., van Meegen, M., Baas, F., Bolhuis, P.A. *et al.* (2000). Identification of mutations in the gene encoding lamins A/C in autosomal dominant limb girdle muscular dystrophy with atrioventricular conduction disturbances (LGMD1B). *Human Molecular Genetics*, **9**, 1453–9.

Muntoni, F., Cau, M., Ganau, A. *et al.* (1993). Brief report, deletion of the dystrophin muscle promoter region associated with X-linked cardiomyopathy. *New England Journal of Medicine*, **329**, 921–5.

Muntoni, F., Wilson, L., Marrosu, G. *et al.* (1995). A mutation in the dystrophin gene selectively affecting dystrophin expression in the heart. *Journal of Clinical Investigation*, **96**, 693–9.

Muntoni, F., Di Lenarda, A., Porcu, M., Sinagra, G., Mateddu, A., Marrosu, G. *et al.* (1997). Dystrophin gene abnormalities in two patients with idiopathic dilated cardiomyopathy. *Heart*, **78**, 608–12.

Nigro, V., de Sa Moreira, E., Piluso, G., Vainzof, M., Belsito, A., Politano, L. *et al.* (1996). Autosomal recessive limb-girdle muscular dystrophy, LGMD2F, is caused by a mutation in the delta-sarcoglycan gene. *Nature Genetics*, **14**, 195–8.

Nigro, V., Okazaki, Y., Belsito, A., Piluso, G., Matsuda, Y., Politano, L. *et al.* (1997). Identification of the Syrian hamster cardiomyopathy gene. *Human Molecular Genetics*, **6**, 601–7.

Nigro, G., Politano, L., Nigro, V., Petretta, V.R., and Comi, L.I. (1994). Mutation of dystrophin gene and cardiomyopathy. *Neuromuscular Disorders*, **4**, 371–9.

Ogata, H., Nakagawa, H., Hamabe, K., Hattori, A., Ishikawa, Y., Ishikawa, Y. *et al.* (2000). A female carrier of Duchenne muscular dystrophy complicated with cardiomyopathy. *Internal Medicine*, **39**, 34–8.

Ohno, Y., Nakata, Y., Sumiyoshi, M., Hisaoka, T., Ogura, S., Nakazato, Y., and Yamaguchi, H. (1991). A case of facioscapulohumeral muscular dystrophy complicated with complete A-V block. *Kokyu To Junkan*, **39**, 491–5.

Padberg, G.W. (1982). Facioscapulohumeral disease. Thesis. Leiden University.

Philips, M.F. and Harper, P.S. (1997). Cardiac disease in myotonic dystrophy. *Cardiovascular Research*, **33**, 13–22.

Piccolo, F., Roberds, S.L., Jeanpierre, M., Leturcq, F., Azibi, K., Beldjord, C. *et al.* (1995). Primary adhalinopathy, a common cause of autosomal recessive muscular dystrophy of variable severity. *Nature Genetics*, **10**, 243–5.

Politano, L., Nigro, V., Nigro, G., Petretta, V.R., Passamano, L., Papparella, S. *et al.* (1996). Development of cardiomyopathy in female carriers of Duchenne and Becker muscular dystrophies. *JAMA*, **275**, 1335–8.

Quinlivan, R.M. and Dubowitz, V. (1992). Cardiac transplantation in Becker muscular dystrophy. *Neuromuscular Disorders*, **2**, 165–7.

Quinlivan, R.M., Lewis, P., Marsden, P., Dundas, R., Robb, S.A., Baker, E., Maisey, M. (1996). Cardiac function, metabolism and perfusion in Duchenne and Becker muscular dystrophy. *Neuromuscular Disorders*, **6**, 237–46.

Reed, U.C., Marie, S.K., Vainzof, M., Salum, P.B., Levy, J.A., Zatz, M., and Diament, A. (1996). Congenital muscular dystrophy with cerebral white matter hypodensity. Correlation of clinical features and merosin deficiency. *Brain Development*, **18**, 53–8.

Rees, W., Schuler, S., Hummel, M., and Hetzer, R. (1993). Heart transplantation in patients with muscular dystrophy associated with end-stage cardiomyopathy. *Journal of Heart and Lung Transplantation*, **12**, 804–7.

Raynolds, M.V., Bristow, M.R., Bush, E.W. *et al.* (1993). Angiotensin-converting enzyme DD genotype in patients with ischaemic or idiopathic dilated cardiomyopathy. *Lancet*, **342**, 1073–5.

Roberds, S.L., Leturcq, F., Allamand, V., Piccolo, F., Jeanpierre, M., Anderson, R.D. (1994). Missense mutations in the adhalin gene linked to autosomal recessive muscular dystrophy. *Cell*, **78**, 625–33.

Ross, J. (1883). On a case of pseudo-hypertrophic paralysis. *British Medical Journal*, **1**, 200–3.

Sakamoto, A., Ono, K., Abe, M., Jasmin, G., Eki, T., Murakami, Y. *et al.* (1997). Both hypertrophic and dilated cardiomyopathies are caused by mutations of the same gene, delta-sarcoglycan, in hamster, an animal model of disrupted dystrophin-associated glycoprotein complex. *Proceedings of the National Academy of Sciences USA*, **194**, 13873–8.

Tamura, T., Shibuya, N., Hashiba, K., Oku, Y., Mori, H., and Yano, K. (1993). Evaluation of myocardial damage in Duchenne's muscular dystrophy with thallium-201 myocardial SPECT. *Jpn Heart J* **34**, 51–61.

Tokgozoglu, L.S., Ashizawa, T., Pacifico, A., Armstrong, R.M., Epstein, H.F., and Zoghbi, W.A. (1995). Cardiac involvement in a large kindred with myotonic dystrophy quantitative assessment and relation to size of CTG repeat expansion. *JAMA*, **274**, 813–9.

Tsubata, S., Bowles, K.R., Vatta, M., Zintz, C., Titus, J., Muhonen, L. *et al.* (2000). Mutations in the human delta-sarcoglycan gene in familial and sporadic dilated cardiomyopathy. *Journal of Clinical Investigation*, **106**, 655–62.

Van der Kooi, A.J., de Voogt, W.G., Barth, P.G., Busch, H.F.M., Jennekens, F.G.I., Jongen P.J.H., and de Visser, M. (1998). The heart in limb girdle muscular dystrophies. *Heart*, **79**, 73–77.

Chapter 12

Medical management and treatment of muscular dystrophy

Adnan Y. Manzur

The last decade has seen major advances in the understanding of the molecular genetics and pathogenesis of the muscular dystrophies (Dubowitz 1998; Emery 1997; 1998), and this in turn has raised expectations of a curative treatment. This is not yet available and symptomatic and palliative treatment is essential to enhance the patient's quality of life. Physical therapy for prevention of contractures and promotion of ambulation is the mainstay of treatment. Judicious surgical intervention may improve or stabilize motor function in carefully selected patients. Early detection and treatment of respiratory and cardiac complications reduces morbidity, improves quality of life and prolongs survival (Vianello 1994; Ishikawa *et al.* 1999; Nigro *et al.* 1995; Bach 1991; Simmonds *et al.* 1998). The potential benefit of pharmacotherapy, especially glucocorticoids in Duchenne muscular dystrophy, has been recognized and is being further evaluated. This chapter addresses the advances in physical and drug therapies aimed at improving function and quality of life. The early detection and treatment of cardiac and respiratory complications, so crucial to improve survival, is covered in Chapters 11 and 13.

Table 12.1 lists some of the muscular dystrophies with brief comments on their course and common complications (Emery 1997; Dubowitz 1995). Knowledge of these is essential to tailor investigations and treatment at various stages of the disease.

Duchenne muscular dystrophy, with an incidence of 1 in 3500 male live births (Emery 1991) is the most common and eventually, uniformly fatal. It is the first dystrophy for which the gene was characterized (Koenig *et al.* 1987), dystrophin (Hoffman *et al.* 1987), the missing gene product, was identified and is currently the subject of maximal therapeutic-oriented research, both in animal models and human subjects. The treatment of Duchenne dystrophy will be discussed in detail, and the principles of treatment of symptoms and complications apply to other muscular dystrophies as well. The awareness of life threatening complications, their early detection, and treatment is important not only for the patients, but also for the asymptomatic carriers (Hoogerwaard *et al.* 1999).

Table 12.1 Clinical features of the various muscular dystrophies

	Gene locus	Loss of walking	Nocturnal hypoventilation, respiratory failure	Cardiac involvement	Survival	Special comments
Duchenne Muscular Dystrophy	Xp21	Invariable by 13 years	Invariable in non-ambulant phase	Cardiomyopathy in 20% in non-ambulant phase	Death in late 2nd or 3rd decade	Treatment of respiratory failure with nocturnal nasal mask ventilation prolongs survival
Becker Muscular Dystrophy	Xp21	Walk beyond 18 years	Unusual	Dilated cardiomyopathy while still ambulant	Dictated by cardiomyopathy	Cardiac transplant may 'normalize' life
α sarcoglycanopathy (Limb Girdle MD Type 2D)	17q12	In teens	In late non-ambulant phase	Rare	Often limited till 3rd decade	
δ sarcoglycanopathy (Limb Girdle MD Type 2F)	5q33	In teens	Uncommon	Cardiomyopathy very common	Limited to teens/twenties	Cardiac failure cause of death
Facioscapulohumeral Dystrophy	4q35	Majority remain ambulant	Rare	Heart not affected	Generally not affected	
Emery–Dreifuss Muscular Dystrophy X-linked	Xq28	Majority remain ambulant	Respiratory failure while still ambulant because of diaphragmatic weakness	Heart block invariable by the 4th decade. Cardiomyopathy may occur	Death by 5th decade unless treated with pacemaker	Pacemaker is life saving
Autosomal dominant	1q11					

Congenital Muscular Dystrophy (Merosin Negative)	6q2	Walking not achieved	Common if survive into 2nd decade	Uncommon	Death by end of 2nd decade	Clinically more severe than Duchenne dystrophy
Oculopharyngeal Muscular dystrophy	14q11	Walking not affected		Heart not affected	Unaffected	Ptosis and dysphagia in 5th decade
Myotonic dystrophy (Adult onset)	19q13	In up to 50% in the 6th decade	Sometimes	Arrhythmias cause of death in 30%	Only 50% survive beyond 60 years	Beware of anaesthetic complications

References: Duchenne muscular dystrophy (Dubowitz 1995; Emery 1993), Becker muscular dystrophy (Finsterer et al. 1999; Quinlivan et al. 1996; Steare et al. 1992), Sarcoglycanopathy (Bushby 1999a; b), Facioscapulohumeral Dystrophy (Fitzsimons 1999; Kissel 1999), Emery Dreifuss Muscular dystrophy (Bonne et al. 1999; Funakoshi et al. 1999), congenital muscular dystrophy (Dubowitz 1997a; 2000a), oculopharyngeal muscular dystrophy (Blumen et al. 1993; Victor et al. 1962), myotonic dystrophy (Die-Smulders et al. 1988; Mathieu et al. 1997; 1999).

Duchenne muscular dystrophy

The presentation of Duchenne muscular dystrophy is with abnormal gait, inability to run and difficulty in rising from the floor in the first five years of life (Emery 1993). A combination of relentless progression of muscle weakness and contractures of the tendo Achilles and iliotibial bands leads to loss of walking at a mean age of 9.5 years. Once these boys become wheelchair bound, there is development of scoliosis in over 90 per cent, and the scoliosis is rapidly progressive through the pubertal years. The late teen years are marked by progression of respiratory muscle weakness, leading to nocturnal hypoventilation, respiratory failure and death in late teens or 20s. The associated cardiomyopathy may become symptomatic in approximately 20 per cent and as early as the teenage years. Feeding difficulties and weight loss are common in the late stages. The leading cause of death is respiratory failure, which may be precipitated by otherwise 'minor' chest infections. No curative treatment for Duchenne muscular dystrophy is known, but the quality of life and comfort of the patient and survival can be enhanced by symptomatic physiotherapeutic and medical treatments.

Physical therapies

Physiotherapy

Physiotherapy assessment protocols have been formulated for comprehensive evaluation of strength and function in Duchenne and other muscular dystrophies (Allsop 1981; Brooke *et al.* 1981; Florence 1984; Florence *et al.* 1992; Personius *et al.* 1994; Scott *et al.* 1982; Smith *et al.* 1991; Tawil *et al.* 1994). These physiotherapy assessment protocols enable accurate charting of disease progression, timing of the therapeutic interventions, and monitoring of the effects of the intervention. The standardized protocols are useful, not only in the management of the individual patient, but also essential for performing multicentre research studies (Brooke *et al.* 1983).

Physiotherapy treatment regimes remain the mainstay of management of muscular dystrophies and are aimed in two directions: promotion of walking and prevention of deformities (Dubowitz and Heckmatt 1980; Heckmatt *et al.* 1989a). In the early ambulant phase of Duchenne dystrophy, the emphasis is on prevention and retardation of lower limb contractures by regular passive stretching of the tendo Achilles and the use of night splints once the ankles cannot be dorsiflexed to beyond the neutral position (Hyde *et al.* 1982; Scott *et al.* 1981a). Though these techniques form the core of most physiotherapy programmes (Bakker *et al.* 1997; Vignos *et al.* 1996), their benefit has been systematically evaluated infrequently. In a prospective study (Scott *et al.* 1981a) of passive stretching and splintage in 59 boys with Duchenne dystrophy, a delay in loss of dorsiflexion was noted in the 23 boys whose families complied with treatment; in the 20 boys who were non-compliant, the deterioration in functional level was most marked. In a review of 283 boys with Duchenne dystrophy, Brooke *et al.* (1989) found no correlation between the use of passive stretching and that of joint contractures; regular use of night splints, however, had a marked effect in reducing contractures of the tendo Achilles. A recent, well designed randomized trial (Hyde *et al.* 2000) compared the effectiveness of regular passive tendo Achilles stretching versus regular tendo Achilles stretching together with the use of below-knee night splints (ankle foot orthoses) in a cohort of 27 ambulant boys with Duchenne muscular dystrophy; boys wearing night splints were found to have an annual delay of 23 per cent in development of contractures. Though it is rational to think that the prevention of leg deformities by physiotherapy may prolong the ambulation, there are no randomized controlled studies to prove it. In a study of 163 patients with Duchenne dystrophy, Demos (1983) reported that the early institution of physiotherapy postponed loss of independent walking by three to four years in the treated as opposed to the untreated patients.

The role of active exercise in improving strength and function is limited. Parents can competently give physical exercise treatment at home (Scott *et al.* 1981b), but no significant benefit of resisted exercise was noted in a study of 18 boys with Duchenne muscular dystrophy over a six-month period (Dubowitz *et al.* 1984). Patients should be encouraged to undertake normal day-to-day physical activities to maintain strength by avoiding disuse atrophy. They are more likely to comply with exercise regimens, which are pleasurable, and an example is swimming which is not only enjoyable but the buoyancy of water also makes exercises easier to perform.

Boys with Duchenne dystrophy should be encouraged to remain ambulant on a daily basis as periods of immobility in minor trauma or illnesses can result in rapid deterioration of muscle strength and loss of ambulation in a previously active boy. Long bone fractures in the legs in such an ambulant boy should preferably be treated with internal fixation with early post-operative mobilization. Alternative orthopaedic techniques like traction in bed, leading to immobility for some 4–6 weeks, may have a major risk of the boy never being able to walk again.

The principles of encouraging physical activity within the limitations of the strength of the affected individual, control of contractures with regular passive stretching and night splints, and avoiding prolonged periods of immobilization are also equally important in the maintenance of mobility in other muscular dystrophies.

Prolongation of walking with orthoses

Prolongation of walking, in Duchenne dystrophy, by fitting leg braces at the time of increasing difficulty in walking was first reported by Spencer and Vignos (1962). Their rehabilitation programme of Achilles tenotomy and provision of steel and leather knee ankle foot orthoses (KAFO) resulted in an average prolongation of walking of two years in 15 boys with Duchenne dystrophy. Similar results were reported by Siegel *et al.* (1968). The technique and orthoses have been refined with time (Heckmatt *et al.* 1985): the appropriate timing of rehabilitation in orthoses is at the time when functional walking is lost, but there is still preserved ability to take a few steps and stand holding on to furniture. A percutaneous Achilles tenotomy is often required for optimal fitting of orthoses, and the patient is mobilized on the second post-operative day. The currently used KAFO are constructed of individually moulded polypropylene and aluminium alloy and have the advantage of being strong, light weight and unobtrusive as they are worn under the trousers (Heckmatt *et al.* 1985). The benefits include a mean prolongation of walking in orthoses of 18 months, psychological benefits, and delay in development of progressive scoliosis (Rodillo *et al.* 1988). It is important to regularly review boys with Duchenne dystrophy at a centre where facilities for rehabilitation at loss of walking ability are available. The advantages include psychological preparation of the family for loss of walking and informing them about the option of rehabilitation in callipers and choosing the appropriate timing of intervention.

The effects of KAFO in the treatment of Duchenne muscular dystrophy have been reviewed systematically (Bakker *et al.* 2000). Of the 35 studies identified, nine were selected for completeness of information: outcome data were available for eight studies and the median for the means of prolongation of independent walking in these studies was 24 months.

Early surgical release of contractures in Duchenne dystrophy

In the late 1980s, Rideau *et al.* described an operation for *early release* of contractures in ambulant boys with Duchenne muscular dystrophy with percutaneous tendo Achilles lengthening, hip and knee flexion contracture release, and bilateral dissection of tensor fascia lata between 4 to 6 years of age (Rideau *et al.* 1987), and claimed that this surgery normalized gait and Gowers' time. Forst *et al.* reported this operation to prolong walking by 12 months in a large non-randomized study (Forst and Forst 1999). A randomized controlled trial of early release of lower limb contractures (Rideau surgery) in Duchenne muscular dystrophy failed to show any benefit (Manzur *et al.* 1992) and this has also been the experience reported from other centres (Granata *et al.* 1994). Early release of lower limb contractures in Duchenne muscular dystrophy as a routine treatment cannot be recommended.

Inspiratory muscle training

In view of the pulmonary morbidity and mortality of muscular dystrophy (Gozal 2000; Melacini *et al.* 1996; Newsom-Davis 1976; 1980; Rideau *et al.* 1981) there has been a lot of interest in respiratory muscle training and the relevant studies have been summarized (McCool and Tzelepis 1995). A randomized double blind crossover study on 22 boys with Duchenne dystrophy showed no benefit (Rodillo *et al.* 1989). Other studies demonstrated some improvement in respiratory muscle endurance and/or strength as assessed by measurement of mouth maximal static inspiratory pressure (PI_{max}) (Martin *et al.* 1986; Wanke *et al.* 1994; Winkler *et al.* 2000), but the improvement was restricted to the individuals who were less severely affected, and there was no improvement in patients who were already retaining CO_2. In any event, forced vital capacity did not improve with respiratory muscle training in any published study of respiratory muscle training, and the role of this therapy is limited.

In contrast, the role of chest physiotherapy in management of respiratory secretions and infections in muscular dystrophy patients with respiratory muscle weakness is very important and well recognized (Mathieu *et al.* 1997; Newsom-Davis 1980; Siegel 1975).

Chronic low frequency electric stimulation

Low frequency electrical stimulation studies in the dystrophic mouse (Dangain and Vrbova 1989; Luthert *et al.* 1980) showed an apparent increase in force output and fatigue resistance of the stimulated muscles. Human studies of chronic low frequency electrical stimulation of quadriceps femoris (Scott *et al.* 1990) or tibialis anterior (Zupan 1992; Zupan *et al.* 1993) muscles on one side with the contralateral muscle serving as control, showed some improvement of strength in the stimulated muscles. Though the authors viewed this technique as having some therapeutic potential, no further studies demonstrating the practicality of electrical stimulation of groups of affected muscles and the functional benefits have been reported.

Pharmacological Therapies

Drug treatment trials in Duchenne muscular dystrophy have been reviewed (Dubowitz and Heckmatt 1980; Emery 1993; Heckmatt *et al.* 1989a). No curative treatment is known as yet but of all the medications studied, glucocorticoids (a sub group of steroids) hold the maximal promise. The terms steroids and glucocorticoids have been used almost interchangeably in this context in neuromuscular literature, though strictly speaking glucocorticoids is the most appropriate descriptive term as it avoids confusion by excluding anabolic and androgenic steroids.

The availability of animal models (Nonaka 1998; and Chapter 16), has opened up the possibility of therapeutic screening of potentially useful drugs. In a programme of pre-clinical screening in the *mdx* mouse, Granchelli *et al.* (2000) reported improvement in whole body strength with prednisolone, glutamine, creatine, and anabolic hormone insulin like growth factor. The study confirms the feasibility of screening studies in animal model of muscular dystrophy prior to launching expensive and ethically difficult human therapeutic trials in the future.

Glucocorticoids

There is now over 25 years of experience in the use of glucocorticoids in Duchenne muscular dystrophy and the individual studies and their key findings are listed in Table 12.2. The steroid preparation used in the initial studies in North America was prednisone, while the preparation available to European researches is its hydroxylated form, prednisolone. Prednisone is broken down in the body to prednisolone and both preparations are equi-potent in glucocorticoid effect (Azarnoff 1975; Frey and Frey 1990). In the last decade, a number of studies reported the use of deflazacort, an oxazoline derivative of

Table 12.2 Glucocorticoid trials in Duchenne muscular dystrophy.

Authors	Design	N=	Age (Years)	Glucocorticoid regimen	Treatment period	Outcome	Comments
Drachman 1974	Open	14	4–10.5	Prednisone 2 mg/kg/day for 3 months Then 2/3rds dose on alternate days	3 weeks–28 months	Improvement	Side effects in 4
Siegel 1974	Double blind	14	6–9	Prednisone 5 mg/kg alternate days	24 months	No benefit	
Brooke 1987	Open	33	5–15	Prednisone 1.5 mg/kg/day	6 months	Improvement	6 drop outs
DeSilva 1987	Open	16	3–10	Prednisone 2 mg/kg/day for 3 months Then 2/3rds dose on alternate days	1–11 years	Walking prolonged by 2 years	Excessive weight gain in 12 Cataracts in 2
Mendell 1989	Randomized double blind	103	5–15	Prednisone 0.75 mg/kg/day Prednisone 1.5 mg/kg/day	6 months	Improved at 3 months then stabilization	30% boys had more than 20% weight gain
Fenichel 1991	Double blind	103	5–15	Prednisone 1.25 mg/kg/alternate day Prednisone 2.5 mg/kg/alternate day	6 months	Improved at 3 months	Similar side effects on daily and alternate day regimes
Fenichel 1991b	Open	92	5–15	Prednisone 0.75 mg/kg/day	2 years	Stabilization for 2 years. Pred 0.65 mg/kg/day least effect dose	Cataracts in 10 Glycosuria in 10 Significant weight gain
Griggs 1991	Randomized	99	5–15	Prednisone 0.3 mg/kg/day Prednisone 0.75 mg/kg/day	6 months	Strength improved at 10 days	30% boys had more than 20% weight gain
Mesa 1991	Double blind	28	5–11	Deflazacort 1 mg/kg/day	9 months	Improved till 6 months, then stable	35% cushingoid No significant weight gain

Study	Design	N	Age	Treatment	Duration	Outcome	Side effects/Notes
Griggs 1993	Randomized	107	5–15	Prednisone 0.75 mg/kg/day Azathioprine 2.5 mg/kg/day	18 months 12 months	Strength and function improved	No additional benefit of Azathioprine
Sansome 1993	Open	32	6–14	Prednisolone 0.75 mg/kg/day, for 10 days/months (10 days on 20 days off)	18 months	Strength improved at 6 months, slow decline at 18 months	Less side effects, but, 26% boys had more than 20% weight gain
Angelini 1994	Randomized	28	6.5–9	Deflazacort 2 mg/kg/alternate days	24 months	Stabilization of strength	70% had >20% weight gain 1 pathological fracture
Backman 1995	Double blind crossover	37	4–19	Prednisone 0.3 mg/kg/day	12 months	Stabilisation for 1 year	Weight gain in 29%
Bonifati 2000	Randomized	18	5–14	Prednisolone 0.75 mg/kg/day Deflazacort 0.9 mg/kg/day	1 year	Prednisolone and deflazacort equally effective	Weight gain more significant in Prednisolone group
Biggar 2001	Open	30	7–15	Deflazacort 0.9 mg/kg/day	3.8 years (±SD 1.5)	Ambulation prolonged, FVC preserved	Cataracts in 30%
Reitter 1995 (Data reported in Dubowitz 2000b)	Double blind	100	5–till ambulant	Prednisolone 0.75 mg/kg/day Deflazacort 0.9 mg/kg/day	2 years	Muscle function stabilized	Excessive weight gain in prednisolone group. Cataracts in 27% of deflazacort group

prednisolone. When deflazacort became available in the United Kingdom in 1998, the manufacturers claimed it to have a lower incidence of side effects compared with prednisolone; this claim was later withdrawn at the request of the UK Medicines Control Agency following its review of the cited data (Committee on Safety of Medicines, 1998). For purposes of comparison, 1 mg prednisone is equivalent in anti-inflammatory (glucocorticoid) effect to 1.2 mg deflazacort (BNF). Deflazacort in the UK is manifoldly more expensive than prednisolone (BNF).

Demos *et al.* (1976) reported remarkable improvement in strength in a boy with Duchenne dystrophy following renal transplant and attributed the improvement to azathioprine and prednisolone used for immunosuppression. The initial open studies of glucocorticoids in Duchenne dystrophy (Brooke *et al.* 1987; DeSilva *et al.* 1987; Drachman *et al.* 1974; Siegel *et al.* 1974) used prednisone in high doses ranging from 1.5 mg/kg/day to 5 mg/kg on alternate days, and suggested some short-term improvement in muscle strength and/or function. The open study by DeSilva *et al.* (1987) used loss of walking ability as the primary end-point, and reported a prolongation of walking by approximately two years. The side effects of steroid treatment in this study were significant: excessive weight gain in 12/16, hyperactivity in 4/16, cataracts in two patients and stress fracture in one. These early open studies documented some possible benefits of glucocorticoid therapy and lead to further randomized controlled trials to assess the efficacy and find the optimal dose regimes to minimize the side effects.

Three sequential randomized controlled studies of prednisone in Duchenne muscular dystrophy (Fenichel *et al.* 1991a, b; Mendell *et al.* 1989) from four collaborating centres in the USA utilized a single cohort of 103 boys. These studies established Prednisone 0.75 mg/kg/day as a suitable starting dose and resulted in improvement in strength at three months followed by stabilization of muscle strength (reported as average muscle score, and compared with natural history controls) for up to a total of three years. The functional benefit to the subjects in these studies is difficult to ascertain, partly because of the wide age range (5–15 years) and because some of them were non-ambulant at entry to the study. The side effects were noted in over half of the patients and further reduction of the drug dose was required. Prednisone 0.65 mg/kg/day was considered to be the minimum effective dose and this could be tolerated only by half the subjects by the end of the study. Though these studies were published a decade ago, the subsequent longer-term outcome of this cohort has not been reported.

The dose response to prednisone and the time course of improvement were further evaluated by Griggs *et al.* (1991). Prednisone 0.75 mg/kg/day was found to be more effective than 0.35 mg/kg/day and the improvement in strength was demonstrable as early as 10 days after initiation of treatment. Though the duration of this study was only six months, 30 per cent of the boys taking prednisone 0.75 mg/kg/day showed a weight gain of more than 20 per cent over the baseline weight. The lower daily dose regime of prednisolone 0.35 mg/kg/day has been assessed in a randomized double blind crossover trial (Backman and Henriksson 1995). The benefit was modest while weight gain still occurred in 29 per cent.

In order to lessen the adverse effects of long-term glucocorticoid treatment, Dubowitz (1991) recommended a regime of Prednisolone 0.75 mg kg day for the first 10 days of every calendar month. An open study of 32 patients demonstrated that this intermittent regime had a positive influence on strength at six months followed by a slow decline at 12 and 18 months (Sansome *et al.* 1993); the weight gain and other side effects were much less than with continuous therapy. Carter and McDonald (2000) reported a patient with Duchenne dystrophy who was treated with intermittent pulse prednisone for severe asthma from age 3 to 17 years and had preservation of motor function, who remains "partially ambulatory" at 20 years of age.

Three recent studies have evaluated deflazacort (Angelini *et al.* 1994; Biggar *et al.* 2001; Bonifati *et al.* 2000) and confirmed the beneficial effect of glucocorticoid therapy, in line with the findings of the previous prednisone studies. High dose deflazacort treatment over 24 months was reported to postpone loss of ambulation by 1.3 years, but weight gain of more than 20 per cent over the base line occurred in 70 per cent and there were some behavioural changes in 54 per cent (Angelini *et al.* 1994). A small randomized comparative study of deflazacort versus prednisolone over the course of one year showed the two drugs to be equally effective, but the weight gain was more significant in the prednisolone group (Bonifati *et al.* 2000). The most impressive long-term functional outcome of deflazacort was reported in a retrospective study by Biggar *et al.* (2001). They used deflazacort 0.9 mg/kg/day in 30 boys with Duchenne dystrophy (age 7–15 years) over 3.8 years (SD 1.5) and reported prolongation of ambulation and remarkable preservation of pulmonary function (forced vital capacity) in some of the treated boys. Interestingly, boys in the treated group weighed less between 9 to 13 years of age as compared to the control group but were shorter and 10 of the 30 developed asymptomatic cataracts.

A multicentre randomized trial comparing prednisolone (0.75 mg/kg/day) with deflazacort (0.9 mg/kg/day) in 100 boys with Duchenne muscular dystrophy has been completed and is awaiting publication (Dubowitz 1997b; 2000b; Reitter 1995). The preliminary data presented at the 75th European Neuromuscular Centre International workshop (Dubowitz 2000b) showed that equipotent anti-inflammatory doses of prednisolone and deflazacort showed equal "effectiveness in almost completely preserving muscle performance" on testing manual muscle strength and timed motor functions. Weight gain was significantly higher in the prednisolone treated group, but 16 out of 44 boys receiving deflazacort developed cataracts (1/36 in the prednisolone group). On longer-term follow-up, cataracts became symptomatic in two boys in the deflazacort group, and these boys required eye surgery for lens replacement (Dubowitz 2000b). Prednisolone and deflazacort therapy of up to four years duration in Duchenne muscular dystrophy was not found to be associated with cardiac side effects (Winter *et al.* 1999).

The precise mechanism by which glucocorticoids increase strength in Duchenne dystrophy is not known but their beneficial effects include inhibition of muscle proteolysis (Elia *et al.* 1981; Rifai *et al.* 1995), stimulatory effect on myoblast proliferation

(Bal and Sanwall 1980), anti-inflammatory/ immunosuppressive effect (Kissel *et al.* 1991) and upregulation of utrophin (Pasquini *et al.* 1995).

In spite of all the data available, the precise role of steroid treatment in clinical management of Duchenne dystrophy is not yet clear. In a recent review of steroid therapy in muscular dystrophy, Dubrovsky *et al.* (1998) listed the then available 14 studies and concluded that "the decision to administer steroids is still individual and depends on the wisdom of the experienced physician to use an appropriate dose and schedule, for which purpose we have been trained". The clinical guidelines are still difficult to formulate in spite of the additional studies available. It is clear that there is stabilization of strength for periods of up to three years and some functional benefit with the use of glucocorticoids in the ambulant phase of Duchenne muscular dystrophy. It is equally clear that the side effects of the effective steroid regimes are significant and may not be tolerable, especially if started at an early age. There are a number of unanswered questions. Do steroids make a significant alteration in the natural history of Duchenne dystrophy? Are the side effects of a long-term successful steroid regime acceptable? What is the best age to start steroid therapy? Is prednisolone better than deflazacort, and vice versa? Deflazacort appears to cause less weight gain, but the incidence of cataracts is very high, and some patients may need cataract surgery. The optimal glucocorticoid regime with maximal efficacy and minimal side effects needs to be formulated and validated in methodologically sound clinical trials.

The intermittent prednisolone regime recommended by Dubowitz (1991; Sansome *et al.* 1993) offers the possibility of long-term use with a lesser risk of pituitary adrenal axis suppression and other side effects. A United Kingdom multicentre randomized trial of intermittent prednisolone schedule (0.75 mg/kg/day, 10 days on, 10 days off) is currently being set up to specifically answer the questions of long-term benefits of prolongation of independent ambulation, and tolerability with acceptable side effects (International Standardized Random Control Trial Number 91883476).

Steroid therapy has also been used for some cases of sarcoglycanopathy (Dubowitz 2000b) with encouraging results, but the data are limited. Steroid therapy is not effective in Facioscapulohumeral dystrophy (Tawil *et al.* 1997).

Oxandrolone

Fenichel *et al.* (1997) reported pilot study of oxandrolone 0.1 mg/kg/day for three months in 10 boys with Duchenne dystrophy. There was an improvement in the average muscle score as compared to natural history controls, and the magnitude of improvement was similar to that after prednisolone administration. No randomized controlled studies are available, and the use of this anabolic steroid is still experimental.

Azathioprine

Improvement in strength in Duchenne dystrophy with prednisolone raised the possibility of immunosuppression as the mode of its action. This hypothesis was tested by a randomized, controlled trial of prednisolone and azathioprine (Griggs *et al.* 1993) to determine whether azathioprine alone, or in combination with prednisone, improves muscle strength. Azathioprine did not have a beneficial effect in this study and this also suggests that prednisone's beneficial effect is not due to immunosuppression.

Cyclosporin

Sharma *et al.* (1993) investigated the effect of cyclosporin in force generation in Duchenne muscular dystrophy. Fifteen boys (age 5–10 years, 5 non-ambulant) were given oral cyclosporin in a dose of 5 mg/kg/day. An increase in tetanic force and maximum voluntary contraction strength in the tibialis anterior muscles was reported after two months of cyclosporin therapy, and this was largely lost following the two month wash-out phase. Functional benefit was not assessed. No further human studies have been reported.

Dehydroepiandrosterone sulphate

The serum adrenal androgen levels in patients with myotonic dystrophy are markedly reduced as compared to healthy controls (Carter and Steinbeck 1985). A pilot study of dehydroepiandrosterone 200 mg/day for eight weeks in 11 adult patients with myotonic dystrophy showed improvement in activities of daily living, muscle strength, and myotonia (Sugino *et al.* 1998). No longer-term or randomized controlled trials have been reported.

Creatine

Creatine, a dietary component in meat-eaters, is also synthesized endogenously and is stored primarily in skeletal muscle. Creatine in the muscle is converted to phosphocreatine to build, and provide energy in the form of adenosine triphosphate (Benzi 2000; Jacobs 1999). Creatine may enhance the performance of high-intensity, short-duration exercise (Kamber *et al.* 1999) but is not useful in endurance sports (Graham and Hatton 1999). Despite this, creatine supplementation is widely taken by athletes to enhance muscular performance (Graham and Hatton 1999). Creatine pre-treatment of *mdx* mice muscle cell cultures increases phosphocreatine levels, myotube formation and survival (Pulido *et al.* 1998). Oral creatine supplementation was reported to improve muscle performance and intracellular creatine levels on gastrocnemius muscle 31P magnetic resonance spectroscopy in a 9-year-old boy with Duchenne dystrophy (Felber *et al.* 2000).

Open trials of creatine supplementation are in progress in many European countries (Dubowitz 2000b). A recent double-blind, crossover trial of creatine monohydrate 36 patients with facioscapulohumeral dystrophy, Becker dystrophy, Duchenne dystrophy, and sarcoglycanopathy showed mild improvement in muscle strength and daily-life activities (Walter *et al.* 2000). Creatine was well tolerated during the study period.

Aminoglycosides

Barton-Davis *et al.* (1999) reported restoration of dystrophin function to skeletal muscles of *mdx* mice with the use of gentamicin. The mechanism of action of this aminoglycoside antibiotic is to cause misreading of the RNA code, allowing insertion of alternative amino acids at the site of the mutated codon, allowing transcription and protein formation (Mankin and Liebman 1999). The application in the human model is limited as this mechanism of action is possible only in patients with point mutation of a stop codon in the dystrophin gene (which comprises only a few per cent of patients) and any potential benefit will have to be weighed against the oto-nephrotoxic side effects of aminoglycosides.

Beta 2 agonists

Beta 2-adrenergic agonists have been shown to induce muscle hypertrophy and prevent atrophy after physical and biochemical insults in animal studies (Agbenyeag and Wareham 1992; Martineau *et al.* 1993). Beta 2 mimetics induce satellite cell prolifcration (Maltin and Delday 1992), inhibit muscle proteolysis (Benson *et al.* 1991), and increase muscle protein production (Hesketh *et al.* 1992). The Facioscapulohumeral dystrophy (FSH-DY) group of North America conducted a pilot trial of albuterol (16.0 mg/day for three months) in 15 patients with facioscapulohumeral dystrophy (Kissel *et al.* 1998). Albuterol improved muscle strength and increased muscle mass as assessed with DEXA (dual energy x-ray absorptiometry bone densitometry) scans. The results of a randomized controlled trial by the FSH-DY group are awaited.

Nutritional aspects

Feeding problems and malnutrition are under-recognized in children and adults with muscular dystrophy as the clinical picture is often overwhelmed by the motor and respiratory difficulties (Aldrich 1993; Perkin and Murray-Lyon 1998; Tilton *et al.* 1998; Willig *et al.* 1994). Malnutrition in individuals with muscular dystrophy (Willig *et al.* 1995) may occur in the form of obesity as a consequence of decreased mobility or chronic under nutrition as a result of swallowing difficulties, and poor appetite secondary to sleep hypoventilation, respiratory failure or cardiac failure.

Dysphagia as a symptom of primary muscle disease may present either in early childhood (congenital myotonic dystrophy, congenital muscular dystrophy) or may become apparent in later years with advancing muscular dystrophy, and further complicated by respiratory distress and abnormal seating posture (Duchenne muscular dystrophy). Dysphagia may be the presenting feature in oculopharyngeal muscular dystrophy, where its severity is disproportionate to any general muscle weakness (Blumen *et al.* 1993; Victor *et al.* 1962).

Children with congenital myotonic dystrophy (Harper 1975; Reardon *et al.* 1993) and congenital muscular dystrophy (Philpot *et al.* 1999) may have chewing and swallowing difficulties, which result in prolonged feeding times, failure to thrive, frequent "chest infections" and wheezing. These children are also more prone to gastroe-sophageal reflux and episodes of aspiration, which may be life threatening (Keller *et al.* 1998; Rutherford *et al.* 1989). Children with these problems need detailed swallowing assessment by speech and language therapists and are investigated by observation at mealtimes and videofluoroscopy (Chen *et al.* 1992; Gilardeau *et al.* 1995). The treatment strategies vary from thickening of feeds, optimal positioning and seating during feeds to nasogastric tube feeding, gastrostomy or fundoplication in more severely affected patients (Gilardeau *et al.* 1995).

In a recent study of 14 children with merosin deficient congenital muscular dystrophy, Philpot *et al.* (1999) reported prolongation of mealtimes to over 30 min, and a high incidence of swallowing abnormalities on videofluoroscopy with frank aspiration and frequent chest infections in some of the cases. Gastrostomy was performed in five of these 14 patients, and this stopped the chest infections and resulted in improved weight gain.

The prevalence of obesity in Duchenne muscular dystrophy becomes noticeable at seven years of age and may reach up to 54 per cent by the age of 13 years (Willig *et al.* 1993). Obesity has negative implications for respiratory function, mobility, post-operative recovery, nursing and caring of non-ambulant patients, and should therefore be avoided. The propensity of boys with Duchenne dystrophy to put on excessive weight is even more important to realize as more and more of them may be treated with glucocorticoids, and this may further aggravate the problem. Families with boys affected by Duchenne dystrophy should be given dietary advice and an early consultation with the dietician may be useful. Specific charts are available to allow the prediction of an ideal weight for boys with Duchenne muscular dystrophy (Griffiths and Edwards 1988; Willig *et al.* 1993). In overweight boys, controlled weight reduction by decreased caloric intake is effective and safe (Edwards *et al.* 1984). In the latter years of non-ambulant phase, under-nutrition becomes a common problem in Duchenne dystrophy, with a prevalence of 54 per cent in patients by the age of 18 years (Willig *et al.* 1993). Weight loss in advanced stages of Duchenne muscular dystrophy is secondary to a high incidence of dysphagia (Jaffe *et al.* 1990), and may be further aggravated by choking episodes (Willig *et al.* 1994), fear of choking, poor posture consequent upon scoliosis, and respiratory or cardiac failure. Weight loss in a non-ambulant patient with Duchenne dystrophy should be investigated for the problems noted above. Treatment may entail optimizing seating posture for feeding times, caloric supplementation and rarely gastrostomy feeding (Gilardeau *et al.* 1995).

Dysphagia is a prominent symptom in oculopharyngeal muscular dystrophy, and often follows ptosis in the course of the disease (Blumen *et al.* 1993; Victor *et al.* 1962). Pharyngeal contraction is depressed with pooling in the hypopharynx and relaxation of the upper oesophageal sphincter is abnormal (Perie *et al.* 1997). Specific surgical procedures like cricopharyngeal myotomy can give significant relief of symptoms (Fradet *et al.* 1997; Perie *et al.* 1997).

Muscular dystrophy patients with poor mobility are prone to develop constipation. In addition, myotonic dystrophy affects the gastrointestinal smooth muscle, and anal sphincter function and predisposing, in particular, children with congenital myotonic dystrophy, to constipation and overflow incontinence (Lenard *et al.* 1977; Fuger *et al.* 1995). This should be pre-empted with patient education, increased fibre content of the diet and appropriate use of laxatives if indicated.

Prevention of anaesthetic complications

All muscular dystrophy patients with respiratory muscle weakness and forced vital capacity below 30 per cent are predisposed to respiratory failure, and are at increased risk for chest infections and post operative respiratory complications (Gozal 2000; Heckmatt *et al.* 1989b; Phillips *et al.* 1999). Patients with myotonic dystrophy are very sensitive to pethidine and general anaesthetics with risk of prolonged sedation, and post-operative retention of bronchial secretions and pneumonia (Die-Smulders *et al.* 1998; Mathieu *et al.* 1997; Moxley 1997). Respiratory complications in the post-operative period should be prevented with early physiotherapy and treated vigorously (Aldridge 1985) as pneumonia is eventually the cause of death in up to 43 per cent of patients with myotonic dystrophy (Mathieu *et al.* 1999). The patients and their treating physicians need to be aware of these risks and published guidelines for the peri-operative surgical care of myotonic dystrophy patients (Moxley 1992) are available.

There is an apparent increased incidence of a hyperpyrexia-like response including cardiac arrest, increased serum creatine phosphokinase concentration, and myoglobinuria during anaesthesia in Duchenne and Becker muscular dystrophy (Breucking *et al.* 2000; Emery 1993; Obata *et al.* 1999; Smith and Bush 1985), and it is prudent to avoid suxamethonium, halothane, isoflurane and sevoflurane in these patients. The group at particular risk is that of young undiagnosed boys, who are inadvertently given suxamethonium (Henderson 1984; Breucking *et al.* 2000).

Summary

The medical management should entail regular follow-up of these patients with anticipation, early detection and treatment of complications of muscular dystrophy. The

Table 12.3 The team for comprehensive management of muscular dystrophy

Doctors	Therapists
• Paediatrician	• Physiotherapist
• Neurologist	• Orthotist
• Geneticist	• Occupational therapist
• Muscle histopathologist	• Speech and language therapist
• Orthopaedic surgeon	• Dietitian
• General surgeon	• Psychologist
• Cardiologist	• Family care officer
• Pulmonologist	
• Intensivist	

comprehensive management of these patients requires a multi-disciplinary team approach (Table 12.3), with one physician co-ordinating the overall care. The principles of promotion of ambulation can be applied to all neuromuscular disorders, with regular passive stretching to prevent contractures. The provision of appropriate orthoses may facilitate and prolong walking. Nutritional management is aimed at avoiding both under-nutrition and obesity. Early detection and prompt treatment of cardiac and respiratory complications is important in effective symptom control and prolongation of survival. The pharmacological therapies, in particular glucocorticoids, hold some promise in Duchenne muscular dystrophy. While waiting for a curative treatment to become available, all symptomatic therapies should be used to ensure optimal condition of the patient.

References

Agbenyeag, E.T. and Wareham, A.C. (1992). Effect of clenbuterol on skeletal muscle atrophy in mice induced by glucocorticoid dexamethasone. *Comparative Biochemistry and Physiology*, **102**, 141–5.

Aldrich, T.K. (1993). Nutritional factors in the pathogenesis and therapy of respiratory insufficiency in neuromuscular diseases. *Monaldi Archives for Chest Diseases*, **48**, 327–30.

Aldridge, L.M. (1985). Anaesthetic problems in myotonic dystrophy. *British Journal of Anaesthesia*, **57**, 1119–30.

Allsop, K.G. and Ziter, F.A. (1981). Loss of strength and functional decline in Duchenne's dystrophy. *Archives of Neurology*, **38**, 406–11.

Angelini, C., Pegoraro, E., Turella, E. *et al.* (1994). Deflazacort in Duchenne dystrophy: Study of long-term effect. *Muscle Nerve*, **17**, 386–91.

Azarnoff, D.L. (1975). Steroid therapy. WB Saunders Co, Philadelphia PA.

Bach, J.R., Campagnolo, D.I., and Hoeman, S. (1991). Life satisfaction of individuals with Duchenne muscular dystrophy using long-term mechanical ventilatory support. *American Journal of Physical and Medical Rehabilitation*, **70**, 129–35.

Backman, E. and Henriksson, K.G. (1995). Low-dose prednisolone treatment in Duchenne and Becker muscular dystrophy. *Neuromuscular Disorders*, **5**(3), 233–41.

Bakker, J.P., de Groot, I.J., Beckerman, H., de Jong, B.A., and Lankhorst, G.J. (2000). The effects of knee-ankle-foot orthoses in the treatment of muscular dystrophy: review of the literature. *Clinical Rehabilitation*, **14**, 343–59.

Bakker, J.P., de Groot, I.J., de Jong, B.A., Van Tol-De Jager. M.A., and Lankhorst, G.J. (1997). Prescription pattern for orthoses in The Netherlands: use and experience in the ambulatory phase of Duchenne muscular dystrophy. *Disability Rehabilitation*, **19**, 318–25.

Bal, E. and Sanwall, W. (1980). A synergistic effect of glucocorticosteroids and insulin on the differention of myoblasts. *Journal of Cell Physiology*, **102**, 27–36.

Barton-Davis, E.R., Cordier, L., Shoturma, D.I. *et al.* (1999). Aminoglycoside antibiotics restore dystrophin function to skeletal muscles of mdx mice. *Journal of Clinical Investigation*, **104**, 375–81.

Benson, D.W., Foley-Nelson, T., Chance, W.T. *et al.* (1991). Decreased myofibrillar protein breakdown following treatment with clenbuterol. *Journal of Surgical Research*, **50**, 1–5.

Benzi, G. (2000). Is there a rationale for the use of creatine either as nutritional supplementation or drug administration in humans participating in sport? *Pharmacological Research*, **41**, 255–64.

Biggar, W.D., Gingras, M., Fehlings, D.L., Harris, V.A., and Steele, C.A. (2001). Deflazacort treatment of Duchenne muscular dystrophy. *Journal of Pediatrics*, **138**(1), 45–50.

Blumen, S.C., Nisipeanu, P., Sadeh, M., Asherov, A., Tome, F.M., and Korczyn, A.D. (1993). Clinical features of oculopharyngeal muscular dystrophy among Bukhara Jews. *Neuromuscular Disorders*, **3**, 575–7.

BNF. British National Formularly (2000), British Medical Association and Royal Pharmaceutical Society of Great Britain. No 40.

Bonifati, M.D., Ruzza, G., Bonometto, P., Berardinelli, A., Gorni, K., Orcesi, S. *et al.* (2000). A multicenter, double-blind, randomized trial of deflazacort versus prednisone in Duchenne muscular dystrophy. *Muscle Nerve*, **23**, 1344–7.

Bonne, G., Di Barletta, M.R., Varnous, S. *et al.* (1999). Mutations in the gene encoding lamin A/C cause autosomal dominant Emery-Dreifuss muscular dystrophy. *Nature genetics*, **21**, 285–8.

Breucking, E., Reimnitz, P., Schara, U., and Mortier, W. (2000). Anesthetic complications. The incidence of severe anesthetic complications in patients and families with progressive muscular dystrophy of the Duchenne and Becker types. *Anaesthesist*, **49**, 187–95.

Brooke, M.H., Fenichel, G.M., Griggs, R.C., Mendell, J.R., Moxley, R., Florence, J. *et al.* (1989). Duchenne muscular dystrophy: patterns of clinical progression and effects of supportive therapy. *Neurology*, **39**, 475–81.

Brooke, M.H., Fenichel, G.M., Griggs, R.C., Mendell, J.R., Moxley, R., Miller, J.P., and Province, M.A. (1983). Clinical investigation in Duchenne dystrophy: 2. Determination of 'power' of therapeutic trials based on the natural history. *Muscle Nerve*, **6**, 91–103.

Brooke, M.H., Fenichel, G.M., Griggs, R.C., Mendell, J.R., Moxley, R.T. 3d, Miller, J.P. *et al.* (1987). Clinical investigation of Duchenne muscular dystrophy. Interesting results in a trial of prednisone. *Archives of Neurology*, **44**, 812–7.

Brooke, M.H., Griggs, R.C., Mendell, J.R., Fenichel, G.M., Shumate, J.B., and Pellegrino, R.J. (1981). Clinical trial in Duchenne dystrophy. I. The design of the protocol. *Muscle Nerve*, **4**, 186–97.

Bushby, K.M.D. (1999a). Making sense of the limb-girdle muscular dystrophies. *Brain*, **122**, 1403–20.

Bushby, K.M.D. (1999b). The limb-girdle muscular dystrophies: diagnostic guidelines. *European Journal of Paediatric Neurology*, **3**, 53–58.

Carter, G.T. and McDonald, C.M. (2000). Preserving function in Duchenne dystrophy with long-term pulse prednisone therapy. *American Journal of Physical and Medical Rehabilitation*, **79**, 455–8.

Carter, J.N. and Steinbeck, K.S. (1985). Reduced adrenal androgens in patients with myotonic dystrophy. *Journal of Clinical Endocrinology and Metabolism*, **60**, 611–4.

Chen, M.Y., Peele, V.N., Donati, D., Ott, D.J., Donofrio, P.D., and Gelfand, D.W. (1992). Clinical and videofluoroscopic evaluation of swallowing in 41 patients with neurologic disease. *Gastrointestinal Radiology*, **17**, 95–8.

Committee on Safety of Medicines, Medicines Control Agency (1998), Calcort (Deflazacort): advertising has been withdrawn. *Current Problems Pharmacovigilance*, **24**:10.

Dangain, J. and Vrbova, G. (1989). Long term effect of low frequency chronic electrical stimulation on the fast hind limb muscles of dystrophic mice. *Journal of Neurology, Neurosurgery and Psychiatry*, **52**, 1382–9.

Demos, J. (1983). Results of the treatment of Duchenne de Boulogne myopathy by early physiotherapy. A comparative study with untreated subjects. *Archives of French Pediatrics*, **40**, 609–13.

Demos, J., Tuil, D., Berthelon, M., Katz, P., Broyer, M., Riberi, P. *et al.* (1976). Progressive muscular dystrophy. Functional improvement after a renal allograft. *Journal of Neurological Science*, **30**, 41–53.

DeSilva, S., Drachman, D.B., Mellits, D., and Kuncl, R.W. (1987). Prednisone treatment in Duchenne muscular dystrophy. Long-term benefit. *Archives of Neurology*, **44**, 818–22.

Die-Smulders, C.E., Howeler, C.J., Thijs, C., Mirandolle, J.F., Anten, H.B., Smeets, H.J., Chandler, K.E., and Geraedts, J.P. (1998). Age and causes of death in adult-onset myotonic dystrophy. *Brain*, **121**, 1557–63.

Drachman, D.B., Toyka, K.V., and Myer, E. (1974). Prednisone in Duchenne muscular dystrophy. *Lancet*, **142**(7894), 1409–12.

Dubowitz, V. (1991). Prednisolone in Duchenne dystrophy. *Neuromuscular Disorders*, **3**, 161–3.

Dubowitz, V. (1995). Muscle disorders. In *Childhood* (2nd edn) W.B. Saunders.

Dubowitz, V. (1997a). 50th ENMC International Workshop: congenital muscular dystrophy. 28 February 1997 to 2 March 1997, Naarden, The Netherlands. *Neuromuscular Disorders*, **7**, 539–47.

Dubowitz, V. (1997b). 47th ENMC International workshop: treatment of muscular dystrophy. 13–15 Dec. 1996, Naarden, The Netherlands. *Neuromuscular Disorders*, **7**, 261–7.

Dubowitz, V. (1998). What's in a name? Muscular dystrophy revisited. *European Journal of Paediatric Neurology*, **2**, 279–84.

Dubowitz, V. (2000a). Congenital muscular dystrophy: An expanding clinical syndrome. *Annals of Neurology*, **47**, 143–4.

Dubowitz, V. (2000b). 75th ENMC International workshop: Treatment of muscular dystrophy, Baarn 10–12 Dec, 1999. *Neuromuscular Disorders*, **10**, 313–320.

Dubowitz, V. and Heckmatt, J. (1980). Management of muscular dystrophy. *British Medical Bulletin*, **36**, 39–144.

Dubowitz, V., Hyde, S.A., Scott, O.M., and Goddard, C. (1984) Controlled trial of exercise in Duchenne muscular dystrophy. In *Neuromuscular diseases* (ed. G. Serratice *et al.*) pp. 571–5. Raven press, New York.

Dubrovsky, A.L., Corrado Angelini, Bonifati, D.M. (1998). Steroids in muscular dystrophy: Where do we stand? *Neuromuscular Disorders*, **8**, 380–4.

Edwards, R.H., Round, J.M., Jackson, M.J., Griffiths, R.D., and Lilburn, M.F. (1984). Weight reduction in boys with muscular dystrophy. *Developmental Medicine and Child neurology*, **26**, 384–90.

Elia, M., Carter, A., Bacon, S. *et al.* (1981). Clinical usefulness of urinary 3-methylhistidine excretion in indicating muscle protein breakdown. *British Medical Journal* (Clin Res Ed) **282**, 351–4.

Emery, A.E.H. (1991). Population frequencies of inherited neuromuscular diseases: a world survey. *Neuromuscular Disorders*, **1**, 19–29.

Emery, A.E.H. (1993). Duchenne muscular dystrophy. (2nd edn) Oxford Monographs on Medical Genetics, Vol 24. Oxford University Press.

Emery, A.E.H. (1997) Diagnostic Criteria for Neuromuscular Disorders. (2nd edn) Royal Society of Medicine Press, London. European Neuromuscular Centre, Baarn, The Netherlands.

Emery, A.E.H. (1998). Neuromuscular Disorders: Clinical and Molecular Genetics. J Wiley & Sons, Chichester.

Felber, S., Skladal, D., Wyss, M., Kremser, C., Koller, A., and Sperl, W. (2000). Oral creatine supplementation in Duchenne muscular dystrophy: a clinical and 31P magneticresonance spectroscopy study. *Neurological Research*, **22**, 145–50.

Fenichel, G., Pestornk, A., Florence, J. *et al.* (1997). A beneficial effect of oxandrolone in the treatment of Duchenne muscular dystrophy: A pilot study. *Neurology*, **48**, 1225–6.

Fenichel, G.M., Florence, J.M., Pestornk, A. *et al.* (1991a). Long-term benefit from prednisolone in Duchenne muscular dystrophy. *Neurology,* **41,** 1874–7.

Fenichel, G.M., Mendell, J.R., Moxley, R.T. 3d, Griggs, R.C., Brooke, M.H., Miller, J.P. *et al.* (1991b). A comparison of daily and alternate-day prednisone therapy in the treatment of Duchenne muscular dystrophy. *Archives of Neurology,* **48,** 575–9.

Finsterer, J., Bittner, R.E., and Grimm, M. (1999). Cardiac involvement in Becker's muscular dystrophy, necessitating heart transplantation, 6 years before apparent skeletal muscle involvement. *Neuromuscular Disorders,* **8,** 598–600.

Fitzsimons, R.B. (1999). Facioscapulohumeral muscular dystrophy. *Current Opinion in Neurology,* **12,** 501–11.

Florence, J.M., Pandya , S., King, W.M., Robison, J.D., Baty, J., Miller, J.P. *et al.* (1992). Intrarater reliability of manual muscle test (Medical Research Council scale) grades in Duchenne's muscular dystrophy. *Physical Therapy,* **72,** 115–22; discussion 122–6.

Florence, J.M., Pandya, S., King, W.M., Robison, J.D., Signore, L.C., Wentzell, M., and Province, M.A. (1984). Clinical trials in Duchenne dystrophy. Standardization and reliability of evaluation procedures. *Physical Therapy,* **64,** 41–5.

Forst, J. and Forst, R. (1999). Lower limb surgery in Duchenne muscular dystrophy. *Neuromuscular Disorders,* **9,** 176–81.

Fradet, G., Pouliot, D., Robichaud, R., St-Pierre, S., and Bouchard, J.P. (1997). Upper esophageal sphincter myotomy in oculopharyngeal muscular dystrophy: long-term clinical results. *Neuromuscular Disorders,* **7**(suppl. 1), S90–5.

Frey, B.M. and Frey, F.J. (1990). Clinical pharmacokinetics of prednisone and prednisolone, **19,** 126–46.

Fuger, K., Barnert, J., Hopfner, W., and Wienbeck, M. (1995). Intestinal pseudoobstruction as a feature of myotonic muscular dystrophy. *Z Gastroenterology,* **33,** 534–8.

Funakoshi, M., Tsuchiya, Y., and Arahata, K. (1999). Emerin and cardiomyopathy in Emery-Dreifuss muscular dystrophy. *Neuromuscular Disorders,* **9,** 108–14.

Gilardeau, C., Kazandjian, M.S., Bach, J.R., Dikeman, K.J., Willig, T.N., and Tucker, L.M. (1995). Evaluation and management of dysphagia. *Seminars in neurology,* **15,** 46–51.

Gozal, D. (2000). Pulmonary manifestations of neuromuscular disease with special reference to Duchenne muscular dystrophy and spinal muscular atrophy. *Pediatric Pulmonology,* **2,** 141–50.

Graham, A.S. and Hatton, R.C. (1999). Creatine: a review of efficacy and safety. *Journal of American Pharmaceutical Association,* (Wash) **39,** 803–10.

Granata, C., Giannini, S., Ballestrazzi, A., and Merlini, L. (1994). Early surgery in Duchenne muscular dystrophy. Experience at Istituto Ortopedico Rizzoli, Bologna, Italy. *Neuromuscular Disorders,* **4,** 87–8.

Granchelli, J.A., Pollina, C., and Hudecki, M.S. (2000). Pre-clinical screening of drugs using the mdx mouse. *Neuromuscular Disorders,* **10,** 235–9.

Griffiths, R.D. and Edwards, R.H. (1988). A new chart for weight control in Duchenne muscular dystrophy. *Archives of Disease in Childhood,* **63,** 1256–8.

Griggs, R.C., Moxley, R.T., Mendell, J.R., *et al.* (1991). Prednisolone in Duchenne dystrophy: a randomised trial defining the time course and dose response. *Archives of Neurology,* **48,** 383–8.

Griggs, R.C., Moxley, R.T., Mendell, J.R., *et al.* (1993). Duchenne dystrophy: randomized, controlled trial of prednisone (18 months) and azathioprine (12 months). *Neurology,* **43,** 520–7.

Harper, P.S. (1975). Congenital myotonic dystrophy in Britain. I. Clinical aspects. *Archives of Disease in Childhood,* **50**(7), 505–13.

Heckmatt, J.Z., Dubowitz, V., Hyde, S.A. *et al.* (1985). Prolongation Of Walking In Duchenne Muscular Dystrophy With Light-Weight Orthoses; Review of 51 Cases. *Developmental Medicine and Child Neurology,* **27,** 149–54.

Heckmatt, J.Z., Rodillo, E., and Dubowitz, E. (1989a). Management of children: Pharmacological and physical. *British Medical Bulletin*, **45**, 788–801.

Heckmatt, J.Z.H., Loh, L., and Dubowitz, V. (1989b). Nocturnal hypoventilation in children with neuromuscular diseases. *Pediatric*, **83**, 250–5.

Henderson, W.A. (1984). Succinylcholine-induced cardiac arrest in unsuspected Duchenne muscular dystrophy. *Canadian Anaesthesia Society Journal*, **31**, 444–6.

Hesketh, J.E., Campbell, G.P., Lobley, G.E. *et al.* (1992). Stimulation of actin and myosin synthesis in rat gastrocnemius muscle by clenbuterol. *Comparative Biochemistry and Physiology*, **102**, 23–7.

Hoffman, E.P., Brown, R.H. Jr, and Kunkel, L.M. (1987). Dystrophin: the protein product of the Duchenne muscular dystrophy locus. *Cell*, **51**, 919–28.

Hoogerwaard, E.M., Bakker, E., Ippel, Pf. *et al.* (1999). Signs and symptoms of Duchenne muscular dystrophy and Becker muscular dystrophy among carriers in the Netherlands. *Lancet*, **353**, 2116–9.

Hyde, S.A., Flytrup, I., Glent, S., Kroksmark, A.K., Salling, B., Steffensen, B.F. *et al.* (2000). A random-ized comparative study of two methods for controlling Tendo Achilles contracture in Duchenne muscular dystrophy. *Neuromuscular Disorders*, **10**, 257–63.

Hyde, S.A., Scott, O.M., Goddard, C.M., and Dubowitz, V. (1982). Prolongation of ambulation in Duchenne muscular dystrophy by appropriate orthoses. *Physiotherapy*, **68**, 105–8.

Ishikawa, Y., Bach, J.R., Minami, R. *et al.* (1999). Cardioprotection for Duchenne's muscular dystrophy. *American Heart Journal*, **137**, 895–902.

Jacobs, I. (1999). Dietary creatine monohydrate supplementation. *Canadian Journal of Applied Physiology*, **24**, 03–14.

Jaffe, K.M., McDonald, C.M., Ingman, E., and Haas, J. (1990). Symptoms of upper gastrointestinal dysfunction in Duchenne muscular dystrophy: case-control study. *Archives of Physical and Medical Rehabilitation*, **71**, 742–4.

Kamber, M., Koster, M., Kreis, R. *et al.* (1999). Creatine supplementation—part I: performance, clinical chemistry, and muscle volume. *Medicine and Science in Sports and Exercise*, **12**, 1763–9.

Keller, C., Reynolds, A., Lee, B., and Garcia-Prats, J. (1998). Congenital myotonic dystrophy requiring prolonged endotracheal and noninvasive assisted ventilation: not a uniformly fatal condition. *Pediatrics*, **101**, 704–6.

Kissel, J.T. (1999). Facioscapulohumeral dystrophy. *Seminars in neurology*, **19**, 35–43.

Kissel, J.T., Burrow, K., Rammohan, K.W. *et al.* (1991). Mononuclear cell analysis of muscle biopsies in prednisolone and azathioprine treated Duchenne muscular dystrophy. *Neurology*, **41**, 667–72.

Kissel, J.T., McDermott, M.P. and Natarajan, R. *et al.* (1998). Pilot trial of albuterol in facioscapulo-humeral muscular dystrophy. *Neurology*, **50**, 1402–6.

Koenig, M., Hoffman, E.P., Bertelson, C.H. *et al.* (1987). Complete cloning of Duchenne muscular dystrophy (DMD) cDNA and preliminary genomic organisation of the, D.M.D gene in normal and affected individuals. *Cell*, **50**, 509–17.

Lenard, H.G., Goebel, H.H., and Weigel, W. (1977). Smooth muscle involvement in congenital myotonic dystrophy. *Neuropadiatrie*, **8**, 42–52.

Luthert, P., Vrbova, G., and Ward, K.M. (1980). Effects of slow frequency electrical stimulation on muscles of dystrophic, mice. *Journal of Neurology, Neurosurgery and Psychiatry*, **43**, 803–9.

Maltin, C.A. and Delday, M.I. (1992). Satellite cells in innervated and denervated muscles treated with clenbuterol. *Muscle Nerve*, **15**, 919–25.

Mankin, A.S. and Liebman, S.W. (1999). Baby, don't stop! *Nature Genetics*, **23**, 8–10.

Manzur, A.Y., Hyde, S.A., Rodillo E. *et al.* (1992). A Randomised Controlled Trial Of Early Surgery In Duchenne Muscular Dystrophy. *Neuromuscular Disorders*, **2**, 379–87.

Martin, A.J., Stern, L., Yeates, J., Lepp, D., and Little, J. (1986). Respiratory muscle training in Duchenne muscular dystrophy. *Developmental Medicine and Child Neurology*, **28**, 314–8.

Martineau, L., Little, R.A., Rothwell, N.J. *et al.* (1993). Clenbuterol, a beta 2 adrenergic agonist, reverses muscle wasting due to scald injury in the rat. *Burns*, **19**, 26–24.

Mathieu, J., Allard, P., Gobeil, G., Girard, M., De Braekeleer, M., and Begin, P. (1997). Anesthetic and surgical complications in 219 cases of myotonic dystrophy. *Neurology*, **49**, 1646–50.

Mathieu, J., Allard, P., Potvin, L., Prevost, C., and Begin, P. (1999). A 10-year study of mortality in a cohort of patients with myotonic dystrophy. *Neurology*, **52**, 1658–62.

McCool, F.D. and Tzelepis, G.E. (1995). Inspiratory muscle training in the patient with neuromuscular disease. *Physical Therapy*, **75**, 1006–14.

Melacini, P., Vianello, A., Villanova, C. *et al.* (1996). Cardiac and respiratory involvement in advanced stage Duchenne muscular dystrophy. *Neuromuscular Disorders*, **6**, 367–76.

Mendell, J.R., Moxley, R.T., Griggs, R.C. *et al.* (1989). Randomized controlled trial of prednisolone in Duchenne's muscular dystrophy. *New England Journal of Medicine*, 320, 1592–7.

Mesa, L.E., Dubrovsky, A.L., Corderi, J., Marco, P., and Flores, D. (1991). Steroids in Duchenne muscular dystrophy—deflazacort trial. *Neuromuscular Disorders*, **1**, 261–6.

Moxley, R.T. III (1992). Myotonic muscular dystrophy. In Handbook of Clinical Neurology, 18(62): Myopathies. Rowland, L.P., DiMauro S, eds. Elsevier Science Publishers, 1992, 209–59.

Moxley, R.T. III (1997). Carrell-Krusen Symposium Invited Lecture-1997. Myotonic disorders in childhood: diagnosis and treatment. *Journal of Child Neurology*, **12**, 116–29.

Newsom-Davis, J., Goldman, M., Loh, L., and Casson, M. (1976). Diaphragm function and alveolar hypoventilation. *Quarterly Journal of Medicine*, 45, 87–100.

Newsom-Davis, J.R. (1980). The respiratory system in muscular dystrophy. *British Medical Bulletin*, **36**, 135–8.

Nigro, G., Comi, L.I., Politano, L. *et al.* (1995). Evaluation of cardiomyopathy in Becker muscular dystrophy. *Muscle Nerve*, 18, 283–91.

Nonaka, I. (1998). Animal models of muscular dystrophies. *Laboratory Animal Science*, **48**, 8–17.

Obata, R., Yasumi, Y., Suzuki, A., Nakajima, Y., and Sato, S. (1999). Rhabdomyolysis in association with Duchenne's muscular dystrophy. *Canadian Journal of Anaesthesia*, **46**, 564–6.

Pasquini, F., Guerin, C., Blake, D. *et al.* (1995). The effect of glucocorticoids on the accumulation of utrophin by cultured normal and dystrophic human skeletal muscle satellite cells. *Neuromuscular Disorders*, **5**, 105–14.

Perie, S., Eymard, B., Laccourreye, L., Chaussade, S., Fardeau, M., Lacau, St. Guily, J. (1997). Dysphagia in oculopharyngeal muscular dystrophy: a series of 22 French cases. *Neuromuscular Disorders*, **7**(suppl.1), S96–9.

Perkin, G.D. and Murray-Lyon, I. (1998). Neurology and the gastrointestinal system. *Journal of Neurology, Neurosurgery and Psychiatry*, **65**, 291–300.

Personius, K.E., Pandya, S., King, W.M., Tawil, R., and McDermott, M.P. (1994). Facioscapulohumeral dystrophy natural history study: standardization of testing procedures and reliability of measurements. The FSHDY Group. *Physical Therapy*, **74**, 253–63.

Phillips, M.F., Smith, P.E., Carroll, N. *et al.* (1999). Nocturnal oxygention and prognosis in Duchenne muscular dystrophy. *American Journal of Respiratory and Critical Care Medicine*, MED, **160**, 198–202.

Philpot-J, Bagnall-A, King-C. *et al.* (1999). Feeding Problems In Merosin Deficient Congenital Muscular Dystrophy. *Archives of Disease in Childhood*, **80**, 542–7.

Pulido-S.M., Passaquin-A.C., Leijendekker-W. *et al.* (1998). Creatine supplementation improves intracellular Ca2+ handling and survival in mdx skeletal muscle cells. *FEBS-Letters* **439**, 357–62.

Quinlivan, R.M., Lewis P, Marsden, P. *et al.* (1996). Cardiac function, metabolism and perfusion in Duchenne and Becker muscular dystrophy. *Neuromuscular Disorders*, **6**, 237–46.

Reardon, W., Newcombe, R., Fenton, I., Sibert, J., and Harper, P.S. (1993). The natural history of congenital myotonic dystrophy: mortality and long term clinical aspects. *Archives of Disease in Childhood*, **68**, 177–81.

Reitter, B. (1995). Deflazacort vs. prednisone in Duchenne muscular dystrophy: trends of an ongoing study. *Brain Development*, **17** suppl, 39–43.

Rideau, Y., Duport, G., and Marie Agnes, Y. (1987). Traitment de dystrophies musculaires. *Sem Hop Paris*, **63**, 438–43.

Rideau, Y., Jankowski, L.W., and Grellet, J. (1981). Respiratory function in the muscular dystrophies. *Muscle Nerve*, **4**, 155–64.

Rifai, Z., Welle, E., Moxley, R.T. *et al.* (1995). Effect of prednisolone on protein metabolism in Duchenne muscular dystrophy. *American Journal of Physiology*, **268**, E67–E74.

Rodillo, E., Noble-Jamieson, C.M., Aber, V., Heckmatt, J.Z., Muntoni, F. and Dubowitz, V. (1989). Respiratory muscle training in Duchenne muscular dystrophy. *Archives of Disease in Childhood*, **64**, 736–8.

Rodillo, E.B., Fernandez-Bermejo, and Heckmatt, J.Z. *et al.* (1988). Prevention Of Rapidly Progressive Scoliosis in Duchenne Muscular Dystrophy by Prolongation Of Walking With Orthosis. *Journal of Child Neurology*, **3**, 269–74.

Rutherford, M.A., Heckmatt, J.Z., and Dubowitz, V. (1989). Congenital myotonic dystrophy: respiratory function at birth determines survival. *Archives of Disease in Childhood*, **64**, 191–5.

Sansome, A., Royston, P., and Dubowitz, V. (1993). Steroids in Duchenne muscular dystropy; Pilot study of a new low-dosage schedule. *Neuromuscular Disorders* **3**, 567–9.

Scott, O.M., Hyde, S.A., Goddard, C., and Dubowitz, V. (1981a). Prevention of deformity in Duchenne muscular dystrophy. A prospective study of passive stretching and splintage. *Physiotherapy*, **67**, 177–80.

Scott, O.M., Hyde, S.A., Goddard, C., and Dubowitz, V. (1982). Quantitation of muscle function in children: a prospective study in Duchenne muscular dystrophy. *Muscle Nerve*, **5**, 291–301.

Scott, O.M., Hyde, S.A., Goddard, C., Jones, R., and Dubowitz, V. (1981b). Effect of exercise in Duchenne muscular dystrophy. *Physiotherapy*, **67**, 174–6.

Scott, O.M., Hyde, S.A., Vrbova, G., and Dubowitz, V. (1990). Therapeutic possibilities of chronic low frequency electrical stimulation in children with Duchenne muscular dystrophy. *Journal of Neurological Science*, **95**, 171–82.

Sharma, K.R., Mynhier, M.A., and Miller, R.G. (1993). Cyclosporine increases muscular force generation in Duchenne musculardystrophy. *Neurology*, **43**, 527–32.

Siegel, I.M. (1975). Pulmonary problems in Duchenne muscular dystrophy. Diagnosis, prophylaxis, and treatment. *Physical Therapy*, **55**, 160–2.

Siegel, I.M., Miller, J.E., and Ray, R.D. (1968). Subcutaneous lower limb tenotomy in the treatment of pseudohypertrophic muscular dystrophy. Description of technique and presentation of twenty-one cases. *The Journal of Bone and Joint Surgery. American Volume*, **50**, 1437–43.

Siegel, I.M., Miller, J.E. and Ray, R.D. (1974). Failure of corticosteroid in the treatment of Duchenne (pseudo-hypertrophic) muscular dystrophy. Report of a clinically matched three year double-blind study. *Illinois Medical Journal*, **145**, 32–3.

Simmonds, A.K., Muntoni, F., Heather, S. *et al.* (1998). Impact Of Nasal Ventilation On Survival In Hypercapnic Duchenne Muscular Dystrophy. *Thorax*, **53**, 949–52.

Smith, C.L. and Bush, G.H. (1985). Anaesthesia and progressive muscular dystrophy. *British Journal of Anaesthesia*, **57**, 1113–8.

Smith, R.A., Newcombe, R.G., Sibert, J.R. and Harper, P.S. (1991). Assessment of locomotor function in young boys with Duchenne muscular dystrophy. *Muscle Nerve*, **14**, 462–9.

Spencer, G.E. and Vignos, P.J. (1962). Bracing for ambulation in childhood progressive muscular dystrophy. *J Bone Joint Surgery*, **44A**, 234–42.

Steare, S.E., Benatar, A., and Dubowitz, V. (1992). Subclinical cardiomyopathy in Becker muscular dystrophy. *British Heart Journal*, 68, 304–8.

Sugino, M., Ohsawa, N., Ito, T., Ishida, S., Yamasaki, H., Kimura, F. and Shinoda, K. (1998). A pilot study of dehydroepiandrosterone sulfate in myotonic dystrophy. *Neurology*, **51**(2), 586–9.

Tawil, R., McDermot, M., Pandya, S. *et al.* (1997). A pilot trial of prednisolone in facioscapulohumeral dystrophy (FSHD). *Neurology*, **48**, 46–9.

Tawil, R., McDermott, M.P., Mendell, J.R., Kissel, J., and Griggs, R.C. (1994). Facioscapulohumeral muscular dystrophy (FSHD): design of natural history study and results of baseline testing. FSH-DY Group. *Neurology*, **44**, 442–6.

Tilton, A.H., Miller, M.D., and Khoshoo, V. (1998). Nutrition and swallowing in pediatric neuromuscular patients. *Seminars in Pediatric Neurology*, **5**, 106–15.

Vianello, A., Bevilaqua, M., Salvador, V. *et al.* (1994). Long term nasal intermittent positive pressure ventilation in Duchenne's muscular dystrophy. *Chest*, **105**, 445–8.

Victor, M., Hayes, R., and Adams, R.D. (1962). Oculopharyngeal muscular dystrophy; familial disease of late life characterised by dysphagia, progressive ptosis of the eyelids. *New England Journal of Medicine*, **267**, 1267–72.

Vignos, P.J., Wagner, M.B., Karlinchak, B., and Katirji, B. (1996). Evaluation of a program for long-term treatment of Duchenne muscular dystrophy. Experience at the University Hospitals of Cleveland. *Journal of Bone and Joint Surgery American*, **78**, 1844–52.

Walter, M.C., Lochmuller, H., Reilich, P., Klopstock, T., Huber, R., Hartard, M. *et al.* (2000). Creatine monohydrate in muscular dystrophies: A double-blind, placebo-controlled clinical study. *Neurology*, **54**, 1848–50.

Wanke, T., Toifl, K., Merkle, M., Formanek, D., Lahrmann, H., and Zwick, H. (1994). Inspiratory muscle training in patients with Duchenne muscular dystrophy. *Chest*, **105**, 475–82.

Willig, T.N., Bach, J.R., Venance, V., and Navarro, J. (1995). Nutritional rehabilitation in neuromuscular disorders. *Seminars in* Neurology, **15**, 18–23.

Willig, T.N., Carlier, L., Legrand, M. *et al.* (1993). Nutritional assessment in Duchenne muscular dystrophy. *Developmental Medicine and Child Neurology*, **35**, 1074–82.

Willig, T.N., Paulus, J., Lacau Saint Guily, J. *et al.* (1994). Swallowing problems in neuromuscular disorders. *Archives of Physical and Medical Rehabilitation*, 75, 1175–81.

Winkler, G., Zifko, U., Nader, A., Frank, W., Zwick, H., Toifl, K., and Wanke, T. (2000). Dose-dependent effects of inspiratory muscle training in neuromuscular disorders. *Muscle Nerve*, **23**, 1257–60.

Winter, K., Schara, U., Mortimer, J., Liersch, R., and Mortier, W. (1999). Duchenne muscular dystrophy with long term steroid therapy. Absence of cardiac side effects. *Acta Myologica*, III, 159–162.

Zupan, A. (1992). Long-term electrical stimulation of muscles in children with Duchenne and Becker muscular dystrophy. *Muscle Nerve*, **15**, 362–7.

Zupan, A., Gregoric, M., Valencic, V., and Vandot, S. (1993). Effects of electrical stimulation on muscles of children with Duchenne and Becker muscular dystrophy. *Neuropediatrics*, **24**, 189–92.

Chapter 13

Respiratory care in muscular dystrophy

Anita K. Simonds

Introduction

Respiratory problems are a major cause of morbidity and mortality in the muscular dystrophies. Indeed, in Duchenne muscular dystrophy (DMD) respiratory complications are the cause of death in over 70 per cent of patients, and virtually all Duchenne patients will develop ventilatory insufficiency if they survive long enough. In the other muscular dystrophies the extent of respiratory compromise will depend on the degree of respiratory muscle involvement, the presence of a thoracic scoliosis and level of bulbar weakness. In congenital muscular dystrophy merosin negative individuals seem more prone to early respiratory failure than merosin positive patients. Ventilatory failure is relatively uncommon, although not unknown in facioscapulohumeral muscular dystrophy, and has a variable prevalence in limb girdle MD. Although ventilatory support has been used sporadically in neuromuscular patients with chronic ventilatory failure for over 50 years, in the last decade the use of non-invasive ventilation has had a significant impact on survival and long-term outcome, particularly in DMD patients. In this chapter the natural history of respiratory problems in the muscular dystrophies is discussed, with particular emphasis on monitoring, identifying high-risk patients, and the outcome of therapeutic interventions.

Natural history of respiratory function

Loss of lung volume in neuromuscular disease is due to a combination of inspiratory muscle weakness and decrease in chest wall and pulmonary compliance, creating a restrictive ventilatory defect. Longitudinal studies (Baydur *et al.* 1990; Rideau *et al.* 1981) of lung volume in DMD patients have shown that absolute values of forced vital capacity (FVC) increase during childhood until around 10 years of age then plateau as the disease advances. The mid to late teenage years are characterized by a fall in FVC as respiratory muscle strength declines and a thoracic scoliosis commonly develops. Plateau FVC values tend to be around 1500 ml. Daytime hypercapnia is likely once vital capacity falls below 500 ms but a fairly wide variation is seen. Brooke *et al.* (1989) have studied patterns of progression of DMD and shown that FVC values in the Duchenne population are not normally distributed—in keeping with the experience that some individuals show much more rapid deterioration than average. This finding is corroborated by the fact that the FVC plateau value is higher in some patients than others and, not surprisingly, those individuals with a higher VC have better respiratory prognosis.

Less predictable trends in lung function are seen in other neuromuscular conditions. An evaluation of the factors predisposing individuals to develop hypercapnia in a heterogenous group including patients with DMD, Becker MD, facioscapulohumeral MD and other disorders found that CO_2 retention was consistently associated with a rapid shallow breathing pattern. This pattern of breathing in turn, was correlated with lower inspiratory and expiratory muscle pressures and an increase in dynamic lung elastance, that is, augmented elastic load on the lungs. In a study focusing exclusively on patients with limb girdle muscular dystrophy, Gigliotti and colleagues (1995) reported moderate decreases in vital capacity (range 37–87 per cent predicted), and inspiratory and expiratory mouth pressures compared to age-matched controls. Hypercapnia was present in 20 per cent of patients, with relatively well-preserved arterial oxygen level (PaO_2). Respiratory muscle strength was inversely proportional to electromyographic (EMG) activity of the diaphragm, and the reduction in respiratory muscle strength was associated with an increase in neural drive indicating that control of breathing was intact. Daytime $PaCO_2$ correlated best with the decrease in vital capacity and duration of illness, rather than respiratory muscle strength—supporting the view that a variety of factors contribute to the development of a restrictive ventilatory defect, not just respiratory muscle strength. The practical extension of this finding is that vital capacity is a more accurate predictor of ventilatory insufficiency in limb girdle muscular dystrophy than measures of respiratory muscle function.

Expiratory muscle function in muscular dystrophies

Most research attention has been paid to the inspiratory muscles in neuromuscular disease because of their central importance for ventilation. However, in many neuromuscular conditions expiratory muscle strength deteriorates at a similar rate to inspiratory muscle strength. This can have serious consequences for cough efficiency. Indeed, chest infections become more problematical in this group not only because inspiratory muscle weakness leads to micro and macroatelectasis, but also because ineffectual coughing limits the clearance of secretions. Bulbar dysfunction will cause aspiration pneumonia in a proportion of affected individuals, but in most DMD patients, significant aspiration is an endstage phenomenon, and occurs long after the development of ventilatory failure.

Sleep disordered breathing

Hypoventilation occurs in normal individuals during sleep, and is most evident during rapid eye movement (REM) sleep periods. This is due to a fall in overall ventilatory drive, and a reduction in intercostal, upper airway, and postural muscle activity. REM sleep in

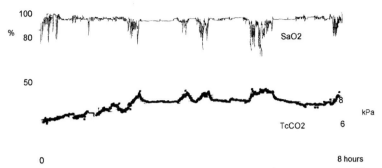

Fig.13. 1 Overnight monitoring of arterial oxygen saturation and transcutaneous CO_2 tension demonstrating REM related nocturnal hypoventilation. (SaO_2—arterial oxygen saturation, $TcCO_2$—transcutaneous carbon dioxide tension)

normals is associated with a rise in CO_2 tension by up to 0.9 kPa and fall in arterial oxygen saturation (SaO_2) by a few percent. In individuals with significant respiratory muscle and bulbar weakness, and/or chest wall restriction due to a thoracic scoliosis, this tendency to alveolar hypoventilation is exaggerated (Fig. 13. 1). Additionally, overt upper airway obstruction in the form of obstructive apnoeas may be precipitated. To further complicate matters, compensatory mechanisms such as the arousal reflex and hypoxic and hypercapnic ventilatory drive, which terminate episodes, may be blunted in individuals with sleep-disordered breathing. As a result of all these physiological changes, sleep is a vulnerable time for patients with muscular dystrophy, and the early manifestations of ventilatory insufficiency will be seen during sleep *before* they become manifest during the day. This provides the rationale for carrying out sleep studies in muscular dystrophy patients, and providing those who have nocturnal hypoventilation with ventilatory support during sleep.

While nocturnal hypoventilation is the commonest form of sleep disordered breathing in Duchenne patients, a proportion present with obstructive apnoeas and hypopnoeas, or a combination of hypoventilation and obstructive sleep apnoea. Khan and Heckmatt (1994) have examined the mechanisms leading to nocturnal hypoxaemia in a group of DMD patients aged 13–23 years, and carried out serial sleep studies in a subgroup to look at the evolution of the respiratory disturbance over time. Over 60 per cent of Duchenne patients had periods of hypoxaemia during sleep with SaO_2 falling below 90 per cent, while none of the age-matched controls experienced hypoxaemia. Approximately two-thirds of the respiratory events were obstructive in aetiology with an average apnoea index of 7.5 h (range 3.5–11.4). Most of the dips in SaO_2 occurred in REM sleep, as expected. The authors found a strong correlation between the severity and frequency of hypoxaemic dips and age ($p < 0.005$), and the number of years of wheelchair use ($p = 0.005$). While all patients over the age of 14 years had hypoxaemic dips, only three of the boys aged 14 years or less experienced nocturnal hypoxaemia. There was no close relationship between the presence and severity of hypoxaemia and vital capacity, or body mass index (average 16 kg/m^2). Ten of the twelve patients with nocturnal hypoxaemia underwent follow-up sleep studies and in virtually all of these hypoxaemia worsened, while the ratio of obstructive events to hypoventilation fell from 60 to 30 per cent. The patient with the most severe nocturnal desaturation during the baseline sleep study died two months after the study was carried out. Clearly, it is now difficult and almost certainly unethical to monitor the natural history of untreated sleep disordered breathing in muscular dystrophy, as treatment with nocturnal ventilatory support is available for those who wish to receive it. However, Phillips *et al.* (1999) followed 18 DMD patients for 10 years after an initial sleep study showing REM related desaturation until death or the introduction of nasal ventilation. Median survival was 50 months from the baseline study and was unrelated to body mass index or respiratory muscle strength, as measured by mouth pressures. Mortality was, however, correlated with daytime $PaCO_2$ ($r = 0.72$, $p < 0.005$), minimum nocturnal SaO_2 ($r = 0.62$, $p < 0.007$) and vital capacity ($r = 0.79$, $p < 0.004$). The best general predictor of mortality was a vital capacity of less than 1 litre.

Barbe *et al.* (1994) looked at sleep-related respiratory disturbances in an older cohort of DMD patients (mean age 18 ± 2 years, mean vital capacity 27 per cent predicted). Sixty seven per cent of these patients had symptoms of daytime somnolence, headache, nightmares, difficulty with sleeping, or snoring. These symptoms correlated well with the number of apnoea and hypopnoeas overnight. Contrary to the findings of Khan and Heckmatt (1994) 85 per cent of the respiratory events were central hypopnoeas, indicating that in some patients obstructive apnoea and hypopnoeas progress to central events with age. In this group too, the apnoea/hypopnoea index (numbers of apnoeas and hypopnoeas per hour) was correlated with daytime CO_2. Only the apnoea/hyponoea index in REM sleep was correlated with age.

Other workers have sought to establish daytime predictors of sleep hypoventilation in DMD. Hukins and Hillman (2000) found that the most consistent factors were FEV1 < 40 per cent, $PaCO_2 > 6.0\,kPa$ and base excess $> 4.0\,mmol/l$. This last factor (as an index of long term CO_2 control) explained 64 per cent of the variation in total sleep time spent at levels of $SaO_2 < 90$ per cent, but in this study, as previously, there was no clear relationship between maximum mouth pressures and sleep desaturation.

A predominance of nocturnal hypoventilation can also be seen in patients with congenital muscular dystrophy, although like DMD patients, younger congenital muscular dystrophy patients may have a mixture of obstructive apnoeas and central hyponoeas. This is especially the case in obese children. This pattern differs from the early form of sleep-disordered breathing seen in children with spinal muscular atrophy (SMA). As diaphragm function is relatively preserved until late in SMA REM related hypoventilation is not an early feature, but recurrent desaturation is often found.

Identifying patients at risk of respiratory complications

What conclusions can we draw from the above information in order to monitor our patients effectively and predict the development of ventilatory complications? Vital capacity is an essential measurement and should be followed serially in all muscular dystrophy patients, particularly in those in whom the VC is less than 50 per cent predicted. Values should be expressed as per cent predicted for span rather than height, which will be affected to a variable extent by the degree of thoracic scoliosis. Patients with a vital capacity of between 20 and 50 per cent predicted are at risk of ventilatory decompensation, especially at the time of chest infections. These individuals should be carefully questioned about symptoms of sleep-disordered breathing such as morning headaches, daytime fatigue and somnolence, breathlessness, sleep fragmentation, nightmares, nocturnal panic attacks or palpitations. School teachers and parents may notice that the child or adolescent is sluggish in the morning, but energy levels increase by the afternoon. Anorexia for breakfast, as a new development, is common in children and adults with sleep disordered breathing.

Sleep studies should be carried out in any patient with sleep related symptoms, a base excess > 4 mmol per litre or daytime hypercapnia. Consideration should also be given to this investigation in all patients with a vital capacity of less than 20 per cent predicted. Many centres merely monitor overnight oximetry. However, this can create problems as the need for nocturnal ventilation is based on the degree of nocturnal hypoventilation which can only be quantitated by CO_2 measurement. At the Royal Brompton Hospital, in addition to oximetry, we use transcutaneous CO_2 ($TcCO_2$) monitoring overnight, which has proved user-friendly in adults and children, and a reliable guide to arterial CO_2 tension (see Fig. 13. 1). While full polysomnography is not essential to make a diagnosis of sleep disordered breathing, the additional use of sensors to monitor oronasal airflow and chest wall effort, will allow respiratory events to be classified into obstructive and central hypopnoeas/apnoeas. This point is not just of academic interest as obstructive sleep apnoea alone (in the absence of CO_2 retention) may respond to continuous positive airway pressure (CPAP) therapy, whereas pure hypoventilation with a marked rise in CO_2 overnight and daytime hypercapnia, is best treated with nocturnal ventilation.

Monitoring of cardiac function by serial clinical assessment, ECG and echocardiogram is also an important part of management and is discussed below.

Ventilatory support in muscular dystrophies
Indications for the initiation of nocturnal ventilatory support

Although ventilatory support using invasive tracheostomy ventilation and negative pressure techniques such as the iron lung and cuirass have been used sporadically for over 50 years, it was the realization by Rideau et al. (1983) that non-invasive nasal ventilation could be used effectively in DMD patients which has revolutionized ventilatory management in patients with respiratory insufficiency due to neuromuscular disease in the last two decades. A recent consensus conference (1999) has now concluded that ventilatory support should be available to all symptomatic patients with confirmed neuromuscular disease and a daytime CO_2 value of $> 6\,kPa$ or significant nocturnal desaturation. These guidelines are not, in fact, based on the results of randomized controlled trials, but such trials would now be unethical as it is has been demonstrated repeatedly that the development of diurnal hypercapania in DMD is a preterminal event, if it is not treated. Vianello *et al.* (1994) reported the outcome in ten DMD patients with daytime hypercapnia. Five received nasal ventilation and five did not. After two years all patients receiving nasal intermittent positive pressure ventilation (NIPPV) were still alive, but 4/5 of the unventilated group had died and the fifth was in severe ventilatory failure. The median time between onset of daytime hypercapnia and death was only 9.7 months.

The issue of whether ventilatory support should be introduced when nocturnal hypercapnia is present *before* the development of diurnal hypercapnia is currently being explored by randomized controlled study. However, it is important to note that the introduction of ventilatory support in *asymptomatic* patients before the development of sleep disordered breathing or daytime hypercapnia is *NOT* recommended. This was demonstrated by Raphael *et al.* (1994) who carried out a trial of preventative NIPPV in an asymptomatic, normocapnic DMD cohort with a vital capacity between 20 and 50 per cent predicted. This early intervention produced no benefit whatsoever, yet there was a small but insignificant excess of deaths in the ventilatory support arm—perhaps partly related to the fact that carers may have delayed seeking hospital treatment for chest infections when ventilatory support was available at home.

Outcome of NIPPV

There is little doubt that the introduction of NIPPV in hypercapnic DMD patients and other groups with ventilatory insufficiency can be lifesaving. The age at which ventilatory failure develops in DMD patients has been consistently shown to be around 20 years. Use of ventilatory support alters the natural history of the condition. A UK study using NIPPV in DMD showed a one-year survival of 85 per cent and five year survival of 73 per cent (Simonds *et al.* 1998) (Fig.13. 2). The probability of continuing NIPPV at three years was lower in a French multicentre study (Leger *et al.* 1994) at 36 per cent, but it is common practice for French patients to be transferred from NIPPV to tracheostomy ventilation, whereas invasive ventilation is less frequently used in the UK. Dependence on ventilatory support tends to increase with time, but most DMD patients can be managed with nocturnal NIPPV for up to five years before additional daytime support is required. In congenital muscular dystrophy and LGMD too, arterial blood gas tensions can be maintained in the normal range long term, using NIPPV solely at night, allowing the recipient to complete schooling, higher education courses, and go to work.

Nasal intermittent positive pressure ventilation is delivered using nasal masks, nasal plugs or a full facemask according to patient preference. The ventilators employed to deliver NIPPV in the home can be broadly classified into volume preset and pressure

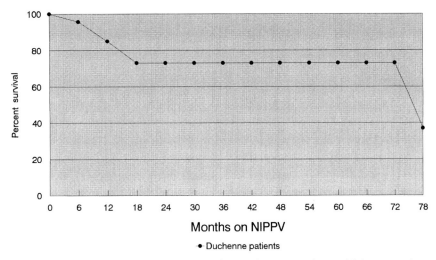

Fig. 13. 2 Survival following the introduction of NIPPV in DMD patients with hypercapnic respiratory failure (Simonds *et al.* 1998)

preset types. There is no evidence at present to suggest that any particular type of ventilator is superior, although in patients with obstructive apnoeas/hyponoeas and/or recurrent atelectasis the use of bilevel pressure support ventilators such as the BiPAP (Respironics Inc.), VPAP (Resmed), or DP90 (Taema) may offer theoretical advantages. These machines provide a background of CPAP during expiration (expiratory positive airway pressure, EPAP) that may help increase functional residual volume, recruit alveoli, and maintain upper airway patency. Ventilator settings should be established during a short hospital stay by monitoring overnight $TcCO_2$ and SaO_2 levels. Long term normalization and stabilization of daytime arterial blood gas tensions should be expected. Supplemental oxygen therapy is rarely required. The capital cost of the home ventilation system is around £2000–£3000. Patients receiving ventilatory support should be routinely followed-up by a centre with experience in this area, which can provide back-up service and maintenance for the equipment and ongoing medical care and family support.

Practitioners who are not familiar with the newer non-invasive ventilatory techniques often question the quality of life of recipients of NIPPV, as there are still concerns that the use of ventilatory support might perpetuate a poor quality existence for the patient. These concerns have been addressed by several studies. Bach *et al.* (1991) found that healthcare practitioners consistently underestimate the quality of life of their patients with DMD. In a series of 82 ventilator dependent individuals, only 12.5 per cent expressed dissatisfaction with their lives, which compares with a dissatisfaction rate of seven per cent in the general population and nine per cent in healthcare workers. In a UK study (Simonds *et al.* 1998) of DMD patients receiving NIPPV the SF36 generic quality of life tool showed that DMD patients had similar levels of health perception and social function to other ventilator users with non-progressive conditions such as poliomyelitis and idiopathic scoliosis. All patients who started NIPPV wished to continue the therapy, and often recommended NIPPV to friends with muscular dystrophy.

Paediatric NIPPV

Previously it has been thought that NIPPV would be unsuccessful in young children as they would be unable to cope with the mask interfaces. Recent experience shows this is not the case (Barois and Estournet-Mathiaud 1993). In 40 consecutive children aged nine months to 16 years with respiratory insufficiency due to neuromusculo-skeletal disease 38 coped well with long term domiciliary NIPPV (Simonds 2000). Around 20 per cent of children had congenital muscular dystrophy. Of these, five were merosin positive and the younger three were merosin negative. For the group as a whole, significant improvements in daytime and nocturnal arterial blood gas tensions were demonstrated. It seems likely that the introduction of ventilatory support in this paediatric population will alter the natural history of some congenital neuromuscular disorders and extend life expectancy, just as has occurred in the adolescent group with DMD.

Tracheostomy ventilation (T-IPPV)

Invasive ventilation is indicated in patients with severe bulbar insufficiency and/or a high level of ventilator dependence. While this situation may pertain in some muscular dystrophy patients, it is the exception to the rule even in DMD patients, as most do not develop intractable bulbar incompetence or extreme ventilator dependence until a very late stage of the disease. However, T-IPPV can be successfully applied if the patients decide on this option. Informed decision-making will always involve a careful discussion of the pros and cons of tracheostomy ventilation, and its likely impact on the quality of life of the individual and his family. As described above, in France a progressive ventilatory care plan is often employed such that patients start on NIPPV when daytime hypercapnia develops and subsequently transfer to T-IPPV if daytime ventilator use exceeds 16 h a day or bulbar problems preclude satisfactory NIPPV use. Currently, in the UK most DMD patients use NIPPV indefinitely, because of the practical problems associated with discharging tracheostomy-ventilated patients into the community. NIPPV is much more user-friendly in this respect.

Negative pressure ventilation

Negative pressure ventilation has been successfully applied in neuromuscular patients for many decades (Thomson 1997). However, it has the disadvantage of provoking upper airway obstruction during sleep, which may seriously limit the efficacy of ventilation. In addition, the equipment is bulky, fairly expensive, and not widely available. For these reasons negative pressure non-invasive ventilation has been superceded by NIPPV in most cases.

Mechanisms of action of ventilatory support in neuromuscular disease

Ventilatory support could improve ventilatory function when the individual breathes spontaneously by three main mechanisms:

- improvement in respiratory muscle strength,
- an increase in lung/chest wall compliance, or
- an increase in ventilatory drive.

Although small increases in respiratory muscle strength may be seen, in most studies these changes are negligible, as are alterations in lung/chest wall mechanics. In a heterogenous group with neuromuscular disease and scoliosis, Annane *et al.* (1999) have shown that improvements in arterial blood gas tensions after starting NIPPV are correlated best with an increase in ventilatory drive. This finding is in keeping with other groups treated with ventilatory support or nasal continuous positive airway pressure (Berthon-Jones and Sullivan 1987). It remains speculative whether this improvement in central chemoreceptor function is due to the ventilator-associated fall in $PaCO_2$ or improvement in sleep quality, as sleep fragmentation is known to decrease the ventilatory response to CO_2 (Cooper and Philips 1982).

General respiratory healthcare and treatment of chest infections

General respiratory advice to patients is largely commonsense. Patients should aim to keep to ideal body weight as respiratory muscle efficiency will be compromised by both obesity and malnourishment. Obesity will also predispose the patient to obstructive sleep apnoea. Dietary advice can be especially helpful when patients become wheelchair bound.

Attention to comfort and support in the wheelchair is also crucial. Customized seating mounds and a slightly tipped back seat position will help avoid wasted energy expenditure in maintaining body position (particularly with accessory muscles maintaining neck position), and allow the diaphragm to work to the best mechanical advantage. Most orthotists take respiratory function fully into account when constructing spinal braces, but bracing can undoubtedly reduce chest wall expansion and compliance so that a careful balance needs to be struck between scoliosis control and respiratory muscle function.

All patients and their families should be taught sensible physiotherapy techniques for clearing bronchial secretions such as assisted coughing (huffing), and the ability to recognize the early signs of a chest infection (increased sputum production, sputum purulence, pyrexia, increased breathlessness etc.). Adults and adolescents with muscular dystrophy should receive the influenza vaccination yearly, and the pneumococcal vaccination unless there are any contraindications. For patients who are subject to regular chest infections, a reserve course of antibiotic kept at home is a wise precaution. In adults and children who tend to wheeze or develop airflow obstruction at the time of a chest infection nebulized bronchodilator (salbutomol, terbutaline or ipratropium) or bronchodilator delivered via a spacer may be helpful, but this is not routinely required in the absence of features of bronchoconstriction, or a history of asthma. In patients with FSH MD, LGMD and CMD long-term survival with or without ventilatory support is often seen. In DMD patients and others with a progressive pathology, the use of ventilatory support will extend life expectancy by 5–10 years on average, but most will ultimately succumb from respiratory failure. Advance directives are helpful in the end-stage situation, as most patients understandably wish to take part in decision-making. The use of respite admissions, opiate infusions, and anticholinergic preparations to reduce secretions all may have a place in the terminal phase and are discussed in detail elsewhere (Simonds 1996; 1998).

Oxygen therapy

In the past oxygen therapy has often been prescribed in muscular dystrophy patients during chest infections and to palliate symptoms. In most cases this is inappropriate as the main problem is alveolar hypoventilation which requires ventilatory support. Oxygen therapy in hypercapnic patients will exacerbate CO_2 retention and may precipitate a ventilatory crisis. Similarly, sleep disordered breathing is most logically treated with CPAP or NIPPV, not oxygen therapy. Oxygen therapy may need to be added to NIPPV at the time of a severe pneumonia, and may also be of value to palliate symptoms in individuals who do not wish to receive ventilatory support. However, at other times the use of oxygen therapy should be carefully questioned.

Cough in-exsufflators

These machines, such as the Emerson in-exsufflator are cough-assist devices. They deliver, via facemask or mouthpiece, a large positive pressure breath during inspiration followed by a swing to negative pressure during expiration. This combination of maneouvres is designed to facilitate sputum clearance in patients with weak inspiratory and expiratory muscles. Studies (Bach 1993; Barach and Beck 1954) in the USA have shown that the cough in-exsufflator can increase peak expiratory cough flow rates compared to conventional physiotherapy, particularly in individuals with a cough peak flow of less than 160 l/min.

Prevalence and management of cardiomyopathy

This subject is discussed here for the sake of completeness, though it is dealt with in greater detail in Chapter 11. Post mortem findings of myocardial atrophy and fibrosis are well described in DMD patients, and it is estimated that about 10 per cent of DMD patients die of cardiac rather than respiratory complications. ECG abnormalities such as septal Q waves and a prominent R wave in the right praecaordial leads are common in the absence of clinical findings. Manning and Cropp (1958) found ECG abnormalities in 20/28 DMD patients, but in all 10 patients with facioscapulohumeral MD the ECG was normal. As with FSHMD, cardiac involvement is unusual in limb girdle muscular dystrophy. The sum of R and S waves may give an indication of abnormality in 80 per cent of DMD patients (Emery 1972). Detailed serial assessment of cardiac function using ECG, echocardiogram and Holter ECG monitoring in DMD has been helpful in establishing the natural history of cardiac disease. Using these measures at six monthly intervals in a cohort of 328 Italian DMD patients, Nigro *et al.* (1990) found evidence of preclinical cardiac involvement in 25 per cent patients under the age of six years. This figure increased to 59 per cent between the ages of six and 10 years. After the age of 10 years the authors described three main clinical types of cardiac abnormality (dilated cardiomyopathy, hypertrophic cardiomyopathy, and conduction defects alone). In all age groups a dilated cardiomyopathy, predominantly affecting the left ventricle was the most frequent finding. Clinically detectable features of cardiomyopathy were first apparent at around the age of 10 years and by 18 years were virtually universal. Two important clinical points are that the decline in cardiac function is not always correlated with the decrease in skeletal muscle function, and many patients do not have typical symptoms of heart failure such as breathlessness on exertion, due to limitations in mobility. It is therefore suggested that regular ECG, echocardiogram assessment ($\pm$ 24 h ECG monitoring) should be considered every 6–12 months in teenage DMD patients.

Cardiac involvement is an important feature of Becker MD and some cases may present with cardiac failure. Cardiomyopathy is also a feature of Emery Dreifuss MD. Here rhythm disturbances may be an early finding with supraventricular dysrhymias progressing to heart block. In patients with severe left ventricular dysfunction, a Cheyne–Stokes pattern of ventilation may be seen during the day and at night. Polysomnography will differentiate this central form of apnoea from obstructive apnoea and hypoventilation syndromes.

In all muscular dystrophy patients with cardiac disease, respiratory insufficiency is likely to reduce myocardial oxygen delivery and exacerbate the situation. Early rhythm disturbances, for example, may be precipitated during episodes of sleep-disordered breathing. It is not clear as yet, whether the provision of ventilatory assistance alters the natural history of cardiac disease in the muscular dystrophies, but early evidence suggest that this may be the case.

Patients with cardiac failure can be treated with diuretic and ACE inhibitor therapy, which should be titrated as in any other patient with heart failure. Good symptom control is usually obtainable. Standard anti arrythmic medication can be used, depending on the arrythmia. Ventilatory support should be considered in any patient with significant sleep-disordered breathing.

Scoliosis and surgical intervention

A thoracolumbar scoliosis is liable to occur in any individual who develops significant respiratory and vertebral muscle weakness before spinal growth is complete. Rideau *et al.* (1983) found that 50 per cent of DMD patients had a severe scoliosis, in 37.5 per cent the scoliosis was moderate and in 12.5 per cent it was mild. Progression usually accompanies the adolescent growth spurt around the age of 10–12 years when the child has just lost ambulation. The aim of surgery in this situation is to stabilize sitting stability and improve comfort. Advances in surgical technique such as the Luque procedure for anchoring vertebrae to metal rods have facilitated early postoperative rehabilitation. A progressive curve with a Cobb angle of 30–40 degrees may be judged as an indication for surgery, but this needs to be balanced against the respiratory reserve of the individual. Some orthopaedic surgeons use a vital capacity of 30 per cent predicted, as a minimum for acceptance for surgery (Leatherman and Dickson 1988), but the use of NIPPV in the preoperative and postoperative phase may allow those with a lower respiratory reserve to undergo surgery safely. Spinal stabilization should not be expected to improve lung volumes, but may slow the loss of vital capacity (Galasko *et al.* 1992).

Respiratory muscle training

Inspiratory muscle training is a controversial issue in neuromuscular disease, as although benefits may potentially accrue, there is also the risk that overtraining weak muscles may lead to fatigue/damage and ultimately, ventilatory failure. Previous studies have shown mixed results possibly due to differences in the training mode and the patient population recruited. It is therefore extremely important to select individuals who are likely to benefit. A controlled study by Wanke *et al.* (1994) has been useful in this respect. Thirty DMD patients took part with half randomized to training and the other half acting as controls. Patients used a resistive training device which produced visual feedback to encourage individuals with their respiratory effort and triggered a videogame reward on completion of the programme. Training consisted of ten loaded breathing cycles at 70 per cent of maximum transdiaphragmatic pressure carried out twice a day at home for six months. The level of resistance was increased in a stepwise manner during the trial as patients became able to sustain higher pressures. Inspiratory muscle strength was assessed serially using maximal sniff oesophageal and transdiaphragmatic pressures. Ten of the fifteen patients were able to increase inspiratory muscle strength and endurance, significantly after one month and improved further at three and six months. After discontinuation of the trial, improvements were maintained for at least six months. There were no changes in inspiratory muscle strength in the control group and both groups showed no change in lung volumes, maximum voluntary ventilation and arterial PaO$_2$ level. Five of the fifteen withdrew after one month when no improvement in inspiratory muscle function was seen. Notably, all these individuals had a vital capacity of less than 25 per cent predicted and were hypercapnic at the start of the trial, indicating that the respiratory muscles were already unable to sustain the normal ventilatory load. One can conclude that either the training intensity in this group was too great, or endstage patients may simply have insufficient functional muscle to take advantage of a training effect. Further, controlled studies are clearly needed, but in the meantime it seems that sensible that patients recruited for studies have a vital capacity in excess of 25 per cent predicted and have not developed ventilatory failure.

Coordinated care

Care for patients with neuromuscular disease in the UK and other European countries tends to be fragmented. It is a particular cause for concern that the transition from paediatric to adult care may be poorly managed. This has potentially disastrous consequences for the Duchenne group as they run into problems with sleep disordered breathing and ventilatory failure at around the time that the transfer to adult care should take place. This issue could be addressed by the development of Adolescent Neuromuscular Clinics (similar to the models of Adolescent Cystic Fibrosis and Congenital Heart disease clinics), with multidisciplinary paediatric/adult neurological, respiratory, cardiological, orthopaedic, physiotherapy and dietetic input. These clinics should also be a valuable resource for the growing number of children with congenital neuromuscular disease who may now be expected to survive to adulthood with more effective treatment of ventilatory insufficiency.

References

Annane, D., Quera-Salva, M.A., Lofaso, F. *et al.* (1999). Mechanisms underlying the effects of nocturnal ventilation on daytime blood gases in neuromuscular diseases. *European Respiratory Journal*, **13**, 157–62.

Bach, J.R. (1993). Mechanical insufflation-exsufflation. Comparison of peak expiratory flows with manually assisted and unassisted coughing techniques. *Chest*, **104**, 1553–62.

Bach, J.R. Campagnolo, D.I., and Hoeman, S. (1991). Life satisfaction of individuals with Duchenne muscular dystrophy using long-term mechanical ventilatory support. *American Journal of Physical and Medical Rehabilitation*, **70**, 129–35.

Barach, A.L. and Beck, G.J. (1954). Exsufflation with negative pressure: physiologic and clinical studies in poliomyelitis, bronchial asthma, pulmonary emphysema and bronchiectsis. *Archives of Internal Medicine*, **93**, 825–41.

Barbe, F., Quera-Salva, M.A., McCann, C. *et al.* (1994). Sleep-related respiratory disturbances in patients with Duchenne muscular dystrophy. *European Respiratory Journal*, **7**, 1403–8.

Barois, A. and Estournet-Mathiaud, B. (1993). Nasal ventilation in congenital myopathies and spinal muscular atrophies. *European Respiratory Journal*, **3**, 275–8.

Baydur, A. Gilgoff, I., Prentice, W., Carlson, M., and Fischer DA. (1990). Decline in respiratory function and experience with long term assisted ventilation in advanced Duchenne's muscular dystrophy. *Chest*, **97**, 884–9.

Berthon-Jones, M. and Sullivan, C.E. (1987). Time course of change in ventilatory response to CO_2 with long-term CPAP therapy for obstructive sleep apnea. *American Review Respiratory Disease*, **135**, 144–7.

Brooke, M.H., Fenichel, G.M., Griggs, R.C., *et al.* (1989). Duchenne muscular dystrophy: Patterns of clinical progression and effects of supportive therapy. *Neurology*, **39**, 475–81.

Consensus Conference. (1999). Clinical Indications for Noninvasive Positive Pressure Ventilation in Chronic Respiratory Failure due to Restrictive Lung Disease, COPD, and nocturnal hypoventilation – a Consensus conference report. *Chest*, **116**, 521–34.

Cooper, K.R. and Philips, B.A. (1982). Effect of short term sleep loss on breathing. *Journal of Applied Physiology*, **53**, 855–8.

Emery, A.E.H. (1972). Abnormalities of the electrocardiogram in hereditary mypathies. *Journal of Medical Genetics*, **9**, 8–12.

Fauroux, B., Sardet, A., and Foret, D. (1995). Home treatment for chronic respiratory failure in children: a prospective study. *European Respiratory Journal*, **8**: 2062–6.

Galasko, G.S., Delaney, C., and Morris, P. (1992). Spinal stabilisation in Duchenne muscular dystrophy. *Journal of Bone and Joint Surgery*, **74**, 210–4.

Gigliotti, F., Pizzi, A., Duranti, R., Gorini, M., Iandelli, I., and Scano, G. (1995). Control of breathing in patients with limb girdle dystrophy: a controlled study. *Thorax*, **50**, 962–8.

Hukins, C.A. and Hillman, D.R. (2000). Daytime predictors of sleep hypoventilation in Duchenne muscular dystrophy. *American journal of Respiratory and Critical Care Medicine*, **161**, 166–70.

Khan, Y. and Heckmatt, J.Z. (1994). Obstructive apnoeas in Duchenne muscular dystrophy. *Thorax*, **49**, 157–61.

Leatherman, K.D. and Dickson, R.A. (1988). Neuromuscular deformities. In *The Management of Spinal Deformities*, (ed. K.D. Leatherman and R.A. Dickson) pp. 211–34. 1st ed. London, Wright.

Leger, P., Bedicam, J.M., Cornette, A., *et al.* (1994). Nasal intermittent positive pressure ventilation. Long term follow-up in patients with severe chronic respiratory insufficiency. *Chest*, **105**, 100–5.

Manning, G.W. and Cropp, G.J. (1958). The electrocardiogram in progressive muscular dystrophy. *British Heart Journal*, **20**, 416–20.

Nigro, G., Coni, L.I., Politano, L., and Bain, R.J.I. (1990). The incidence and evolution of cardiomyopthy in Duchenne muscular dystrophy. *International Journal of Cardiology*, **26**, 271–7.

Phillips, M.F., Smith, P.E., Carroll, N., Edwards, R.H., and Calverley, P.M. (1999). Nocturnal oxygenation and prognosis in Duchenne muscular dystrophy. *American journal of Respiratory and Critical Care Medicine*, **160**, 198–202.

Raphael, J-C., Chevret, S., Chastang, C., and Bouvet, F. (1994). Randomised trial of preventive nasal ventilation in Duchenne muscular dystrophy. *Lancet*, **343**, 1600–4.

Rideau, Y., Gatin, G., Bach, J., and Gines, G. (1983). Prolongation of life in Duchenne's muscular dystrophy. *Acta Neurologica*, **5**, 118–24.

Rideau, Y., Janoski, L.W., and Grellet, G. (1981). Respiratory function in the muscular dystrophies. *Muscle and Nerve*, **4**, 155–64.

Simonds, A.K., Muntoni, F., Heather, S., and Fielding, S. (1998). Impact of nasal ventilation on survival in hypercapnic Duchenne muscular dystrophy. *Thorax*, **53**, 949–52.

Simonds, A.K. (1996). Non-invasive ventilation in progressive neuromuscular disease and patients with multiple handicaps. In *Non-invasive respiratory support*, (ed. A.K. Simonds) 1st ed. pp. 96–101. London, Chapman & Hall Medical.

Simonds, A.K. (2000). Nasal ventilation in progressive neuromuscular disease: experience in adults and adolescents. *Monaldi Archives Chest Disease*, **55**, 237–41.

Simonds, A.K., Ward, S., Heather, S., Bush, A.B., and Muntoni, F. (2000). Outcome of paediatric domiciliary mask ventilation in neuromuscular and skeletal disease. *European Respiratory Journal*, **16**, 476–81.

Thomson, A. (1997). The role of negative pressure ventilation. *Archives of Disease in Childhood*, **77**, 454–8.

Vianello, A., Bevilacqua, M., Salvador, V., Cardaioli, C., and Vincenti, E. (1994). Long-term nasal intermittent positive pressure ventilation in advanced Duchenne's Muscular Dystrophy. *Chest*, **105**, 445–8.

Wanke, T., Toifl, K., Merkle, M., Formanek, D., Lahrmann, H., Zwick, H. (1994). Inspiratory muscle training in patients with Duchenne muscular dystrophy. *Chest*, **105**, 475–82.

Chapter 14

Gene and cell therapy for primary myopathies

Giulio Cossu and Paula R. Clemens

Introduction

During the last 15 years, following the identification of dystrophin as the gene responsible for Duchenne Muscular Dystrophy (Hoffmann *et al.* 1987), the genes responsible for the large majority of primary myopathies have been identified. Most of these genes encode for proteins that form a supra-molecular link between the cytoskeleton and the extra-cellular matrix (Nawrotzki *et al.* 1996). In the absence of one of these proteins, the mechanical stress associated with contraction progressively leads to degeneration of the muscle fibre, though the molecular mechanism is not yet understood in detail. Death of the muscle fibres is followed by an inflammatory reaction, mainly composed of monocytes and lymphocytes (Arahata and Engel 1984), that results in a reactive sclerosis and reduced local micro-vasculature. In the first phase of the disease, new muscle fibres are formed by fusion of satellite cells, myogenic precursors that reside beneath the basal lamina (Seale and Rudnicki 2000) and possibly by blood-born progenitors (see below). In both cases the newly formed fibres share the molecular defect of the fibres they replace and consequently they also undergo degeneration. Once the proliferation potential of myogenic cells is exhausted, there is no further regeneration and the skeletal muscle is replaced by connective tissue.

Current therapeutic approaches involve pharmacological suppression of the inflammatory and the immune response and have met with modest beneficial effects (Urtizberea 2000). Future approaches foresee different strategies such as pharmacological up-regulation of utrophin synthesis, a cognate protein that compensates for dystrophin absence when over-expressed in dystrophic mice (Deconinck *et al.* 1997). Much hope is directed towards design of more efficient and less antigenic vectors and to optimization of myoblast transplantation. This chapter will deal with past and current attempts at gene and cell transfer for primary myopathies.

Gene and cell therapy: basic concepts

Gene therapy entails the delivery of genes to somatic cells using vectors derived from viruses (viral vectors) or constructed using non-viral elements (non-viral vectors).

The rationale for using gene transfer strategies to treat inherited disorders is most easily understood in recessive conditions in which a critical protein is missing due to a mutation in a single gene. A vector is used as a vehicle to transport a normal copy of the mutant gene to the nucleus of cells, either targeting the desired cell type by some mechanism or limiting expression to the desired cell type by appropriate selection of gene promoter.

Gene transfer can be accomplished both in cells *in vitro* and in tissues *in vivo*. The *in vitro* application involves culturing cells in a dish, transducing them with the vector of choice that delivers a gene encoding a new protein to be expressed. The engineered cells are then available for cell therapy (see below). Gene transfer can also be approached *in vivo*. The gene vector is introduced to an intact organism by injection into a blood vessel or directly into a target tissue, such as muscle, liver or brain. The recessively inherited muscular dystrophies, DMD and the limb-girdle muscular dystrophies due to sarcoglycan deficiency, are excellent models with which to test muscle gene therapy since each is due to a mutation in a single gene and results in primary deficiency of a single protein. In each of these muscular dystrophies, the other muscle proteins that are lost on a secondary basis are restored by provision of a gene coding for the primary deficiency.

Cell therapy is a procedure where the active therapeutic agent is represented by cells and not by molecules. Blood transfusion is the oldest and still most common form of cell therapy: erythrocytes from a compatible donor are transferred to a recipient patient who has a reduced content of these cells. Since the cells are derived from another individual of the same species the donor cells are considered heterologous and the transplant is defined as allogenic. In rare cases, not considered here, cells may derive from another species and the transplant is thus called xenogenic.

Donor cells derived from the same patient are considered autologous. The best example of this form of cell therapy is auto-transplantation of keratinocytes in patients suffering from major burns. Cells are isolated from a skin biopsy, expanded *in vitro* and then re-implanted on the dermis of the same patient. Auto-transplantation of keratinocytes differs from blood transfusion also because cells are extensively manipulated *in vitro* before being re-introduced in the patient.

If cells are also genetically manipulated during their *in vitro* expansion (e.g. to introduce a normal copy of the mutated gene though a viral vector), the procedure represents a form of *in vitro* or *ex-vivo* gene therapy (see above). In the case of primary myopathies, cell therapy offers two main options: transplantation of normal cells from a compatible donor or auto-transplantation of the patient cells, after gene replacement *in vitro*.

Novel, pre-clinical approaches of cell and gene therapy are strictly dependent upon availability of animal models that allow testing of efficacy and toxicity. Most of these studies have been carried out on the *mdx* mouse that, like patients with DMD, has a dystrophin gene mutation that results in the production of an unstable, truncated dystrophin protein. There is also a large animal model for DMD, the Golden Retriever

Muscular Dystrophy (GRMD) dog (Valentine *et al.* 1992), that will become invaluable for pre-clinical studies because of the large size and of the clinically severe phenotype. Naturally-occurring and knock-out rodent models are also available for the four sarco-glycan genes *(α, β, γ, δ)* (Allamand *et al.* 2000; Araishi *et al.* 1999; Coral-Vazquez *et al.* 1999; Duclos *et al.* 1998; Hack *et al.* 1998; Liu and Engvall 1999). A detailed description of all animal models can be found in Chapter 16.

Viral vectors

Viral vectors exploit the natural biology of viruses in which the viral DNA is delivered to the nucleus of an infected cell. Viruses are genetically modified to generate vectors for gene therapy. These modifications are designed to reduce viral pathogenicity and to encode the desired therapeutic gene. Skeletal and cardiac muscles are two tissues primarily affected in the muscular dystrophies and both tissues are composed of post-mitotic, non-dividing cells. This has focused the choice of viral vectors for *in vivo* muscle gene transfer to adenovirus (Ad), adeno-associated virus (AAV) and herpes simplex virus (HSV). Although retroviral vectors based on the Moloney murine leukemia virus require actively dividing cells for effective gene transfer, they have potential for myoblast transduction *ex vivo* with subsequent delivery of engineered cells into muscle tissue. Lentiviral vectors, engineered from HIV-1, have been studied more recently for their potential for gene delivery to both dividing and non-dividing cells (Table 14.1).

Table 14.1 Viral vectors for muscle gene therapy

Vector	Particle diameter (nm)	Genome size (kb)	Genome type	Insert capacity (kb)
Adenoviral (replication-defective)	100	36	ds-DNA	8
Adenoviral (high-capacity)	100	36	ds-DNA	30
Adeno-associated	20	4.7	ss-DNA	4.7
Herpes simplex (replication-defective)	200	152	ds-DNA	44
Herpes simplex (amplicon)	200	152	ds-DNA	Concatamers of transgene expression cassette to generate total of 150 kb
Retroviral	100	8	ss-RNA	8
Lentiviral	100	9.4	ss-RNA	8

Abbreviations: nm: nanometer, kb: kilobase, ds: double-stranded, ss: single-stranded

Adenoviral vectors

Several of the over 40 serotypes of human Ad have been extensively studied over the past several decades. The extensive knowledge of Ad life cycle that was derived from these studies resulted in genetic manipulation of Ad to generate non-lytic Ad vectors. Some of the advantages of Ad vectors include relative ease of manipulation in the laboratory, the ability to attain high viral titers, the stability of recombinant Ad vectors in mammalian cells and the ability to transduce non-dividing cells (Berkner 1988). The 36 kb linear, double-stranded Ad DNA is packaged in a 100 nm diameter capsid. In first-generation Ad vectors, the early region 1 (E1) gene was deleted to generate a replication-defective vector and to create space for an inserted gene coding for a marker or therapeutic protein. A cell line that complements the E1 gene deletion allows propagation of the viral vector in cultured cells. Graham and colleagues pioneered the development of simple methods to generate recombinant Ad vectors (Bett *et al.* 1994; McGrory *et al.* 1988). These first-generation Ad vectors can accommodate up to approximately 8 kb of insert DNA (Bett *et al.* 1994).

Delivery of a reporter gene to skeletal muscle using first-generation Ad vectors was accomplished both in cultured cells and in intact animals (Quantin *et al.* 1992; Stratford-Perricaudet *et al.* 1992). Ad vectors encoding internally deleted dystrophin cDNAs were generated and tested by direct intra-muscular injection of *mdx* mice. The ability to deliver dystrophin to neonatal skeletal muscle *in vivo* (Ragot *et al.* 1993) permitted the demonstration of protection against dystrophic change in transduced muscle fibres (Vincent *et al.* 1993).

However, it was soon recognized that there were limitations to the use of first-generation Ad vectors for gene transfer in general and gene transfer to muscle specifically. Important general limitations to the use of first-generation Ad vectors are the cellular and humoral immune responses induced in the gene transfer recipient. In the setting of Ad vector-mediated gene transfer, a cellular immune response could be directed at any of a number of antigens, including viral, marker and therapeutic proteins. The deletion of Ad E1 sequences from first-generation Ad vectors was shown to be insufficient to completely eliminate the expression of other early and late viral genes or to prevent replication of viral DNA. Cytotoxic T lymphocyte (CTL) assays *in vitro* showed that the viral proteins produced from first-generation Ad vectors induced a T cell-mediated immune response. This was first studied in liver gene transfer models in which the T cell-mediated immune response resulted in the elimination of vector transduced liver cells (Yang *et al.* 1994; 1995a,b). A similar phenomenon was observed in Ad vector-mediated muscle gene transfer (Yang *et al.* 1996). In one study of muscle gene transfer, an intra-muscular injection of a first-generation Ad vector encoding the canine factor IX cDNA under muscle-specific control resulted in late viral gene expression from the vector and a subsequent cellular immune response to viral antigens (Dai *et al.* 1995). Furthermore, a humoral immune response to both canine factor IX and viral proteins was observed. Neutralizing antibody responses to Ad proteins preclude effective re-administration of an Ad vector of the same serotype.

A second limitation to the use of first-generation Ad vectors was the insert capacity limit of 8 kb. Although this is sufficient to encode many therapeutic genes, the 14 kb dystrophin cDNA could not be accommodated. Use of first-generation Ad vectors for DMD gene transfer was, therefore, limited to truncated, internally-deleted dystrophin cDNAs. Transgenic studies have demonstrated therapeutic benefit to these shortened dystrophin genes, but not to the same degree as full-length dystrophin (Phelps *et al.* 1995).

High-capacity Ad vectors provide the potential to circumvent barriers of immunity and insert size limitation (Kochanek 1999). The development of high-capacity Ad vector technology arose from the observation that the only viral elements required for proper packaging of the Ad that could not be provided by trans-complementation were the inverted terminal repeats (ITR) and the packaging signal. Therefore, the entire Ad vector genome could be 'gutted' (hence the alternative name, 'gutted Ad vector') removing all viral genes and providing 30 kb of insert cloning capacity. Unlike first-generation Ad vectors, high-capacity Ad vectors cannot express immunogenic late viral proteins since they do not encode any viral genes. To rescue and propagate high-capacity Ad vectors, the packaging cell line is co-transduced with (1) the vector DNA cloned into a single plasmid and (2) a 'helper' first-generation vector (Kochanek *et al.* 1996; Kumar-Singh and Chamberlain 1996). Novel approaches to favour packaging of vector over packaging of helper virus have been developed. The presence of 'helper' virus in the final vector preparation is limited to less than 0.1 per cent, which significantly limits the immunogenicity of the vector (Parks *et al.* 1996). Cytotoxicity of high-capacity Ad vectors also has been shown to be less in liver gene transfer studies (Scheidner *et al.* 1998).

Some of the first applications of high-capacity Ad vector technology were applied to DMD studies. The high-capacity Ad vector provided the opportunity to transduce skeletal muscle fibres with the full-length dystrophin gene with relatively high efficiency. By delivering the vector through an intra-muscular injection to neonatal *mdx* hindlimb muscle, significant protection of muscle fibres from the damage of the dystrophic process could be demonstrated (Fig. 14.1). Furthermore, as predicted from transgenic studies, gene delivery of dystrophin to *mdx* muscle restored the full dystrophin-glycoprotein complex at the muscle cell membrane indicating the functional potential of recombinant dystrophin provided to post-mitotic somatic cells (Clemens *et al.* 1996).

However, as with first-generation Ad vector gene delivery to muscle, gene-delivered protein expression provided by high-capacity Ad vectors is lost over time. This loss of expression is more rapid in animals treated as adults as compared to those treated as neonates, suggesting involvement of the immune system. Many studies have explored the antigen specificity of induced immunity to Ad vector gene transfer. Foreign transgene proteins, such as β-galactosidase, are profoundly immunogenic when delivered by an Ad vector (Chen *et al.* 1997). Evidence regarding the immunity of therapeutic

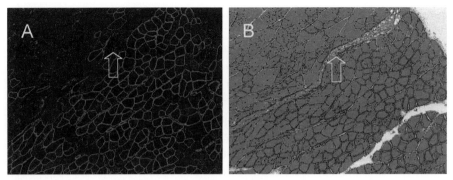

Fig. 14.1 High-capacity adenoviral vector-mediated dystrophin gene transfer to neonatal *mdx* muscle prevents the histopathological changes associated with muscular dystrophy. Serial sections of muscle collected 40 weeks following an intramuscular injection of a high-capacity adenoviral vector encoding the full-length murine dystrophin cDNA controlled by the murine muscle creatine kinase promoter were immunostained for dystrophin (A) and stained with hematoxylin and eosin (B). Preservation of normal muscle fibre architecture correlates with dystrophin expression in the lower right-hand aspect of the section below a connective tissue band (arrow). Dystrophic pathology, observed in the upper left-hand aspect of the section, correlates with a region that does not express recombinant dystrophin.

proteins that may be recognized as non-self in null mutant recipients such as muscular dystrophy patients or animal models is only now emerging (Braun *et al.* 2000; Ferrer *et al.* 2000; Ohtsuka *et al.* 1998). The presence of "revertant" fibres or homologous proteins such as utrophin may blunt the immunity induced by dystrophin. Revertant fibres represent a very small percentage of muscle fibres in DMD patients and *mdx* mice that express a truncated dystrophin, often due to a second somatic dystrophin gene mutation that reverts the DNA sequence to the proper reading frame for protein translation (Hoffman *et al.* 1990). The immunity due to Ad antigens in response to high-capacity Ad vector gene delivery is largely limited to input capsids. The neutralizing antibody response to Ad prevents effective vector re-administration (Dai *et al.* 1995; Yang *et al.* 1995b).

When immune barriers are eliminated, it is observed that Ad vector DNA resides in muscle nuclei without loss of vector genomes or integrity (Chen *et al.* 1999). Therefore, it appears that the primary barrier to long-term gene expression or vector re-administration is immune-mediated. To be therapeutically effective it may be that some form of immune suppression will be required in conjunction with Ad vector-mediated muscle gene delivery.

A third limitation to the use of Ad vectors for muscle gene transfer is that the efficiency of gene transfer decreases with the maturation of muscle fibres. This phenomenon was demonstrated both *in vitro* (Acsadi *et al.* 1994a) and *in vivo* (Acsadi *et al.* 1994b). Classical adenoviral attachment (Coxsackie-Adenovirus Receptor) and internalization receptors ($\alpha_v\beta_3$ and $\alpha_v\beta_5$ integrins) are down-regulated with muscle maturation

(Acsadi *et al.* 1994a,b). Furthermore, development of the basal lamina with muscle maturation may present a physical barrier to Ad vector-mediated gene delivery (Feero *et al.* 1997).

One strategy to increase the efficiency of gene delivery to muscle is to intentionally modify the means of vector attachment to its target cell. Muscle-specific vector tropism has the potential to facilitate both an increase in gene uptake by muscle cells and a decrease in gene uptake by non-target cells. Ultimately, this could provide a vector suitable for systemic gene delivery, which will likely be required to reach a clinically significant fraction of skeletal muscle. Recent research demonstrates the potential to genetically modify the Ad fibre protein that mediates vector attachment to the target cell or to use antibody conjugates to re-direct vector attachment (Douglas *et al.* 1996; Krasnykh *et al.* 1996; 2000; Wickham *et al.* 1996a,b). Such strategies have been demonstrated in several systems, although not yet using muscle-specific ligands. Proof-of-principle experiments in muscle demonstrate that the transduction of muscle cells *in vitro* and *in vivo* can be enhanced by targeting heparan sulphate that is abundantly present on multiple cell types including skeletal muscle (Bouri *et al.* 1999). For muscle gene transfer, the challenge will be to identify target moieties that are abundant and specific.

Adeno-associated viral vectors

AAV vectors are derived from a non-pathogenic parvovirus that has a single-stranded DNA genome. AAV are thought to be naturally defective because of their requirement for co-infection with a helper virus such as Ad or HSV for a productive infection. Furthermore, AAV is not associated with any known disease and induces very little immune reaction when used as a vector (Grimm and Kleinschmidt 1999). Surprisingly, especially when compared with parallel observations using Ad vectors, even foreign proteins such as β-galactosidase do not induce significant immunity when delivered by an AAV vector to skeletal muscle. Long-term gene expression following gene transfer into skeletal muscle is achieved using AAV (Fisher *et al.* 1997; Xiao *et al.* 1996).

For muscle disease application, AAV vector-mediated muscle gene delivery was initially tested in rodent models for limb-girdle muscular dystrophy (LGMD). Four of the autosomal recessive forms of LGMD are due to primary deficiencies of the four sarcoglycan proteins, α, β, γ and δ. The cDNAs encoding these proteins are each approximately 1 kb in length and therefore, could be accommodated by the limited cloning capacity of AAV vectors. Direct intramuscular injection of an AAV vector encoding δ-sarcoglycan into tibialis anterior muscle of the δ-sarcoglycan deficient BIO14.6 hamster resulted in a high level of gene transfer and functional correction as demonstrated by muscle weight, histology and *in vitro* force measurements (Xiao *et al.* 2000). Furthermore, other experiments demonstrate the potential of regional delivery through the vasculature of the BIO14.6 hamster hind limb of AAV encoding the δ-sarcoglycan cDNA (Greelish *et al.* 1999). The rapid successes in these early studies applying AAV vector gene delivery to dystrophic skeletal muscle has resulted in the initiation of the first muscle gene transfer human clinical trial toward the ultimate gene transfer treatment of an inherited muscle disorder. This initial trial is designed to explore the safety of direct intra-muscular injection of an AAV vector encoding a sarcoglycan gene in a small muscle of several sarcoglycan-deficient LGMD patients (Stedman *et al.* 2000).

The application of AAV vectors to muscle gene transfer for DMD patients is significantly limited by the small cloning capacity of these vectors. The maximum length of DNA that can be accommodated by AAV is approximately 5 kb. Experiments are underway to test highly truncated, internally deleted dystrophin cDNAs (Wang B. *et al.* 2000) and strategies of delivering the desired gene in segments for subsequent splicing within the target cell (Sun *et al.* 2000; Yan *et al.* 2000). Although the small cloning capacity of AAV is a limitation, the resulting small size of the vector may be an important part of the reason why this vector transduces mature skeletal muscle efficiently (Pruchnic *et al.* 2000).

Herpes simplex vectors

HSV, a human pathogen that causes the common cold sore and infections of the conjunctiva, is a double-stranded DNA virus with a capsid and a surrounding tegument and envelope. HSV has a 152 kb genome and HSV vectors can potentially accommodate up to approximately 44 kb of DNA insert (Glorioso 2000). Both full-length and truncated forms of the dystrophin cDNA are easily accommodated into HSV vectors (Akkaraju *et al.* 1999). HSV has undergone numerous manipulations to generate HSV replication-defective vectors designed for gene delivery. One strategy has been to delete essential immediate early genes, a process that renders the vector replication-incompetent. The first replication-incompetent HSV vector was generated by removing the ICP (infected cell polypeptide) 4 gene (DeLuca *et al.* 1985). Analogous to Ad vectors, growth of replication-incompetent HSV vectors in cultured cells is accomplished using cell lines that complement any gene product that is removed from the vector genome (Glorioso 2000). Further immediate early gene deletions have been made in the HSV vector resulting in non-toxic vectors (Hobbs and DeLuca 1999). Like Ad, the HSV vector genome remains as an episome in the nucleus of the transduced cell. A unique aspect of HSV vectors, which are neurotrophic, is that HSV can establish latency in neurons. Therefore, the majority of gene transfer applications of HSV vectors have been directed toward the nervous system.

The application of replication-deficient HSV for muscle gene transfer met with some early success. In cultured cells, HSV vectors transduced both myoblasts, muscle precursor cells, and myotubes, syncytia of fused myoblasts generated by exposing myoblasts in culture to media conditions that promote differentiation (Huard *et al.* 1995). Unfortunately, after an intra-muscular injection *in vivo*, HSV vector transduction resulted in significant toxicity as well as vector-induced immunity (Huard *et al.* 1997). Furthermore, a significant proportion of the HSV vector that was injected directly into skeletal muscle, remained in the extra-cellular space. The simplest explanation for this is that HSV is excluded at the level of the muscle fibre basal lamina due to its large size (Huard *et al.* 1996).

Another application of HSV vector technology is the development of HSV amplicon vectors. HSV amplicon vectors lack all viral genes. The proteins necessary for replication and packaging to produce the vector *in vitro* are provided by cloned helper DNA (in overlapping cosmid clones or as a bacterial artificial chromosome) comprising replication-competent, packaging-defective HSV-1 genomes (Sena-Esteves *et al.* 2000). These vectors could potentially accommodate 150 kb of insert DNA; the largest insert packaged to date in an HSV amplicon vector is 51 kb (Wang X. *et al.* 2000). Amplicon HSV vectors have been used for gene transfer of muscle cells in culture (Wang Y. *et al.* 2000).

Retroviral vectors

Retroviral vectors are engineered from murine retroviruses, enveloped single-stranded RNA viruses. The most commonly employed retroviral vectors are derived from the Moloney murine leukemia virus. Retroviral vectors are rendered replication-defective due to deletion of the three viral genes, *gag*, *pol*, and *env*, encoding structural, enzymatic and envelope proteins of the retrovirus. These proteins are supplied *in trans* by the packaging cell line (Cornetta *et al.* 1991). Over the last 10 years there have been multiple enhancements in retroviral vector design to improve safety, expand tropism and increase transgene expression (Daly and Chernajovsky 2000). For efficient gene transduction, retroviral vectors require actively dividing cells. This restriction limits their use for *in vivo* muscle applications because muscle fibres are post-mitotic and therefore, not susceptible to retroviral infection. However, a potential advantage of retroviral vectors is their ability to integrate into the host cell genome providing stability of transgene expression. Ideally, transduction of myogenic precursor cells *in vivo* would provide a stable reservoir of therapeutic transgene as muscle undergoes regeneration.

Experimentation directed toward the use of muscle gene transfer has made use of the *mdx* mouse as a therapeutic target. Since retroviral vectors have an insert capacity limited to approximately 8 kb, a vector encoding an internally-deleted dystrophin cDNA was generated and used to deliver dystrophin to proliferating myoblasts, *in vitro* (Dunckley *et al.* 1992). Direct injection of this vector into skeletal muscle resulted in a low percentage of myofibres expressing a truncated dystrophin protein, indicating that direct retroviral gene transfer to myoblasts in regenerating muscle was feasible but not an efficient strategy to transduce post-mitotic muscle (Dunckley *et al.* 1993).

Further work with the use of retroviral vectors for muscle gene transfer demonstrated that both murine and human primary myogenic cells could be infected with a retroviral vector *in vitro*, followed by intra-muscular injection of transduced cells resulting in transgene-expressing muscle fibres (Salvatori *et al.* 1993). Inclusion of muscle-specific promoters provides the potentially desirable effect of limiting vector transgene expression to muscle cells (Ferrari *et al.* 1995; Naffakh *et al.* 1996). Another strategy is to directly inject retroviral producer cell lines in skeletal muscle with the goal of infection of myogenic precursor cells *in vivo* (Fassati *et al.* 1996; 1997). Advances in retroviral vector technology, currently applied to tissues other than muscle, may benefit muscle gene transfer in the future as the understanding of myogenic precursor cells increases.

Lentiviral vectors

The newest development in vector development from the *Retroviridae* family are lentiviral vectors, derived from HIV-1. Like retroviral vectors based on the Moloney murine leukemia virus, lentiviral vectors integrate into the host cell genome providing permanent gene transfer for a transduced cell and all of its progeny. However, lentiviral vectors infect non-dividing, as well as dividing, cells (Daly and Chernajovsky 2000). This feature enhances their attractiveness for muscle gene transfer applications. The potential of successful muscle gene transfer using lentiviral vectors has been demonstrated (Kafri *et al.* 1997). Over the last several years, significant effort has been directed toward increasing the safety of lentiviral vectors and maximizing vector titers and levels of transgene expression (Daly and Chernajovsky 2000; Dull *et al.* 1998; Kafri *et al.* 1999; Miyoshi *et al.* 1998; Naldini *et al.* 1996a,b; Zufferey *et al.* 1998).

Non-viral vectors

In 1990, Wolff and colleagues first demonstrated direct gene transfer of naked plasmid DNA or RNA resulting in transgene expression in skeletal muscle fibres (Wolff *et al.* 1990). This fundamental observation suggested the possibility of a simple gene transfer strategy for muscle that could facilitate (1) the use of muscle as a gene depot for the production of secreted proteins, and (2) gene delivery for primary muscle disorders. The mechanism of uptake of naked DNA by skeletal muscle is not entirely clear, but several hypotheses have emerged (Budker *et al.* 2000; Dowty *et al.* 1995; Hagstrom *et al.* 1996; Wolff *et al.* 1992). The feasibility of dystrophin gene transfer using direct intramuscular DNA injection was demonstrated (Acsadi *et al.* 1991). Direct DNA gene transfer can be modulated by manipulating injection conditions (Davis *et al.* 1993; Wolff *et al.* 1991). Furthermore, recent advances in naked DNA gene transfer efficiency are encouraging for the potential application to the treatment of a primary muscle disorder (Budker *et al.* 2000). In addition, the use of adjuncts to plasmid DNA demonstrate additional potential to improve the gene transfer efficiency of DNA (Lemieux *et al.* 2000; Liang *et al.* 2000; Vitiello *et al.* 1996).

Gene correction of point mutations

For diseases caused by point mutations, an alternative to gene replacement is to change the mutant nucleotide to the correct one *in vivo*. A recently described strategy employs chimeric RNA/DNA oligonucleotides, called chimeraplasts, to target and change single nucleotides in genomic DNA of somatic cells of intact animals (Cole-Strauss *et al.* 1996). This strategy uses genetic mismatch repair mechanisms within the cell to accomplish the desired base change. The potential feasibility of this approach to treat muscular dystrophy patients was demonstrated in both the *mdx* mouse and the GRMD dog (Bartlett *et al.* 2000; Rando *et al.* 2000). Both of these DMD animal models are appropriate for these studies as the mutation resulting in absence of dystrophin protein is a point mutation. The successful implementation of this strategy will depend on the development of mechanisms for widespread muscle gene delivery and high levels of gene correction.

Myoblast transplantation from compatible donors

In 1989 Partridge and colleagues showed that intra-muscular injection of C2 cells, an immortal myogenic cell line derived from adult satellite cells, would reconstitute with high efficiency dystrophin positive, apparently normal fibres in dystrophic *mdx* mice. Several clinical trials followed in the next two years: myogenic cells were isolated from immune compatible donors, expanded *in vitro* and injected in a specific muscle of the patient. These clinical trials failed (for a review see Partridge 1996), even though they did not cause any adverse effects with disillusion following prematurely raised hopes. Failure was due to a number of reasons, some of which may have been predicted (C2 have unlimited lifespan and are singeneic with mdx mice) while others became apparent long after the start of the trials. It was later shown that most injected cells (up to 99 per cent) succumb first to an inflammatory response and then to an immune reaction (Beauchamps *et al.* 1997). This latter is directed against donor cell antigens but also against the therapeutic gene (which is often a new antigen for the patient) and, as discussed above, against the viral vector antigens (Yang *et al.* 1996). Furthermore the few surviving cells do not migrate more than few mm away from the injection site, indicating that numberless injection sites would be needed to provide a homogeneous distribution of donor cells.

   Through the years, the work of several laboratories has focused on these problems and in a stepwise manner has produced progressive increase in the survival success of injected myoblasts and in their colonization efficiency. Immune-suppression and injection of neutralizing antibodies, pretreatment of myoblasts *in vitro* with growth factors and modification of the muscle connective tissue (Kinoshita *et al.* 1994; Guerette *et al.* 1997) all contributed to this improvement. Recent extension of this protocol to primates (Kinoshita *et al.* 1996) opens up the possibility of a new clinical trial in the not too distant future and with much more information available than in the trials which failed 10 years ago.

Ex vivo therapy with autologous, engineered myoblasts

The *ex vivo* approach to gene therapy of primary myopathies was designed to overcome at least some of the immunological problems linked to myoblast transplantation. In this case cells of the patients are isolated from a muscle biopsy, expanded *in vitro*, transduced with an appropriate vector encoding the therapeutic gene and finally re-injected into one or (hopefully) more muscles of the patient from which they had been initially isolated (Blau and Springer 1997). In this case, however, two additional problems occur: (a) the difficulty of producing an appropriate integrating vector that would accommodate the very large cDNA of dystrophin (this is not a problem for other myopathies such as sarcoglycanopathies where the gene is relatively small); (b) the limited lifespan of myogenic cells isolated from myopathic patients. The proliferation potential of human myogenic precursors declines considerably during early post-natal growth (Webster and Blau 1990), in parallel with the progressive reduction in telomere length which occurs in the first two decades of life (Decary et al. 1997). Given the extra number of cell divisions that myogenic cells from DMD patients must undergo in vivo during the various cycles of fibre degeneration and regeneration, their replication capacity is already dramatically decreased during childhood, and continues to fall during the first decade of life. These cells are recovered in low number from muscle biopsies, grow poorly in vitro, and rapidly undergo senescence, even though they can be transduced by retroviral vectors with an efficiency comparable to that of normal cells (Huard et al. 1994; Salvatori et al. 1993). This problem makes it very difficult to obtain reasonable numbers of genetically modified cells ex vivo, and consequently lowered the expectation that such type of experimental strategy might become practical.

Attempts to solve this problem have focused on two main strategies: first, immortalization of myogenic cells and, second, recruitment of multipotent mesodermal cells. Immortalization of mammalian cells by oncogenes has been successfully obtained for decades (Bryan and Reddel 1994) and in the case of molecules such as the large T antigen of SV40 or polyoma virus, immortalization is not incompatible with a certain degree of differentiation (Mouly et al. 1996; Salvatori et al. 1997; Simon et al. 1996). Nevertheless the persistence of an active oncogene inside the genome of immortalized cells, has so far precluded any clinical application of this protocol. As an alternative, several laboratories have devised strategies, such as expressing active telomerase (Wright and Shay 1995) or inhibiting the expression of anti-oncogenes such as p53 (Gao et al. 1996) or producing a retroviral vector expressing the wild type SV40 T antigen excisable by the cre recombinase (Berghella et al. 1999). All these strategies have produced promising results but seem still quite far away from clinical application.

As an alternative strategy, two groups reported that expression of MyoD (a myogenic determination gene) from an adenoviral vector caused myogenic differentiation in non-muscle, autologous cells such as skin fibroblasts that are compromised in primary myopathies. These data (Lattanzi et al. 1998) support the feasibility of an alternative approach to gene therapy for primary myopathies, based on implantation of large numbers of genetically-modified primary fibroblasts converted to myoblasts by adenoviral delivery of MyoD ex vivo.

However, even after the possible solution of the problems related to the source and quantity of myogenic cells, future clinical protocols await the solution of the problems related to delivery and survival of donor cells.

Blood born myogenic progenitors

Myogenic conversion, i.e. spontaneous activation of myogenesis in various cells when co-cultured with muscle cells or injected into regenerating muscle *in vivo* has been reported by several groups (Breton *et al.* 1995; Gibson *et al.* 1995; Salvatori *et al.* 1995). This occurs rarely under normal conditions, although it has been observed in cells derived from many tissues, such as the CNS, the dermis or the bone marrow (reviewed in Cossu 1997). These studies were carried out using a transgenic mouse line in which a *lacZ* gene encoding a nuclearly-targeted β-galactosidase is expressed under the control of muscle-specific regulatory elements (MLC3F-n*lacZ*). In these animals, the *lacZ* reporter is expressed only in striated muscle (Kelly *et al.* 1995), thus representing a cell-autonomous, heritable and sensitive marker of myogenic differentiation, both *in vitro* and *in vivo*. When cells from MLC3F-n*lacZ* mice are injected into regenerating muscle of immune-deficient mice, myogenic conversion is evidenced by the formation of muscle fibres with β-gal-positive nuclei. By this type of assay, it was observed that unfractionated bone marrow gives rise to labelled muscle fibres with an unexpectedly high efficiency, suggesting the existence of progenitor cells endowed with myogenic potential in the bone marrow. Therefore, bone marrow from MLC3F-n*lacZ* mice was transplanted into lethally-irradiated *scid/bg* mice. When the latter were fully reconstituted with donor bone marrow, regeneration was induced in a leg muscle. Histochemical analysis unequivocally showed the presence of β-gal-staining nuclei at the centre and periphery of regenerated fibres, demonstrating for the first time that murine bone marrow contains transplantable progenitors that can be recruited to an injured muscle through the peripheral circulation, and participate in muscle repair (Ferrari *et al.* 1998). The publication of this report in 1998 renewed interest in myogenic progenitors, and raised expectations as to their possible clinical use.

Bone marrow is a special tissue composed of different cell types that include the hematopoietic stem cell (and their differentiated derivatives), the stroma-derived mesenchymal stem cell (a long-lasting precursor of bone, cartilage and adipocytes: Horwitz *et al.* 1999; Prockop 1997) as well as the endothelial and perithelial cells that comprise the wall of the sinuosids. In principle the myogenic progenitor may originate from one or more of these cell types. Even before investigating these important biological issues, the practical possibility appeared that bone marrow transplantation may represent a potential alternative to local injection of autologous or heterologous myogenic cells.

In 1999 Gussoni and colleagues (Gussoni *et al.* 1999) reported that dystrophin-deficient, *mdx* mice transplanted with the bone marrow of syngeneic normal mice develop a small number of dystrophin-positive fibres containing donor nuclei. The efficiency of muscle reconstitution by marrow-derived progenitors appeared to be slightly higher in this model, but the number of fibres carrying both dystrophin and the Y chromosome never exceeded 1 per cent of the total fibres in the average muscle. Thus, even in a chronically regenerating environment marrow-derived progenitors are unable to give rise to new muscle fibres in clinically relevant numbers.

These studies clearly indicated that clinical efficacy could not be reached. This may be due to: (1) the small number of myogenic progenitors present in the bone marrow; (2) inefficient transplantation under conditions that have been optimized for hematopoietic progenitors; (3) lack of a selective advantage for donor cells in the *mdx* background, where resident myogenic cells continue to generate new fibres throughout most of the adult life of the animal. Indeed the same mutation results in a much milder phenotype in the mouse when compared with human DMD where the repair potential of muscle satellite cells is lost in the first years of a patients' life. In this situation, dystrophin-positive fibres made by transplanted bone marrow progenitors might have a selective advantage, resist degeneration, and progressively replace dystrophin-negative fibres. This situation calls for further experimentation in a different animal model: the dog muscular dystrophy, currently treated with BMT, may provide this additional evidence.

Pluripotent stem cells and their possible use in cell transplantation

The original demonstration of myogenic potential in bone marrow cells, was soon followed by other observations that suggested that such plasticity is not limited to skeletal myogenesis. Neural stem cells were shown to be able to generate hematopoietic cells (Bjornson *et al.* 1999) and more recently skeletal muscle cells (Galli *et al.* 2000). Moreover, skeletal muscle and probably many other tissues contain a population of 'stem' cells (identified by a number of different criteria) that are capable of long-term hematopoietic reconstitution upon transplantation (Gussoni *et al.* 1999; Jackson *et al.* 1999). Studies aimed at defining the embryological origin of bone marrow-derived myogenic progenitors revealed that they originate from the embryonic vessels (De Angelis *et al.* 1999), probably from endothelial cells; however, it remains to be investigated in quantitative terms what may be their contribution to tissue growth and repair.

Together these data provide the rather unexpected evidence that stem cells resident in a given adult tissue, when naturally or experimentally transferred to a different tissue (even of a different germ layer) can produce differentiated cells typical of tissue they have reached (Lemishka 1999). The term 'plasticity', used for the occasion, would thus indicate the capacity of pluripotent stem cells to differentiate along alternative pathways depending on local cues provided by different tissue environments, and/or in response to specific recruitment signals. These findings may provide the basis for an entirely new concept of cell therapy, based on transplantation of adult pluripotent stem cells. These cells may be isolated from the most convenient source (likely unaffected by the disease) and then induced to differentiate into specific tissues. However, if these cells represent only a very minor population, they may never be obtained in numbers meaningful for practical purposes. More experimental work on the biology of pluripotent stem cells is needed before an answer can be provided to this question. Myogenic stem cells derived from blastocysts or umbilical blood are other possibilities being considered.

Future clinical perspectives for gene and cell therapies

At the time of writing, only one gene therapy clinical trial with adeno-associated vectors is under way and there are no immediate perspectives for cell therapy trials. However, given the speed at which research proceeds it may be possible that novel trials may begin in the near future, based on data produced in this period. Indeed all the experiments and failures reported above have certainly increased our knowledge and thus the chances that future attempts may be met with better outcomes.

In the case of gene therapy, the principal problems to be overcome include gene delivery and immunogenic and cytotoxic effects that limit therapeutic benefit and long term gene expression. Designing efficient gene delivery strategies must be tailored to a specific application and target tissue type. For gene therapy treatment of inherited myopathies, where large amounts of muscle must be transduced, targeted systemic forms of gene delivery are likely to be required. The immunogenic and cytotoxic effects are specific for each vector system in the context of a specific target tissue. Each of these effects must be appreciated and addressed. A further hurdle to clinical application involves the issues of scaling up for large human application including the development of technologies to produce adequate amounts of gene therapy vector of sufficient quality.

Similarly, several perspectives remain ahead for cell therapy (Table 14.2): (1) bone marrow transplantation may be a therapeutic possibility if procedures for isolation, expansion and transplantation of the responsible stem cell population can be significantly improved; (2) autologous stem cells may alternatively be considered: they would then be genetically corrected by insertion of a functional, appropriately regulated copy of the missing gene (but dystrophin and large proteins represent an additional problem) and then transplanted in sufficient numbers by an appropriate delivery route. In both cases 1

Table 14.2 Cellular sources for muscle cell therapy

Cell type	Availability	Gene transfer	Delivery	Immune-suppression
Heterologous myoblasts	Yes	No	Intra-muscular injection	Essential
Autologous myoblasts	limited or no	Yes	Intra-muscular injection	No
Autologous fibroblasts + MyoD	Yes	Yes	Intra-muscular injection	No
Bone marrow transplantation	Yes	No	Circulation	No
Heterologous isolated progenitors	Yes	No	Intra-vascular	Essential
Autologous isolated progenitors	?	Yes	Intra-vascular	No

and 2, myogenic differentiation and self-renewing capacity should be maintained *in vivo*. Finally, direct myoblast, myogenically converted fibroblasts or even bone marrow derived stem cells may be directly injected into the muscle, once problems related to cell survival and distribution are solved. Although less fascinating, this possibility should not be ignored and in fact, although probably the most limited in long lasting effect, it is also the simplest to be translated into a clinical trial.

References

Acsadi, G., Dickson, G., Love, D.R., Jani, A., Walsh, F.S., Gurusinghe, A. *et al.* (1991). Human dystrophin expression in mdx mice after intramuscular injection of DNA constructs. *Nature*, 352, 815–8.

Acsadi, G., Jani, A., Huard, J., Blaschuk, K., Massie, B., Holland, P. *et al.* (1994a). Cultured human myoblasts and myotubes show markedly different transducibility by replication-defective adenovirus recombinants. *Gene Therapy*, 1, 338–40.

Acsadi, G., Jani, A., Massie, B., Simoneau, M., Holland, P., Blaschuk, K. *et al.* (1994b). A differential efficiency of adenovirus-mediated *in vivo* gene transfer into skeletal muscle cells of different maturity. *Human Molecular. Genetics*, 3, 579–84.

Akkaraju, G.R., Huard, J., Hoffman, E.P., Goins, W.F., Pruchnic, R., Watkins, S.C. *et al.* (1999). Herpes simplex virus vector-mediated dystrophin gene transfer and expression in MDX mouse skeletal muscle. *Journal of Gene Medicine*, 1, 280–9.

Allamand, V., Donahue, K.M., Straub, V., Davisson, R.L., Davidson, B.L., and Campbell, K.P. (2000). Early adenovirus-mediated gene transfer effectively prevents muscular dystrophy in alpha-sarcoglycan-deficient mice. *Gene Therapy*, 7, 1385–91.

Arahata, K. and Engel, A.G. (1984). Monoclonal antibody analysis of mononuclear cells in myopathies. I: quantitation of subsets according to diagnosis and sites of accumulation and demonstration and counts of muscle fibres invaded by T cells. *Annals of Neurology*, 16, 193–208.

Araishi, K., Sasaoka, T., Imamura, M., Noguchi, S., Hama, H., and Wakabayashi, E. (1999). Loss of the sarcoglycan complex and sarcospan leads to muscular dystrophy in beta-sarcoglycan-deficient mice. *Human Molecular Genetics*, 8, 1589–98.

Bartlett, R.J., Stockinger, S., Denis, M.M., Bartlett, W.T., Inverardi, L., Le, T.T. *et al.* (2000). *In vivo* targeted repair of a point mutation in the canine dystrophin gene by a chimeric RNA/DNA oligonucleotide. *Nature Biotechnology*, 18, 615–22.

Beauchamp, J.R., Pagel, C.N., and Partridge, T.A. (1997). A dual-marker system for quantitative studies of myoblast transplantation in the mouse. *Transplantation*, 63: 1794–7.

Berghella, L., De Angelis, L., Coletta, M., Berarducci, B. , Sonnino, C., Salvatori, G. *et al.* (1999). Reversible immortalization of human myogenic cells by site-specific excision of a retrovirally-transferred oncogene. *Human Gene Therapy*, 10, 1607–18.

Berkner, K.L. (1988). Development of adenovirus vectors for the expression of heterologous genes. *Biotechniques*, 6, 616–29.

Bett, A.J., Haddara, W., Prevec, L., and Graham, F.L. (1994). An efficient and flexible system for construction of adenovirus vectors with insertions or deletions in early regions 1 and 3. *Proceedings of the National Academy of Sciences, USA*, 91, 8802–6.

Bjornson, C.R., Rietze, R.L., Reynolds, B.A., Magli, M.C., and Vescovi, A.L. (1999). Turning brain into blood: a hematopoietic fate adopted by adult neural stem cells *in vivo* (see comments). *Science*, 283, 534–7.

Blau, H.M. and Springer, M.L. (1997). Muscle-mediated gene therapy. *New England Journal of Medicine*, **333**, 1554–6.

Bouri, K., Feero, W.G., Myerburg, M.M., Wickham, T.J., Kovesdi, I., Hoffman, E.P. *et al.* (1999). Poly-lysine modification of adenoviral fibre protein enhances muscle cell transduction. *Human Gene Therapy*, **10**, 1633–40.

Breton, M., Li, Z., Paulin, D., Harris, J.A., Rieger, F., Pincon-Raymond, M. *et al.* (1995). Myotube driven myogenic recruitment of cells during *in vitro* myogenesis. *Developmental Dynamics*, **202**, 126–36.

Braun, S., Thioudellet, C., Rodriguez, P., Ali-Hadji, D., Perraud, F., Accart, N. *et al.* (2000). Immune rejection of human dystrophin following intramuscular injections of naked DNA in mdx mice. *Gene Therapy*, **7**, 1447–57.

Bryan, T.M. and Reddel, R.R. (1994). SV40-induced immortalization of human cells. *Critical Reviews on. Oncogenes*, **5**, 331–7.

Budker, V., Budker, T., Zhang, G., Subbotin, V., Loomis, A., and Wolff, J.A. (2000). Hypothesis: naked plasmid DNA is taken up by cells *in vivo* by a receptor-mediated process. *Journal of Gene Medicine*, **2**, 76–88.

Chen, H.-H., Mack, L.M., Choi, S.Y., Ontell, M., Kochanek, S., and Clemens, P.R. (1999). DNA from both high-capacity and first-generation adenoviral vectors remains intact in skeletal muscle. *Human Gene Therapy*, **10**, 365–73.

Chen, H.-H., Mack, L.M., Kelly, R., Ontell, M., Kochanek, S., and Clemens, P.R. (1997). Persistence in muscle of an adenoviral vector that lacks all viral genes. *Proceedings of the National Academy of Sciences, USA*, **94**, 1645–50.

Clemens, P.R., Kochanek, S., Sunada, Y., Chan, S., Chen, H.-H., Campbell, K.P. *et al.* (1996). *In vivo* muscle gene transfer of full-length dystrophin with an adenoviral vector that lacks all viral genes. *Gene Therapy*, **3**, 965–72.

Cole-Strauss, A., Yoon, K., Xiang, Y., Byrne, B.C., Rice, M.C., Gryn, J. *et al.* (1996). Correction of the mutation responsible for sickle cell anemia by an RNA- DNA oligonucleotide. *Science*, **273**, 1386–9.

Coral-Vazquez, R., Cohn, R.D., Moore, S.A., Hill, J.A., Weiss, R.M., Davisson, R.L. *et al.* (1999). Disruption of the sarcoglycan-sarcospan complex in vascular smooth muscle: a novel mechanism for cardiomyopathy and muscular dystrophy. *Cell*, **98**, 465–74.

Cornetta, K., Morgan, R.A., and Anderson, W.F. (1991). Safety issues related to retroviral-mediated gene transfer in humans. *Human Gene Therapy*, **2**, 5–14.

Cossu, G. (1997). Unorthodox myogenesis: possible developmental significance and implications for tissue histogenesis and regeneration. *Histology Histopathology*, **12**: 755–60.

Dai, Y., Schwarz, E.M., Gu, D., Zhang, W.-W., Sarvetnick, N., and Verma, I.M. (1995). Cellular and humoral immune responses to adenoviral vectors containing factor IX gene: tolerization of factor IX and vector antigens allows for long-term expression. *Proceedings of the National Academy of Sciences, USA*, **92**, 1401–5.

Daly, G. and Chernajovsky, Y. (2000). Recent Developments in Retroviral-Mediated Gene Transduction. *Molecular Therapy*, **2**, 423–34.

Davis, H. L., Whalen, R. G., and Demeneix, B.A. (1993). Direct gene transfer into skeletal muscle in vivo: factors affecting efficiency of transfer and stability of expression. *Human Gene Therapy*, **4**, 151–9.

De Angelis, L, Berghella, L, Coletta, Cusella De Angelis, M.G., Lattanzi, L, Ponzetto, C. and Cossu, G. (1999). Skeletal myogenic progenitors originating from embryonic dorsal aorta co-express endothelial and myogenic markers and contribute to post-natal muscle growth and regeneration *Journal of Cell Biology*, **147**, 869–78.

Decary, S., Mouly, V., Ben Hamida, C., Sautet, A., Barbet, J.P., and Butler-Browne, G.S. (1997). Replicative Potential And Telomere Length In Human Skeletal Muscle: Implications For Myogenic Cell-Mediated Gene Therapy. *Human Gene Therapy*, 8, 1429–38.

Deconinck, N., Tinsley, J., De Backer, F., Fisher, R., Kahn, D., Phelps, S. *et al.* (1997). Expression of truncated utrophin leads to major functional improvements in dystrophin-deficient muscles of mice. *Nature Medicine*, 3, 1216–21.

DeLuca, N.A., McCarthy, A.M., and Schaffer, P.A. (1985). Isolation and characterization of deletion mutants of herpes simplex virus type 1 in the gene encoding immediate-early regulatory protein ICP4. *Journal of Virology*, 56, 558–70.

Douglas, J.T., Rogers, B.E., Rosenfeld, M.E., Michael, S.I., Feng, M., and Curiel, D.T. (1996). Targeted gene delivery by tropism-modified adenoviral vectors. *Nature Biotechnology*, 14, 1574–8.

Dowty, M.E., Williams, P., Zhang, G., Hagstrom, J.E., and Wolff, J.A. (1995). Plasmid DNA entry into postmitotic nuclei of primary rat myotubes. *Proceedings of the National Academy of Sciences, USA*, 92, 4572–6.

Duclos, F., Straub, V., Moore, S.A., Venzke, D.P., Hrstka, R.F., Crosbie, R.H. *et al.* (1998). Progressive muscular dystrophy in alpha-sarcoglycan-deficient mice. *Journal of Cell Biology*, 142, 1461–71.

Dull, T., Zufferey, R., Kelly, M., Mandel, R.J., Nguyen, M., Trono, D. *et al.* (1998). A third-generation lentivirus vector with a conditional packaging system. *Journal of Virology*, 72, 8463–71.

Dunckley, M.G., Love, D.R., Davies, K.E., Walsh, F.S., Morris, G.E., and Dickson, G. (1992). Retroviral-mediated transfer of a dystrophin minigene into mdx mouse myoblasts *in vitro*. *FEBS Letters*, 296, 128–34.

Dunckley, M.G., Wells, D.J., Walsh, F.S., and Dickson, G. (1993). Direct retroviral-mediated transfer of a dystrophin minigene into mdx mouse muscle *in vivo*. *Human Molecular Genetics*, 2, 717–23.

Fassati, A., Wells, D.J., Sgro Serpente, P.A., Walsh, F.S., Brown, S.C., Strong, P.N., and Dickson, G. (1997). Genetic correction of dystrophin deficiency and skeletal muscle remodeling in adult MDX mouse via transplantation of retroviral producer cells. *Journal of Clinical Investigation*, 100, 620–8.

Fassati, A., Wells, D.J., Walsh, F.S., and Dickson, G. (1996). Transplantation of retroviral producer cells for *in vivo* gene transfer into mouse skeletal muscle. *Human Gene Therapy*, 7, 595–02.

Feero, W.G., Rosenblatt, J.D., Huard, J., Watkins, S.C., Epperly, M., Clemens, P.R. *et al.* (1997). Viral gene delivery to skeletal muscle: insights on maturation-dependent loss of fibre infectivity for adenovirus and herpes simplex type 1 viral vectors. *Human Gene Therapy*, 8, 371–80.

Ferrari, G., Salvatori, G., Rossi, C., Cossu, G., and Mavilio, F. (1995). A retroviral vector containing a muscle-specific enhancer drives gene expression only in differentiated muscle fibres. *Human Gene Therapy*, 6, 733–42.

Ferrari, G., Cusella-De Angelis, G., Coletta, M., Paolucci, E., Stornaiuolo, A., Cossu, G. *et al.* (1998). Muscle regeneration by bone marrow-derived myogenic progenitors. *Science*, 279, 1528–30.

Ferrer, A., Wells, K.E., and Wells, D.J. (2000). Immune responses to dystropin: implications for gene therapy of Duchenne muscular dystrophy. *Gene Therapy*, 7, 1439–46.

Fisher, K.J., Jooss, K., Alston, J., Yang, Y., Haecker, S.E., High, K. *et al.* (1997). Recombinant adeno-associated virus for muscle directed gene therapy. *Nature Medicine*, 3, 306–12.

Galli, R., Borello U., Gritti, A., Giulia Minasi, M.G., Bjornson, C., Coletta, M. *et al.* (2000). Skeletal Myogenic Potential of Adult Neural Stem Cells. *Nature Neurosciences*, 3, 986–91.

Gao, Q., Hauser, S.H., Liu, X.L., Wazer, D.E., Madoc-Jones, H., and Band, V. (1996). Mutant p53-induced immortalization of primary human mammary epithelial cells. *Cancer Research*, 56: 3129–33.

Gibson, A.J., Karasinski, J., Relvas, J., Moss, J., Sherratt, T.G., Strong, P.N. *et al.* (1995). Dermal fibroblasts convert to a myogenic lineage in *mdx* mouse muscle. *Journal of Cell Science*, **108**: 207–14.

Glorioso, J.C. (2000). Perspectives on viral vector design and applications. *Advances in Virus Research* **55**, 403–7.

Greelish, J.P., Su, L.T., Lankford, E.B., Burkman, J.M., Chen, H., Konig, S.K. *et al.* (1999). Stable restoration of the sarcoglycan complex in dystrophic muscle perfused with histamine and a recombinant adeno-associated viral vector. *Nature Medicine*, **5**, 439–43.

Grimm, D. and Kleinschmidt, J.A. (1999). Progress in adeno-associated virus type 2 vector production: promises and prospects for clinical use. *Human Gene Therapy*, **10**, 2445–50.

Guerette, B.D., Skuk, F., Celestin, J.C., Huard, F., Tardif, I., Asselin, B. *et al.* (1997). Prevention by anti-LFA-1 of acute myoblast death following transplantation. *Journal of Immunology*, **159**, 2522–31.

Gussoni, E., Soneoka, Y., Strickland, C.D., Buzney, E.A., Khan, M.K., Flint, A.F. *et al.* (1999). Dystrophin expression in the *mdx* mouse restored by stem cell transplantation. *Nature*, **401**, 390–4.

Hack, A.A., Ly, C.T., Jiang, F., Clendenin, C.J., Sigrist, K.S., Wollmann, R.L., and McNally, E.M. (1998). Gamma-sarcoglycan deficiency leads to muscle membrane defects and apoptosis independent of dystrophin. *Journal of Cell Biology*, **142**, 1279–87.

Hagstrom, J.E., Rybakova, I.N., Staeva, T., Wolff, J.A., and Ervasti, J.M. (1996). Nonnuclear DNA Binding Proteins in Striated Muscle. *Biochemical Molecular Medicine*, **58**, 113–21.

Hobbs, W.E. and DeLuca, N.A. (1999). Perturbation of cell cycle progression and cellular gene expression as a function of herpes simplex virus ICP0. *Journal of Virology*, **73**, 8245–55.

Hoffman, E.P., Morgan, J.E., Watkins, S.C., and Partridge, T.A. (1990). Somatic reversion/suppression of the mouse *mdx* phenotype *in vivo*. *Journal of Neurological Sciences*, **99**, 9–25.

Hoffman, E.P., Brown, R.H. Jr., and Kunkel, L.M. (1987). Dystrophin: the protein product of the Duchenne muscular dystrophy locus. *Cell*, **24**, 919–28.

Horwitz, E.M., Prockop, D.J., Fitzpatrick, L.A., Koo, W.W.K., Gordon, P.L., Neel, M. *et al.* (1999). Transplantability and therapeutic effects of bone marrow-derived mesenchymal cells in children with osteogenesis imperfecta. *Nature Medicine*, **5**, 309–13.

Huard, J., Akkaraju, G., Watkins, S.C., Pike-Cavalcoli, M., and Glorioso, J.C. (1997). LacZ gene transfer to skeletal muscle using a replication-defective herpes simplex virus type 1 mutant vector. *Human Gene Therapy*, **8**, 439–52.

Huard, J., Feero, W.G., Watkins, S.C., Hoffman, E.P., Rosenblatt, D.J., and Glorioso, J.C. (1996). The basal lamina is a physical barrier to herpes simplex virus-mediated gene delivery to mature muscle fibres. *Journal of Virology*, **70**, 8117–23.

Huard, J., Goins, W.F., and Glorioso, J.C. (1995). Herpes simplex virus type 1 vector mediated gene transfer to muscle. *Gene Therapy*, **2**, 385–92.

Huard, J., Verreault, S., Roy, R., Tremblay, M., and Tremblay, J.P. (1994). High efficiency of muscle regeneration after human myoblast clone transplantation in SCID mice. *Journal of Clinical Investigation*, **93**, 586–99.

Jackson, K.A., Mi, T., and Goodell, M.A. (1999). Hematopoietic potential of stem cells isolated from murine skeletal muscle. *Proceedings of the National Academy of Sciences, USA, A* **96**, 14482–6.

Kafri, T., Blomer, U., Peterson, D. A., Gage, F. H., and Verma, I. M. (1997). Sustained expression of genes delivered directly into liver and muscle by lentiviral vectors. *Nature Genetics*, **17**, 314–7.

Kafri, T., van Praag, H., Ouyang, L., Gage, F. H., and Verma, I.M. (1999). A packaging cell line for lentivirus vectors. *Journal of Virology*, **73**, 576–84.

Kelly, R., Alonso, S., Tajbakhsh, S., Cossu, G., and Buckingham, M. (1995). Myosin light chain 3F regulatory sequences confer regionalized cardiac and skeletal muscle expression in transgenic mice. *Journal of Cell Biology*, **129**, 383–96.

Kinoshita, I., Vilquin, J.T., Guerette,B., Asselin, I., Roy, R., and Tremblay, J.P. (1994). Very Efficient Myoblast Allotransplantation In Mice Under Fk-506 Immunosuppression. *Muscle & Nerve*, **17**, 1407–15.

Kinoshita, I., Roy, R., Dugre, F.J., Gravel, C, Goulet, M., Asselin, I. *et al.* (1996). Myoblast transplantation in monkeys: control of immune response by FK506. *Journal of Neuropathology and Experimental Neurology*, **55**, 687–97.

Kochanek, S. (1999). High-capacity adenoviral vectors for gene transfer and somatic gene therapy. *Human Gene Therapy*, **10**, 2451–9.

Kochanek, S., Clemens, P.R., Mitani, K., Chen, H.-H., Chan, S., and Caskey, C.T. (1996). A new adenoviral vector: Replacement of all viral coding sequences with 28 kb of DNA independently expressing both full-length dystrophin and -galactosidase. *Proceedings of the National Academy of Sciences, USA*, **93**, 5731–6.

Krasnykh, V.N., Douglas, J.T., and van Beusechem V.W. (2000). Genetic targeting of adenoviral vectors. *Molecular Therapy*, **1**, 391–05.

Krasnykh, V.N., Mikheeva, G.V., Douglas, J.T., and Curiel, D.T. (1996). Generation of recombinant adenovirus vectors with modified fibres for altering viral tropism. *Journal of Virology*, **70**, 6839–46.

Kumar-Singh, R. and Chamberlain, J.S. (1996). Encapsidated adenovirus minichromosomes allow delivery and expression of a 14 kb dystrophin cDNA to muscle cells. *Human Molecular Genetics*, **5**, 913–21.

Lattanzi, L., Salvatori, G., Coletta, M., Sonnino, C., Cusella De Angelis, M.G., Gioglio, L. *et al.* (1998). High efficiency myogenic conversion of human fibroblasts by adenoviral vector-mediated MyoD gene transfer. An alternative strategy for *ex vivo* gene therapy of primary myopathies. *Journal of Clinical Investigation*, **101**, 2119–28.

Lemieux, P., Guerin, N., Pacadis, G., Provix, R., Chistyakova, A., and Alakhov, V. (2000). A combination poloxamers increases gene expression of plasmid DNA in skeletal muscle. *Gene Therapy*, **7**, 986–91.

Lemischka, I. (1999). The power of stem cells reconsidered? *Proceedings of the National Academy of Sciences, USA*, **96**, 14193–5.

Liang, K.W., Hoffman, E.P., and Huang, L. (2000). Targeted delivery of plasmid DNA to myogenic cells via transferrin-conjugated peptide nucleic acid. *Molecular Therapy*, **1**, 236–43.

Liu, L.A. and Engvall, E. (1999). Sarcoglycan isoforms in skeletal muscle. *Journal of Biolgical Chemistry*, **274**, 38171–6.

McGrory, W.J., Bautista, D.S., and Graham, F.L. (1988). A simple technique for the rescue of early region I mutations into infectious human adenovirus type 5. *Virology*, **163**, 614–7.

Miyoshi, H., Blomer, U., Takahashi, M., Gage, F.H., and Verma, I.M. (1998). Development of a self-inactivating lentivirus vector. *Journal of Virology*, **72**, 8150–7.

Mouly, V., Edom, S., Decary, P., Vicart, P., Barbet, J.P., and Butler Browne, G.S. (1996). SV40 large T antigen interferes with adult myosin heavy chain expression, but not with differentiation of human satellite cells. *Experimental Cell Research*, **225**, 268–76.

Naffakh, N., Pinset, C., Montarras, D., Li, Z., Paulin, D., Danos, O., and Heard, J.M. (1996). Long-term secretion of therapeutic proteins from genetically modified skeletal muscles. *Human Gene Therapy*, **7**, 11–21.

Naldini, L., Blomer, U., Gage, F.H., Trono, D., and Verma, I.M. (1996a). Efficient transfer, integration, and sustained long-term expression of the transgene in adult rat brains injected with a lentiviral vector. *Proceedings of the National Academy of Sciences, USA*, **93**, 11382–8.

Naldini, L., Blomer, U., Gallay, P., Ory, D., Mulligan, R., Gage, F.H., Verma, I.M., and Trono, D. (1996b). *In vivo* gene delivery and stable transduction of nondividing cells by a lentiviral vector. *Science*, **272**, 263–7.

Nawrotzki, R., Blake, D.J., and Davies, K.E. (1996). The genetic basis of neuromuscular disorders. *Trends in Genetics*, **12**, 294–8.

Ohtsuka, Y., Udaka, K., Yamashiro, Y., Yagita, H., and Okumura, K. (1998). Dystrophin acts as a transplantation rejection antigen in dystrophin-deficient mice: Implication for gene therapy. *Journal of Immunology*, **160**, 4635–40.

Parks, R.J., Chen, L., Anton, M., Sankar, U., Rudnicki, M.A., and Graham, F.L. (1996). A helper-dependent adenovirus vector system-removal of helper virus by cre-mediated excision of the viral packaging signal. *Proceedings of the National Academy of Sciences, USA*, **93**, 13565–70.

Partridge TA, Beauchamp, J.R., and Morgan, J.E. (1989). Conversion of *mdx* myofibres from dystrophin-negative to -positive by injection of normal myoblasts. *Nature*, **337**, 176–9.

Partridge, T.A. (1996). Myoblast transplantation. In *Yearbook of Cell and Tissue Transplantation*. (R.P. Lanza and W.L. Chick ed.). Kluwer Academic Publishing, pp. 53–9.

Phelps, S.F., Hauser, M.A., Cole, N.M., Rafael, J.A., Hinkle, R.T., Faulkner, J.A., and Chamberlain, J.S. (1995). Expression of full-length and truncated dystrophin mini-genes in transgenic mdx mice. *Human Molecular Genetics*, **4**, 1251–8.

Prockop, D.J. (1997). Marrow stromal cells as stem cells for nonhematopoietic tissues. *Science*, **276**, 71–4.

Pruchnic, R., Cao, B., Peterson, Z.Q., Xiao, X., Li, J., Samulski, R.J. *et al.* (2000). The use of adeno-associated virus to circumvent the maturation-dependent viral transduction of muscle fibres. *Human Gene Therapy*, **11**, 521–36.

Quantin, B., Perricaudet, L.D., Tajbakhsh, S., and Mandel, J.L. (1992). Adenovirus as an expression vector in muscle cells *in vivo*. *Proceedings of the National Academy of Sciences, USA*, **89**, 2581–4.

Ragot, T., Vincent, N., Chafey, P., Vigne, E., Gilgenkrantz, H., Couton, D. *et al.* (1993). Efficient adenovirus-mediated transfer of a human minidystrophin gene to skeletal muscle. *Nature*, **361**, 647–50.

Rando, T.A., Disatnik, M.H., and Zhou, L.Z. (2000). Rescue of dystrophin expression in mdx mouse muscle by RNA/DNA oligonucleotides. *Proceedings of the National Academy of Sciences, USA*, **97**, 5363–8.

Salvatori, G., Ferrari, G., Mezzogiorno, A., Servidei, S., Coletta, M., Tonali, P. *et al.* (1993). Retroviral vector-mediated gene transfer into human primary myogenic cells leads to expression in muscle fibres *in vivo*. *Human Gene Therapy*, **4**, 713–23.

Salvatori, G., Lattanzi, L., Coletta, M., Aguanno, S., Vivarelli, E., Kelly, R. *et al.* (1995). Myogenic conversion of mammalian fibroblasts induced by differentiating muscle cells. *Journal of Cell Science*, **108**: 2733–9.

Salvatori, G, Lattanzi, L., Puri, P.L., Melchionna, R., Fieri, C., Levrero, M. *et al.* (1997). A temperature conditional mutant of SV40 Large T Antigen requires serum to inhibit myogenesis and does not induce DNA synthesis in myotubes. *Cell Growth and Differentiation*, **8**, 157–64.

Scheidner, G., Morral, N., Parks, R.J., Wu, Y., Koopmans, S.C., Langston, C. *et al.* (1998). Genomic DNA transfer with a high-capacity adenovirus vector results in improved *in vivo* gene expression and decreased toxicity. *Nature Genetics*, **18**, 180–3.

Seale, P., and Rudnicki, M.A (2000). A new look at the origin, function, and "stem-cell" status of muscle satellite cells. *Developmental Biology*, 218, 115–24.

Sena-Esteves, M., Saeki, Y., Fraefel, C., and Breakefield, X.O. (2000). ics. HSV-1 amplicon vectors – simplicity and versatility. *Molecular Therapy*, 2, 9–15.

Simon, L.V., Beuchamps, J.R., O'Hare, M., and Olsen. I. (1996). Establishment of long-term myogenic cultures from patients with Duchenne muscular dystrophy by retroviral transduction of a temperature-sensitive SV40 large T antigen. *Experimental Cell Research*, 224, 264–71.

Stedman, H., Wilson, J.M., Finke, R., Kleckner, A.L., and Mendell, J. (2000). Phase I clinical trial utilizing gene therapy for limb girdle muscular dystrophy: alpha-, beta-, gamma-, or delta-sarcoglycan gene delivered with intramuscular instillations of adeno-associated vectors. *Human Gene Therapy*, 11, 777–90.

Stratford-Perricaudet, L.D., Makeh, I., Perricaudet, M., and Briand, P. (1992). Widespread long-term gene transfer to mouse skeletal muscles and heart. *Proceedings of the National Academy of Sciences, USA*, 90, 626–30.

Sun, L., Li, J. and Xiao, X. (2000). Overcoming adeno-associated virus vector size limitation through viral DNA heterodimerization. *Nature Medicine*, 6, 599–602.

Urtizberea, J.A. (2000). Therapies in muscular dystrophy: current concepts and future prospects. *European Neurology*, 43, 127–32.

Valentine, B.A., Winand, N.J., Pradhan, D., Moise, N.S., de Lahunta, A., Kornegay, J.N. *et al.* (1992). Canine X-linked muscular dystrophy as an animal model of duchenne muscular dystrophy: A review. *American Journal of Medical Genetics*, 42, 352–6.

Vincent, N., Ragot, T., Gilgenkrantz, H., Couton, D., Chafey, P., Gregoire, A. *et al.* (1993). Long-term correction of mouse dystrophic degeneration by adenovirus-mediated transfer of a minidystrophin gene. *Nature Genetics*, 5, 130–4.

Vitiello, L., Chonn, A., Wasserman, J.D., Duff, C., and Worton, R.G. (1996). Condensation of plasmid DNA with polylysine improves liposome-mediated gene transfer into established and primary muscle cells. *Gene Therapy*, 3, 396–404.

Wang, B., Li, J., and Xiao, X. (2000). AAV vector carrying human mini-dystrophin genes effectively ameliorates muscular dystrophy in mdx mouse model. *Proceedings of the National Academy of Sciences, USA*, 97, 13714–9.

Wang, X., Zhang, G.R., Yang, T., Zhang, W., and Geller, A.I. (2000). Fifty-one kilobase HSV-1 plasmid vector can be packaged using a helper virus-free system and supports expression in the rat brain. *Biotechniques*, 28, 102–7.

Wang, Y., Fraefel, C., Protasi, F., Moore, R.A., Fessenden, J.D., Pessah, I.N. *et al.* (2000). HSV-1 amplicon vectors are a highly efficient gene delivery system for skeletal muscle myoblasts and myotubes. *American Journal of Physiology*, 278, C619–C26.

Webster, C. and Blau, H.M. (1990). Accelerated age-related decline in replicative life span of Duchenne muscular dystrophy myoblasts: implication for cell and gene therapy. *Somatic Cellular and Molecular Genetics*, 16, 557–65.

Wickham, T.J., Roelvink, P.W., Brough, D.E., and Kovesdi, I. (1996b). Adenovirus targeted to heparan-containing receptors increases its gene delivery efficiency to multiple cell types. *Nature Biotechnology*, 14, 1570–3.

Wickham, T.J., Segal, D.M., Roelvink, P.W., Carrion, M.E., Lizonova, A., Lee, G.-M. *et al.* (1996a). Targeted adenovirus gene transfer to endothelial and smooth muscle cells by using bispecific antibodies. *Journal of Virology*, 70, 6831–8.

Wolff, J.A., Dowty, M.E., Jiao, S., Repetto, G., Berg, R.K., Ludtke, J.J. *et al.* (1992). Expression of naked plasmids by cultured myotubes and entry of plasmids into T tubules and caveolae of mammalian skeletal muscle. *Journal of Cell Science*, 103 (Pt 4), 1249–59.

Wolff, J.A., Malone, R.W., Williams, P., Chong, W., Acsadi, G., Jani, A., and Felgner, P.L. (1990). Direct gene transfer into mouse muscle *in vivo. Science*, **247**, 1465–8.

Wolff, J.A., Williams, P., Acsadi, G., Jiao, S., Jani, A., and Chong, W. (1991). Conditions affecting direct gene transfer into rodent muscle *in vivo. Biotechniques*, **11**, 474–85.

Wright, W.E. and Shay, K. (1995). Time, telomeres and tumours: Is cellular senescence more than an anticancer mechanism? *Trends in Cell Biology*, **5**, 293–6.

Xiao, X., Li, J., and Samulski, R.J. (1996). Efficient long-term gene transfer into muscle tissue of immunocompetent mice by adeno-associated virus vector. *Journal of Virology*, **70**, 8098–08.

Xiao, X., Li, J., Tsao, Y.P., Dressman, D., Hoffman, E.P., and Watchko, J.F. (2000). Full functional rescue of a complete muscle (TA) in dystrophic hamsters by adeno-associated virus vector-directed gene therapy. *Journal of Virology*, **74**, 1436–42.

Yan, Z., Zhang, Y., Duan, D., and Engelhardt, J.F. (2000). Trans-splicing vectors expand the utility of adeno-associated virus for gene therapy. *Proceedings of the National Academy of Sciences, USA*, **97**, 6716–21.

Yang, Y., Haecker, S.E., Su, Q., and Wilson, J.M. (1996). Immunology of gene therapy with adenoviral vectors in mouse skeletal muscle. *Human Molecular Genetics*, **5**, 1703–12.

Yang, Y., Li, Q., Ertl, H.C.J., and Wilson, J.M. (1995b). Cellular and humoral immune responses to viral antigens create barriers to lung-directed gene therapy with recombinant adenoviruses. *Journal of Virology*, **69**, 2004–15.

Yang, Y., Nunes, F.A., Berencsi, K., Furth, E.E., Gonczol, E., and Wilson, J.M. (1994). Cellular immunity to viral antigens limits E1-deleted adenoviruses for gene therapy. *Proceedings of the National Academy of Sciences, USA*, **91**, 4407–11.

Yang, Y., Xiang, Z., Ertl, H.C.J., and Wilson, J.M. (1995a). Upregulation of class I major histocompatibility complex antigens by interferon is necessary for T-cell-mediated elimination of recombinant adenovirus-infected hepatocytes *in vivo. Proceedings of the National Academy of Sciences, USA*, **92**, 7257–61.

Zufferey, R., Dull, T., Mandel, R.J., Bukovsky, A., Quiroz, D., Naldini, L., and Trono, D. (1998). Self-inactivating lentivirus vector for safe and efficient *in vivo* gene delivery. *Journal of Virology*, **72**, 9873–80.

Chapter 15

Surgical management of muscular dystrophy

Luciano Merlini and Jürgen Forst

Proper management can only be achieved if the natural history of the disease is precisely known. This principle pertains to all diseases, particularly neuromuscular disorders. In Duchenne muscular dystrophy (DMD), strength is near normal in the early stages; a rapid downhill progression follows with loss of the ability to walk, respiratory involvement, and eventual cardiac failure. We have subdivided orthopaedic treatment in DMD according to the stage of the disease; early lower limb surgery, combined limb surgery and orthosis in the late stage of walking ability, and spinal surgery for scoliosis. In addition, two other orthopaedic interventions are mentioned: scapular fixation in facioscapulohumeral muscular dystrophy (FSH) and neck hyperextension correction in rigid spine syndrome.

Early lower limb surgery

Early lower limb surgery in DMD aims to correct the initial contractures that, if carefully sought, invariably occur in the initial phase of the disease, generally between 4 and 6 years of age. To correct these early contractures, Rideau (Rideau *et al.* 1986) suggested a new three-step surgical approach consisting of bilateral tenotomy of the superficial hip flexors, aponeurectomy of the ilio-tibial band, subcutaneous tenotomies of the knee and foot. The Rideau protocol of early lower limb surgery has been modified by a German group (Forst and Forst 1999) and entails bilateral open release of iliac spine muscles (m. sartorious, m. tensor fasciae latae, both heads of the m. rectus femoris), resection of the gluteal fascia, a complete aponeurectomy of the iliotibial band as well as septum intermusculare, the incision of m. biceps femoris, a subcutaneous tenotomy of medial knee flexors, and a lengthening of Achilles tendon. As this surgery is performed long before the incapacitating stage of the disease' that starts after the age of 6, patients ambulate unassisted and without exception 10–14 days after surgery and need no daily physical therapy.

In an open and prospective study at the Orthopaedic University Clinic in Aachen and later in Erlangen (Forst and Forst 1995; 1999), 280 DMD-patients have undergone lower limb surgery since 1988, 87 in an early stage (mean age 6.5 years, range 4.8 to 7.6). The treatment protocol was as follows: Day 1: preoperative check, Day 2: surgery, Day 3: starting with mobilization (standing) and if possible, walking (usually day 4–6). Patients are discharged from hospital if they can walk unassisted (mean duration 11.3 days, range 7 to 14). Since 1995 the anaesthetic management has included one administration of caudal anaesthesia with bupivacaine (0.2 ml/kg BW 0.5 per cent bupivacaine, 0.8 ml/kg BW 0.25 per cent bupivacaine, maximum volume 20 ml). In a control group loss of walking ability occurred at an average age of 9.29 years (5.8–13.6, SD 1.97). In the early surgical group loss occurred at an average of 10.5 years (8.2–14.4, SD 1.76). It is evident that early lower limb surgery significantly prolongs the ability to walk unassisted about 1.25 years on average ($P<0.05$). Long-term correction of contractures was an additional benefit of this surgery, also after walking ability was lost. In short, early intervention enables boys to have a longer period of normal life.

The primary reason' early lower limb surgery has such a high rate of success can be attributed to the fact that deterioration in DMD doesn't usually start until after the age of 6 (Brooke et al. 1981; Rideau et al. 1995). The linear decrease of general muscle strength usually begins between the ages of 5 and 6, after a plateau phase. At the same time, a limitation or loss of the physiological extension capacity of the lower limb joints, as well as an asymmetric retraction of the iliotibial band, is present. The latter leads to instability when standing and an unsteady gait with frequent falls. Furthermore, the increased time of Gower's manoeuvre can be observed at about 6 to 7 years indicating deteriorating function in the pelvic girdle muscles. These factors dictate that the best time to perform early lower limb surgery is usually before the age of 6.

There is not a universal consensus regarding early lower limb surgery. Some surgeons are more likely to consider it a viable alternative treatment, particularly those with a high success rate such as the German group (Bach and McKeon 1991; Forst and Forst 1999; Riccio et al. 1991). Manzur et al. (1992) however, showed negative results in a randomized controlled trial involving 20 patients, 10 of whom underwent early surgery. In this trial, follow-up was only one year. Granata et al. (1994) reported some benefit in 7 patients who were operated at a mean age of 6.7 years (range 5.0 to 7.5 years). However, the gain in ambulation time was only 0.4 years; all eventually lost the ability to walk at a mean age of 10.1 years (SD 0.8, range 8–11), which was found not statistically different ($P>0.5$) from their natural history control group of 67 DMD patients (mean age of walking loss 9.7 years, SD 1.5, range 6.3 to 13.7 years). The reasons for this lack of general consensus may be summarised as follows: (a) the clinical preoperative evaluation requires specialized training, (b) the rigorous surgery is quite long and potentially risky, involving patients with possible cardiomyopathy and anaesthetic susceptibility, (c) number of incisions; at least four bilaterally with frequent keloid formation, (d) transient benefit, (e) requires a specialized dedicated team which may not be easily assembled. In addition, non-invasive steroids treatment does prolong walking for a comparable period of time (Angelini et al. 1994).

Limb surgery and orthosis

Walking and standing ability can be extended for a few years by the use of long leg orthosis in Duchenne boys who reach the critical phase of loss of independent walking ability (Granata *et al.* 1988; Heckmatt *et al.* 1985; Scheuerbrandt *et al.* 1998; Smith *et al.* 1993). In most cases, orthopaedic intervention will be necessary before the use of the orthosis. Surgery consists of subcutaneous tenotomy of the Achilles tendon only (Heckmatt *et al.* 1985), or of the Achilles tendon, the superficial flexors of the hip, and the medial knee flexors (Bonnet *et al.* 1991; Granata *et al.* 1988; Smith *et al.* 1993). Open surgery is also an option (Williams *et al.* 1984). In our experience, the outcome of this treatment, which should be performed at the time walking is lost or within 3–6 months afterwards, is very successful (Merlini and Granata 1994).

At the Istituto Ortopedico Rizzoli in Bologna between 1982 and 1996, 59 patients were provided with long-leg orthosis when they lost their ability to walk (mean age 10.1 years, range 7.2 to 13.9). Any contractures at the hip or ankles were released by tenotomy in order to have the patient in a functional position for fitting the orthosis (Granata *et al.* 1988; Scheuerbrandt *et al.* 1998). Treatment protocol: Day 1: admission to the hospital and moulding for preparation of the orthosis; Day 2: bilateral percutaneous tenotomy of the Achilles tendon and hip flexors; Days 3–5: bed rest; Day 6: fitting and standing with the orthosis; Days 7 and 8: assisted and unassisted walking in orthosis; Day 9: discharge from the hospital. Prolonged bed rest during the day should be discouraged. Post-operative pain, minimal and primarily in the heel, can be easily controlled with the usual drugs. The mean period of prolongation of walking/standing with orthosis in the Rizzoli experience (Scheuerbrandt *et al.* 1998) of 59 patients was 3.9 years (range 0.9 to 11.3). The orthosis stabilizes the ankle and the knee, and provides a posterior support on which the child 'sits'. This is important for maintaining balance. The children walk in orthosis with locked knees and only on flat surfaces: they can wear them most of the day, and they are able to sit comfortably after unlocking the knee device.

This rehabilitation procedure is rather simple, yet requires close collaboration between the clinician, orthopaedic surgeon, anaesthesiologist, and the orthotist. If such a team is available, we recommend performing this simple and successful treatment as soon as the child ceases to walk.

Scoliosis treatment in Duchenne muscular dystrophy

Scoliosis is a very common complication of DMD. (Furderer *et al.* 2000; Rideau *et al.* 1984; Smith *et al.* 1989). Scoliosis in DMD develops 1–3 year after the child is wheelchair-bound, which happens around age 9.5 on average, and progresses relentlessly at a rate of 1–2° per month (Hsu 1983; Smith *et al.* 1989). Three patterns of spinal deformity have been observed (Granata *et al.* 1982): kyphoscoliosis with collapse of the spine, lordoscoliosis, and hyperlordosis with rigid spine. Kyphoscoliosis is the most frequent deformity and is caused by paralysis of the axial muscles combined with the asymmetrical contractures of the pelvis and lower limbs. Occurring during the pubertal growth spurt, this deformity evolves rapidly. It is a large 'C' shaped thoraco-lumbar scoliosis with pelvic obliquity. Scoliosis is aesthetically unpleasant, affects comfort in the sitting position, and may contribute to deterioration of respiratory function.

Conservative treatment is not effective. Spinal support systems and braces may delay, but do not prevent progression of scoliosis (Colbert and Craig 1987), are badly toler-ated (Robin 1977), and limit lung function (Noble-Jamieson et al. 1986). The use of a corset, however, can only be taken into consideration as a compromise either for young patients who have refused surgery or are unsuitable, or for older patients who have reached an inoperable stage (Forst et al. 1997). Usually, patients older than 16 who have not undergone surgery need a corset to help them sit.

Effective treatment of a severe neuromuscular spinal deformity currently involves sur-gical instrumentation and arthrodesis (Yazici et al. 2000). In the 1970s, the Harrington rod was used (Gibson et al. 1978; Sakai et al. 1977) for surgical correction and stabiliza-tion, and although fusion was usually achieved, about half the cases suffered mechanical complications. Lengthy immobilization in a cast also caused problems. During the 1980s, the use of the multiple sublaminar wiring technique of Luque, and of intrailiac (Galveston) posts (Allen and Ferguson 1982), provided an efficient immediate internal support and reduced or eliminated post-operative immobilization in cast. Treatment evolution continued in the following decade. Implant systems were designed with inte-gration in a posterior spinal implant system of spinal hooks, wires, screws, and post anchors (Yazici et al. 2000). Fusion from the upper thoracic spine to the sacrum is rec-ommended because fusion limited to L5 is accompanied by an increase in pelvic obliqui-ty and difficulty in sitting (Alman and Kim 1999; LaPrade and Rowe 1992).

With both the Luque and the new techniques, a 50–60 per cent long-lasting correc-tion of the spine is obtained. Patients with surgically stabilized spines are more comfortable later in life and are easier to care for (Miller et al. 1992). The majority of operated Duchenne patients (Granata et al. 1996) believed that the operation was ben-eficial with regard to correcting the deformity and the sitting position. Well-being and physical appearance were also considered to be improved (Granata et al. 1996).

Nevertheless, it has been established that spinal stabilization in DMD neither improves nor alters the decline in pulmonary function, which is related primarily to muscle weakness (Chataigner et al. 1998; Granata et al. 1996; Kennedy et al. 1995; Miller et al. 1992; Shapiro et al. 1992). In addition, spinal surgery does not improve survival rate (Chataigner et al. 1998; Kennedy et al. 1995).

Poor head control has been found in 30 per cent of operated patients at follow-up (Bellen et al. 1992; Cambridge and Drennan 1987; Granata et al. 1996; Miller et al. 1992). A disabling tilt of the head may manifest itself a few years after spinal surgery, requiring a difficult adjustment of the headrest (Bellen et al. 1992). Another occurrence is neck hyperextension due to contractures of the posterior neck muscles (Granata et al. 1996;

Scheuerbrandt *et al.* 1998). In this situation, the patient needs to lean forward against the chest belts in order to look straight ahead, compensating for the extension of the neck. A combination of tilt and hyperextension is particularly disabling. These two situations, head tilt and neck extension, are the consequence of the growth of the spine outside the instrumentation. The upper thoracic and cervical spine outside the instrumentation are still subjected to the effects of the disease, i.e. muscle weakness (neck flexors particularly), contractures (neck extensors), and imbalance on the sagittal and axial planes caused by the incomplete correction of the curves below, hip flexion, and pelvic tilt.

It is now well recognized that the risk of major postoperative complications is significant in DMD patients with scoliosis who undergo spinal instrumentation and fusion (Ramirez *et al.* 1997). Perioperative mortality may be around 6 per cent (Galasko and Delaney 1993), although this should have improved now that the significance of vital capacity compromise is fully understood. Of the 338 patients operated on (Alman and Kim 1999; Bellen *et al.* 1992; Chataigner *et al.* 1998; Fox *et al.* 1997; Galasko *et al.* 1992; Gayet 1999; Granata *et al.* 1996; Miller *et al.* 1992; Ramirez *et al.* 1997; Shapiro *et al.* 1992) 25 per cent were dead at a 4-year follow up, 6 per cent within the first 2 years. Major intraoperative or postoperative complication rates between 32, and 61 per cent have been reported involving one, or a combination of, three areas: cardiopulmonary compromise, infection, and instrumentation failure (Ramirez *et al.* 1997). These risks must be recognized by the surgeon and discussed thoroughly with the patient's family before surgery (Ramirez *et al.* 1997).

The blood loss in patients with DMD who undergo spinal surgery is significantly higher than that in patients with spinal muscular atrophy (Forst *et al.* 1998). The excessive blood loss may be because of defective muscle vaso-constrictive response due to a lack of dystrophin in the smooth muscle (Noorden *et al.* 1999). Duchenne patients have a platelet function defect in spite of a normal bleeding time and therefore need extensive blood transfusion during surgery (Forst *et al.* 1998).

In order to reduce preventable risks and obtain a well-informed consent for spinal surgery, the following steps should be considered. The diagnosis of DMD should be clearly established clinically and with dystrophin or gene analysis. Preoperative planning for spinal surgery should include appropriate cardiac and pulmonary evaluations. Timing for spine surgery is crucial in DMD. With the concern of the declining respiratory function, a "prophylactic" (Rideau 1986) or "early" surgery (Galasko and Delaney 1993; Shapiro *et al.* 1992; Smith *et al.* 1989; Sussman 1984), when the curve is less than 40° and vital capacity is more than 35–40 per cent, is recommended (Granata *et al.* 1996; Merlini and Granata 1994). Good cardiac function, i.e. a left ejection fraction of more than 45 per cent, and a cardiac frequency below 110, are prerequisites for surgery of the spine (Bellen *et al.* 1992; Gayet 1999).

Orthotic treatment may offer an acceptable compromise in exceptional cases if the patient rejects surgical intervention, or is in the late (inoperable) stages of the disease. A double plaster cast has emerged as the best method to optimize adaptation (especially in severe curvatures) and the time needed for manufacturing the orthosis (Heller *et al.* 1997).

In idiopathic scoliosis, surgery is usually done when the curve is more than 40°. In contrast, DMD patients obtain better and safer results when scoliosis is less than 40° (Granata *et al.* 1996; Marchesi *et al.* 1997). DMD patients operated for scoliosis when the curve was less than 40° were younger (12.6 vs 14.1) and had a significantly better forced vital capacity (65 per cent vs 48 per cent) compared to the group with a preoperative curve of more than 40° (Granata *et al.* 1996). There is, therefore, a window of opportunity for surgery after which the patient becomes unsafe to anaesthetize (Fox *et al.* 1997).

We reviewed 30 patients with DMD who underwent spine surgery at the Istituto Ortopedico Rizzoli, Bologna, Italy, from 1985 to 1991 (Granata *et al.* 1996). The surgical instrumentation used was Luque in 22 cases (Fig. 15.1), Cotrel-Dubousset in one case, and Hartshill in seven cases. In all, fusion was performed from the upper thoracic spine to the sacrum, using back bone. Mean age at surgery was 13.3 (range 10.0 to 15.9). The mean follow-up was 3.9 (1.6–8.5). The mean preoperative curve was 42° (10°–92°). The mean postoperative curve was 17° (0°–43°). The mean curve at follow-up was 23° (0°–60°). The mean preoperative vital capacity was 57 per cent (22–87 per cent). The mean postoperative vital capacity was 50 per cent (15–86 per cent). The mean vital capacity at follow-up was 34 per cent (5–59 per cent). The majority of patients and parents have positively evaluated the sitting position, cosmetic improvement, and the quality of life after spinal fusion. More than 90 per cent would have the operation or give their consent again (Granata *et al.* 1996).

The survival rate at December 2000 in the 30 patients operated at Rizzoli (Granata *et al.* 1996) was as follows: 17 patients died with a mean postoperative survival of 7.5 years (0.1–13), and mean age of death of 20.8 (12.3–28). Thirteen patients were living 11.3 years after surgery (8.3–16), at a mean age of 24.8 (21–29) (Fig. 15.1).

It is evident that this useful treatment should only be considered in facilities where an experienced surgical/anaesthesiologist team is in place.

Neck hyperextension

Extension contractures of the neck are a rather common feature in myopathies with congenital or childhood onset, including congenital muscular dystrophy, congenital myopathies, rigid spine syndrome, and Emery–Dreifuss muscular dystrophy (Merlini *et al.* 1989). All these myopathies have weakness of the axial muscles (particularly the neck flexors) and a marked tendency to muscle shortening or contracture. In the neck, the extensor muscles are shortened and the flexor muscles are very weak, with resulting limitation in flexion of the cervical spine. During childhood and adolescence the spine elongates, but the shortened muscles are not able to accommodate the increase in length. The shortened neck extensors will hyperextend the cervical spine like an archer's bow. When limitation of neck flexion is mild to moderate, the patient stands leaning forward in order to maintain a level vision. In this case, X-rays of the cervical spine show a flexion

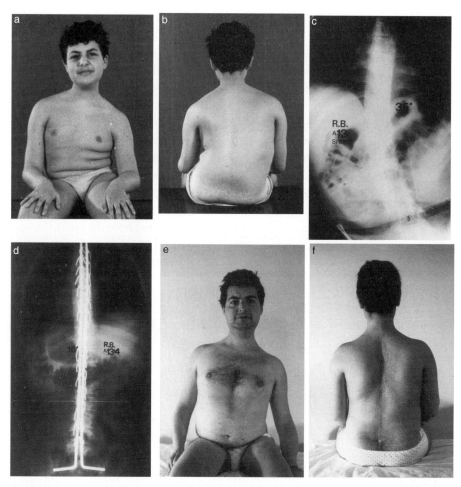

Fig. 15.1 Duchenne muscular dystrophy. A 13-year-old boy (a, b) who lost the ability to walk at age 10 and developed a progressive scoliosis at age 12. Dystrophin was absent in his muscle biopsy. His younger brother also lost ambulation at the same age. Spinal X-rays (c) showing a thoraco-lumbar scoliosis of 35°, kyphosis of 40°, and pelvic obliquity. He underwent Luque segmental spinal instrumentation plus fusion (d) with good correction of the deformity (postoperative scoliosis 16°, kyphosis 10°). Preoperative vital capacity was 1500 cc (56 per cent). He started mechanical ventilation at age 14 after having shown oxygen desaturation at night. At age of 29 (e, f) he is still able to sit upright and retains good head control. His forced vital capacity is 400 ml (10 per cent of normal), and ejection fraction is 35 per cent.

posture of the upper cervical spine (C1–C2) combined with extension below (C3–C8). In severe cases, hyperextension of the neck combines with lordotic posture of the thoraco-lumbar spine. In this situation, when standing, the head, unsupported by the weak flexor muscles, falls backward and the patient must support it with his hand.

The surgical technique devised by Giannini (Giannini *et al.* 1988) corrects the neck hyperextension by opening the interspinous spaces from C2 to C7 through a capsulotomy. The correction is stabilized with bone grafts fixed to the spinous processes.

Neck hyperextension may also develop after spinal surgery for scoliosis in patients with Duchenne muscular dystrophy. This is a rather disabling late complication of this surgery, particularly when combined with neck tilt. In this surgery, correction and fixation extend from the sacrum to the upper thoracic spine, usually T3. In the mobile upper segment, contractures of the extensor muscles combined with growth of the unfixed spine may produce neck hyperextension, sometime with tilt.

Scapular fixation in Facioscapulohumeral muscular dystrophy (FSH)

Facioscapulohumeral muscular dystrophy is an autosomal dominant myopathy with predominant involvement of the face, shoulder girdle, and upper arms (See Chapter 8). FSH involves muscles of the scapulothoracic joint (serratus anterior, trapezius, teres major and teres minus muscles) resulting in unstable scapula with anterior shoulder drop and scapular winging. The deltoid muscle is usually spared. When the deltoid contracts, the arm attempts to move in a normal fashion, but because the scapula is no longer stable, it wings and rotates under the forces of the long lever arm of the upper limb and scapula complex. Mechanical fixation of the scapula to the thoracic wall provides a stable fulcrum on which the deltoid can exert its powerful action on the humerus and abduct the arm without rotation of the scapula.

Several surgical procedures have been attempted in FSH patients to increase scapular abduction and improve cosmetics. The different procedures can be divided into two major types: arthrodesis of the scapula to the thoracic wall using fascia, screws, wires, or plates, with or without bone graft, and interscapular fixation or scapuloplexy. The arthrodesis produces a solid fusion; however, it is thought to reduce respiratory function and requires long immobilization in cast that may result in muscle atrophy. Scapuloplexy does not have these limitations, however, the fascia slings tend to stretch, resulting in a less satisfactory outcome. In addition, scapuloplexy may cause compression on the vascular and nerve supplies, and is no longer considered a treatment option.

Copeland and Howard in 1978 performed 11 thoracoscapular fusions on six patients using tibial cortical graft and screws and achieving firm fusion and improving function. We also reported (Toni *et al.* 1986) on the results of this procedure. Letournel (Letournel *et al.* 1990) used a three-plate construct to fix scapula to the ribs with screws and wires, and without bone grafts. Bunch and Siegel (1993) obtained scapulothoracic arthrodesis with iliac grafts and screws in 12 patients with FSH. They performed 17 procedures with a 3–21-year follow-up. Abduction was greatly improved; all of the patients but one, were pleased with the result. Complications were a brachial plexus palsy that resolved, and a frozen shoulder. Good results were reported using a similar technique for scapulocostal fusion (Jakab and Gledhill 1993). The long-term

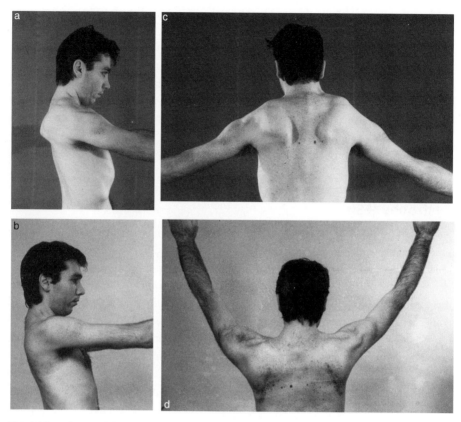

Fig. 15.2 Facioscapulohumeral muscular dystrophy. A 26-year-old man showing limited arm anterior flexion and abduction with scapular winging and upward rotation. Six years after bilateral scapulothoracic fixation with wires without arthrodesis, according to the technique of Giannini (Girolami *et al.* 1990), a good correction of the deformity and an evident gain in function is maintained.

results of scapulothoracic fusions with screws (Copeland *et al.* 1999) suggest that this operation is successful in achieving stability of the scapula, while greatly improving function and cosmetics. Although the course of this type of muscular dystrophy is variable, the benefits of surgery have not deteriorated despite progression of the disease during a maximum follow-up of 44 years (Copeland *et al.* 1999). In our experience a stable scapulothoracic fixation can be achieved with wires without arthrodesis (Girolami *et al.* 1990). This technique is easy and quick to perform, does not need grafts, reduces post surgical complication such as pneumothorax, and ensures good results over time (Fig. 15. 2).

Good long-standing results have been reported with these techniques. However, complications of this surgery were relevant (Andrews *et al.* 1998; Bunch and Siegel

1993; Copeland and Howard 1978; Letournel *et al.* 1990; Twyman *et al.* 1996) and included pneumothorax, pleural effusion, atelectasis, fracture of the scapula, brachial plexus lesion, and pseudarthrosis. Some loss of vital capacity, particularly after bilateral fusions, has been observed (Copeland *et al.* 1999; Copeland and Howard 1978; Jakab and Gledhill 1993). However, none of the patients complained of respiratory symptoms immediately following, or after surgery.

Scapular fusion is recommended both for improving function and for cosmetic reasons (Fig. 15.2). Young adults may consider the latter the main reason for surgery. Scapulothoracic arthrodesis is a major procedure with inherent risks. In the indication for scapular fixation, the function of the deltoid muscle should be tested. The patient is asked to raise both arms forward and maintain this position with the arms horizontal until fatigue causes them to drop. The test then is repeated with the scapula manually pushed downward to the chest wall by the examiner to prevent winging (Copeland and Howard 1978). If maintenance of flexion or abduction improves significantly and the fatigue test is prolonged, then scapular fusion may be indicated. In addition, manually pushing the shoulder back and upward indicates to what degree the shoulder drop could be corrected, and how much this could improve the cosmetic outcome.

References

Allen, B.L. and Ferguson, R.L. (1982). The Galveston technique for L rod instrumentation of the scoliotic spine. *Spine*, 7, 276–84.

Alman, B.A. and Kim, H.K. (1999). Pelvic obliquity after fusion of the spine in Duchenne muscular dystrophy. *Journal of Bone and Joint Surgery British*, 81, 821–4.

Andrews, C.T., Taylor, T.C., and Patterson, V.H. (1998). Scapulothoracic arthrodesis for patients with facioscapulohumeral muscular dystrophy. *Neuromuscular Disorders*, 8, 580–4.

Angelini, C., Pegoraro, E., Turella, E., Intino, M.T., Pini, A., and Costa, C. (1994). Deflazacort in Duchenne dystrophy: study of long-term effect. *Muscle Nerve*, 17, 386–91.

Bach, J.R. and McKeon, J. (1991). Orthopedic surgery and rehabilitation for the prolongation of brace-free ambulation of patients with Duchenne muscular dystrophy. *American Journal of Physical Medicine & Rehabilitation*, 70, 323–31.

Bellen, P., Hody, J.L., Clairbois, J., Denis, N., and Soudon, P. (1992). Surgical treatment of spinal deformities in Duchenne muscular dystrophy. *Revue de Chirurgie Orthopedique et Reparatrice de l'Appareil Moteur*, 78, 470–9.

Bonnet, I., Burgot, D., Bonnard, C., and Glorion, B. (1991). Surgical management of lower limbs contractures in Duchenne muscular dystrophy. *Revue de Chirurgie Orthopedique et Reparatrice de l'Appareil Moteur*, 77, 189–97.

Brooke, M.H., Griggs, R.C., Mendell, J.R., Fenichel, G.M., Shumate, J.B., and Pellegrino, R.J. (1981). Clinical trial in Duchenne dystrophy. I. The design of the protocol. *Muscle Nerve*, 4, 186–97.

Bunch., W.H. and Siegel, I.M. (1993). Scapulothoracic arthrodesis in facioscapulohumeral muscular dystrophy. Review of seventeen procedures with three to twenty-one-year follow-up. *Journal of Bone and Joint Surgery American*, 75 (3) 372–6.

Cambridge, W. and Drennan, J.C. (1987). Scoliosis associated with Duchenne muscular dystrophy. *Journal of Pediatric Orthopedics*, 7, 436–40.

Chataigner, H., Grelet, V. and Onimus, M. (1988). Surgery of the spine in Duchenne's muscular dystrophy. *Revue de Chirurgie Orthopedique et Reparatrice de l'Appareil Moteur*, 84, 224–30.

Colbert, A.P. and Craig, C. (1987). Scoliosis management in Duchenne muscular dystrophy: prospective study of modified Jewett hyperextension brace. *Archives of Physical and Medical Rehabilitation*, 68, 302–4.

Copeland, S.A. and Howard, R.C. (1978). Thoracoscapular fusion for facioscapulohumeral dystrophy. *Journal of Bone and Joint Surgery British*, 60B, 4, 547–51.

Copeland, S.A., Levy, O., Warner, G.C., and Dodenhoff, R.M. (1999). The shoulder in patients with muscular dystrophy. *Clinical Orthopaedics & Related Research*, 368, 80–91.

Forst, J., Forst, R., Leithe, H., and Maurin, N. (1998). Platelet function deficiency in Duchenne muscular dystrophy. *Neuromuscular Disorders*, 8, 46–49.

Forst, R., Forst, J., Heller, K.D., and Hengstler, K.(1997). Characteristics in the treatment of scoliosis in muscular diseases. *Zeitschrift für Orthopadie Und Ihre Grenzgebiete*, 135, 95–105.

Forst, R. and Forst, J. (1995). Importance of lower limb surgery in Duchenne muscular dystrophy. *Archives of Orthopaedic and Trauma Surgery*, 114, 106–11.

Forst, R. and Forst, J. (1999). Lower limb surgery in Duchenne muscular dystrophy. *Neuromuscular Disorders*, 9, 176–81.

Fox, H.J., Thomas, C.H. and Thompson, A.G. (1997). Spinal instrumentation for Duchenne's muscular dystrophy: experience of hypotensive anaesthesia to minimise blood loss. *Journal of Pediatric Orthopedics*, 17, 750–3.

Furderer, S., Hopf, C., Zollner, J. and Eysel, P. (2000). Scoliosis and hip flexion contracture in Duchenne muscular dystrophy. *Zeitschrift für Orthopadie Und Ihre Grenzgebiete*, 138, 131–5.

Galasko, C.S., Delaney, C. and Morris, P. (1992). Spinal stabilisation in Duchenne muscular dystrophy. *Journal of Bone and Joint Surgery British*, 74, 210–4.

Galasko, C.S. and Delaney, C.M. (1993). Severity of scoliosis in patients with Duchenne muscular dystrophy at the time of referral to an orthopedic clinic. *Muscle Nerve*, 16, 433–4.

Gayet, L.E. (1999). Surgical treatment of scoliosis due to Duchenne muscular dystrophy. *Chirurgie*, 124, 423–31.

Giannini, S., Ceccarelli, F., Granata, C., Capelli, T., and Merlini, L. (1988). Surgical correction of cervical hyperextension in rigid spine syndrome. *Neuropediatrics*, 19, 105–8.

Gibson, D.A., Koreska, J., Robertson, D., Kahn, A., and Albisser, A.M. (1978). The management of spinal deformity in Duchenne's muscular dystrophy. *The Orthopedic Clinics of North America*, 9, 437–50.

Girolami, M., Merlini, L., Ballestrazzi, A., Granata, C. and Giannini S. (1990). New technique of fixation of the scapula in facioscapulohumeral muscular dystrophy (FSH). *Journal of the Neurological Sciences*, 98, 428.

Granata, C., Giannini, S., Rubbini, L., Curbascio, M., Bonfiglioli, S., Sabattini, L., and Merlini L. (1988). Orthopedic surgery to prolong walking in Duchenne muscular dystrophy. *Le Chirurgia Degree Organisational Movements*, 73, 237–48.

Granata, C., Merlini, L., Cervellati, S., Ballestrazzi, A., Giannini, S., Curbascio, M., and Lari, S. (1996). Long-term results of spine surgery in Duchenne muscular dystrophy. *Neuromuscular Disorders*, 6, 61–8.

Granata, C., Merlini, L., Parigini, P., and Savini, R. (1982). Spinal deformity in Duchenne muscular dystrophy. *Cardiomiology*, 1, 117–26.

Granata, C., Giannini, S., Ballestrazzi, A., and Merlini, L. (1994). Early surgery in Duchenne muscular dystrophy. Experience at Istituto Ortopedico Rizzoli, Bologna, Italy. *Neuromuscular Disorders*, 4, 87–8.

Heckmatt, J.Z., Dubowitz, V., Hyde, S.A., Florence, J., Gabain, A.C., and Thompson, N. (1985). Prolongation of walking in Duchenne muscular dystrophy with lightweight orthoses: review of 57 cases. *Developmental Medicine and Child Neurology*, 27, 149–54.

Heller, K.D., Forst, R., Forst, J., and Hengstler, K. (1997). Scoliosis in Duchenne muscular dystrophy: aspects of orthotic treatment. *Prosthetics and Orthotics International*, 21, 202–9.

Hsu, J.D. (1983). The natural history of spine curvature progression in the nonambulatory Duchenne muscular dystrophy patient. *Spine*, 8, 771–5.

Jakab, E. and Gledhill, R.B. (1993). Simplified technique for scapulocostal fusion in facioscapulo-humeral dystrophy. *Journal of Pediatric Orthopaedics*, 13, 749–51.

Kennedy, J.D., Staples, A.J., Brook, P.D., Parsons, D.W., Sutherland, A.D., Martin, A .J. *et al.* (1995). Effect of spinal surgery on lung function in Duchenne muscular dystrophy. *Thorax*, 50, 1173–8.

LaPrade, R.F. and Rowe, D.E. (1992). The operative treatment of scoliosis in Duchenne muscular dystrophy. *Orthopedic Reviews*, 21, 39–45.

Letournel, E., Fardeau, M., Lytle, J.O., Serrault, M., and Gosselin, R.A. (1990). Scapulothoracic arthrodesis for patients who have fascioscapulohumeral muscular dystrophy. *Journal of Bone and Joint Surgery American*, 72, 78–84.

Manzur, A.Y., Hyde, S.A., Rodillo, E., Heckmatt, J.Z., Bentley, G., and Dubowitz, V. (1992). A randomized controlled trial of early surgery in Duchenne muscular dystrophy. *Neuromuscular Disorders*, 2, 379–87.

Marchesi, D., Arlet, V., Stricker, U., and Aebi, M. (1997). Modification of the original Luque technique in the treatment of Duchenne's neuromuscular scoliosis. *Journal of Pediatric Orthopedics*, 17, 743–9.

Merlini, L., Granata, C., Ballestrazzi, A., and Marini, M.L. (1989). Rigid spine syndrome and rigid spine sign in myopathies. *Journal of Child Neurology*, 4, 274–82.

Merlini, L. and Granata, C. (1994). Management of Children with Neuromuscular disorders. In *Neurological Rehabilitation* (ed. L. Illis), pp. 295–312. Blackwell Scientific Publications, Inc., Cambridge, MA.

Miller, F., Moseley, C.F., and Koreska, J. (1992). Spinal fusion in Duchenne muscular dystrophy. *Developmental Medicine and Child Neurology*, 34, 775–86.

Noble-Jamieson, C.M., Heckmatt, J.Z., Dubowitz, V., and Silverman, M. (1986). Effects of posture and spinal bracing on respiratory function in neuromuscular disease. *Archives of Disease in Childhood*, 61, 178–81.

Noordeen, M.H., Haddad, F.S., Muntoni, F., Gobbi, P., Hollyer, J.S., and Bentley, G. (1999). Blood loss in Duchenne muscular dystrophy: vascular smooth muscle dysfunction? *Journal of Pediatric Orthopedics B*, 8, 212–5.

Ramirez, N., Richards, B.S., Warren, P.D., and Williams, G.R. (1997). Complications after posterior spinal fusion in Duchenne's muscular dystrophy. *Journal of Pediatric Orthopedics*, 17, 109–14.

Riccio, V., Riccardi, G., Cervone de Martino, M., Stanzione, P., and Marrone, G. (1991). Early treatment of lower limb deformities and preliminary muscular studies with ultrasound in Duchenne muscular distrophyes. *Acta Cardiomiologica*, 3, 149–54.

Rideau, Y., Duport, G., and Delaubier, A. (1986). The 1st reproducible remissions in the evolution of Duchenne's muscular dystrophy. *Bulletin of the Academy of National Medicine*, 170, 605–10.

Rideau, Y. (1986). Prophylactic surgery for scoliosis in Duchenne muscular dystrophy. *Developmental Medicine and Child Neurology*, 28, 398–9.

Rideau, Y., Duport, G., Delaubier, A., Guillou, C., Renardel Irani, A., and Bach J.R. (1995). Early treatment to preserve quality of locomotion for children with Duchenne muscular dystrophy. *Seminar in Neurology*, 15, 9–17.

Rideau, Y., Glorion, B., Delaubier, A., Tarle, O., and Bach, J. (1984). The treatment of scoliosis in Duchenne muscular dystrophy. *Muscle Nerve*, 7, 281–6.

Robin, G.C. (1977). Scoliosis in Duchenne muscular *Developmental Medicine and Child Neurology* strophy. *Israel Journal of Medical Sciences*, 13, 203–6.

Sakai, D.N., Hsu, J.D., Bonnett, C.A., and Brown, J.C. (1977). Stabilization of the collapsing spine in Duchenne muscular dystrophy. *Clinical Orthopaedics and Related Research*, 128, 256–60.

Scheuerbrandt, G. (1998). First meeting of the Duchenne Parent Project in Europe: Treatment of Duchenne Muscular Dystrophy. 7–8 November 1997, Rotterdam, The Netherlands. *Neuromuscular Disorders*, 8, 213–9.

Shapiro, F., Sethna, N., Colan, S., Wohl, M. E., and Specht, L. (1992). Spinal fusion in Duchenne muscular dystrophy: a multidisciplinary approach. *Muscle Nerve*, 15, 604–14.

Smith, S.E., Green, N.E., Cole, R.J., Robison, J.D., and Fenichel, G.M. (1993). Prolongation of ambulation in children with Duchenne muscular dystrophy by subcutaneous lower limb tenotomy. *Journal of Pediatric Orthopedics*, 13, 336–40.

Smith, A.D., Koreska, J., and Moseley, C.F. (1989). Progression of scoliosis in Duchenne muscular dystrophy. *Journal of Bone and Joint Surgery American*, 71, 1066–74.

Sussman, M.D. (1984). Advantage of early spinal stabilization and fusion in patients with Duchenne muscular dystrophy. *Journal of Pediatric Orthopedics*, 4, 532–7.

Toni, A., Merlini, L., Sudanese, A., Baldini, N., and Granata, C. (1986). Thoraco-scapular arthrodesis in facioscapulohumeral dystrophy. *La Chirurgia degli Organi di Movimento*, 71, 127–31.

Twyman, R.S., Harper, G.D., and Edgar, M.A. (1996). Thoracoscapular fusion in facioscapulohumeral dystrophy: clinical review of a new surgical method. *Journal of Shoulder and Elbow Surgery*, 5, 201–5.

Williams, E.A., Read, L., Ellis, A., Morris, P,. and Galasko, C.S. (1984). The management of equinus deformity in Duchenne muscular dystrophy. *Journal of Bone and Joint Surgery British*, 66, 546–50.

Yazici, M., Asher, M.A., and Hardacker, J.W. (2000). The safety and efficacy of Isola-Galveston instrumentation and arthrodesis in the treatment of neuromuscular spinal deformities. *Journal of Bone and Joint Surgery American*, 82, 524–43.

Chapter 16

Animal models of muscular dystrophy

Satoru Noguchi and Yukiko K. Hayashi

Introduction

Scientists have employed animal models for research into muscular dystrophy over the last two decades. These models have been used for pathophysiological analysis as well as for biochemical studies. The clinical symptoms and pathological features observed in animal models are somewhat different from those in human patients. However, they provide us with valuable information and experimental material, and contribute to our progress in understanding human diseases and help in devising possible therapies. There is no doubt about the benefits of animal models.

Spontaneous models had been used for a long time, until the mutated genes in muscular dystrophy were identified. Following recent progress in molecular biology, several responsible genes for human muscular dystrophies have been cloned as shown in Fig. 16.1, and the mutations of the genes in the spontaneous models have also been identified and these models have proved genetically similar to human cases. On the other hand, new animal models have been generated soon after a novel mutation responsible gene for a muscular dystrophy has been identified.

There are several benefits in studying animal models: (1) Animals can be analysed as an affected group instead of as affected individuals in human cases. Temporal observations of the pathological changes from the embryo and throughout later life can provide information on the course of a disease. (2) Samples from age-matched animals can be obtained and permit studies of *in vitro* systems such as biochemical analyses and cell culture. (3) Particularly in model mice, the animal strain with a homogeneous genetic background can be obtained by repeated inbreeding. The effects of other genetic 'modifier' factors, beside the responsible gene, on the phenotype of the models can be excluded. On the other hand, modifier genes that may influence the pathological phenotype could be identified by inbreeding with strains with different genetic backgrounds. (4) Detailed molecular analyses at the amino acid residue level or time or site-specific functions of the involved proteins can be performed by using developmental biological techniques, as 'knocked-in' and conditional 'knocked-out' methods. (5) Furthermore, they can be used in basic research into possibilities of pharmacotherapy or gene therapy.

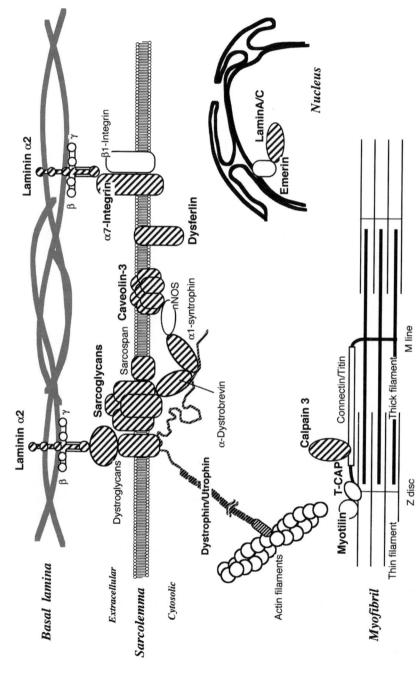

Fig. 16.1 Schema of protein molecules at the sarcolemma, myofibril and nucleus involved in muscular dystrophy. The protein products of the genes responsible for muscular dystrophies are shown in bold characters. The protein molecules indicated by hatched are where muscular dystrophic animal models possessing the relevant gene mutation occurred spontaneously or been obtained inductively. The β1-integrin null and nNOS null mice have been generated by gene-targeting technique (Huang et al. 1993; Stephens et al. 1995), however the former mouse is lethal during early postimplantation development and the latter does not exhibit any muscular dystrophic signs in its muscle. The mice deficient in both of nNOS and dystrophin show pathological changes similar to those in the mdx mouse (Chao et al. 1998; Crosbie et al. 1998)

Animal models of muscular dystrophy

There are now many animal models of muscular dystrophy which include both spontaneous and induced models. Many spontaneous models have been identified including the *mdx* mouse (Bulfield *et al.* 1984; Sicinski *et al.* 1989) and golden retriever dog (GRMD) (Cooper *et al.* 1988; Kornegay *et al.* 1988; Valentine *et al.* 1986) with a deficiency of *dystrophin* gene product, *dy* and *dy²ᴶ* mice with a deficiency of laminin α2 chain of merosin (Michelson *et al.* 1955; Xu *et al.* 1994a;b), BIO 14.6 hamster with a *sgcd* (δ-sarcoglycan) gene mutation (Homburger 1979; Nigro *et al.* 1997; Sakamoto *et al.* 1997), *SJL* mouse with a mutation in *dysferlin* gene (Bittner *et al.* 1999), *myd* mouse with a mutation in a gene of a glycosyl transferase, Large (Grewal *et al.* 2001), and the Japanese quail with an α-*glucosidase* gene mutation (Murakami *et al.* 1980).

On the other hand, there are considerable numbers of the induced animal models associated with the increasing number of identified responsible genes for muscular dystrophy as shown in Table 16.1. In this chapter, we shall focus on animal models for dystrophinopathy, sarcoglycanopathy and congenital muscular dystrophy and discuss their various benefits.

Models of dystrophinopathy (DMD/BMD)

mdx mouse

This spontaneous mouse model of human DMD was established by Bulfield (Bulfield *et al.* 1984) and the mutation (C to T replacement at the nucleotide position of 3185) in the *dystrophin* gene was identified (Sicinski *et al.* 1989). Unlike human DMD patients, the *mdx* mouse exhibits a milder muscular dystrophic phenotype and is fertile. There is no abnormality at birth. Muscle weakness has been described at 3–4 weeks when there is extensive muscle fibre degeneration (Muntoni *et al.* 1993), however after this period, no obvious clinical weakness is apparent until 18 months when these older mice show lumbar kyphosis, dropped head, and hindlimb contractures. Life span is shorter than normal C57BL/10 mice (Lefaucheur *et al.* 1995; Pastoret and Sebille 1995). Serum creatine kinase levels are elevated. Histopathologically, necrotic and regenerating muscle fibres are observed from 15 days of age, and are most prominent around 3–9 weeks. Multifocal grouped necrosis and regeneration are often observed. After two months of age, most of the muscle fibres contain central nuclei. Focal necrosis becomes less frequent. The regenerating process can compensate for the necrosis especially in young and adult mice, however after 65 weeks, replacement by connective and fatty tissue increases. In this mouse, the diaphragm is more severely affected than the limb muscles (Stedman *et al.* 1991). Despite the differences between the *mdx* mouse and human DMD, this mouse model has been widely used as a pathological model of DMD and for trials of gene therapy.

Table 16.1 The induced animal models for muscular dystrophy

Mouse	Method	Product of affected gene	Reference
mdx^{2-4cv}	mutagen	dystrophin, all short forms	(Cox et al. 1993; Chapman et al. 1989)
mdx52	knock out	dystrophin, DP260	(Araki et al. 1997)
utrn −/−	knoct out	utrophin	(Grady et al. 1997a Deconinck et al. 1997a)
mdx/utrn−/−	inbreeding	Dystrophin, utrophin	(Deconinck et al. 1997b Grady et al. 1997b)
MyoD/mdx	inbreeding	Dystrophin, MyoD	(Megeney et al. 1999)
sgca −/−	knock out	α-sarcoglycan	(Duclos et al. 1998; Liu and Engvall, 1999)
sgcb −/−	knock out	β-sarcoglycan	(Araishi et al. 1999; Durbeej et al. 2000)
sgcg −/−	knock out	γ-sarcoglycan	(Hack et al. 1998; Sosaoka 1998)
sgcd −/−	knock out	δ-sarcoglycan	(Coral et al. 1999; Hack et al. 2000)
sspn −/−	knock out	sarcospan	(Lebakken et al. 2000)
adbn −/−	knock out	α-dystrobrevin	(Grady et al. 1999)
syna −/−	knock out	α-syntrophin	(Adams et al. 2000; Kameya et al. 1999)
cav3 overexpression	transgene	caveolin-3	(Galbiati et al. 2000)
cav3 Pro104Leu	transgene	caveolin-3	(Sunada et al. 2001)
cav3 −/−	knock out	caveolin-3	(Hagiwara et al. 2000)
P94:C129S	transgene	P94/calpain 3	(Tagawa et al. 2000)
capn −/−	Knock out	calpain 3	(Richard et al. 2000)
Dag1 −/−	Knock out	α/β-dystroglycan	(Williamson et al. 1997)
Dag1 −/− chimcaera	Dag1−/− ES cell injection	α/β-dystroglycan	(Cote et al. 1999)
Dy^{3k}, Dy^{w}	knock out	laminin α2 chain	(Miyagoe et al. 1997; Kuang et al. 1999)
Itgn7 −/−	knock out	integrinα7	(Mayer et al. 1997)
MTPK-long repeat	transgene	MTPK	(Mankodi et al. 2000)
Lmna −/−	knock out	laminA/C	(Sullivan et al. 1999)

Dystrophin gene-disrupted mice

Mouse models with disruption of the *dystrophin* gene have been generated and called mdx^{2-4Cv} (Chapman *et al.* 1989; Cox *et al.* 1993) and *mdx*52 (Araki *et al.*, 1997). These mice lack both dystrophin and its C-terminal isoform (Dp70 and Dp260, respectively).

The pathological features of the skeletal muscles of these mice resemble those of the original *mdx* mouse. However, the *mdx*52 mouse, in which exon 52 in the dystrophin gene is disrupted by the gene knockout technique, exhibits hypertrophy in limb muscles that which is not seen in the *mdx* mouse. Abnormal electroretinograms have also been reported in *mdx*[3Cv] and *mdx*52 mice (Cox *et al.* 1993; Kameya *et al.* 1997).

GRMD dog

The Golden Retriever muscular dystrophy (GRMD) dog is now established as the most appropriate animal model of human DMD. This dog was identified and characterized by Valentine *et al.* and Kornegay *et al.* (Kornegay *et al.* 1988; Valentine *et al.*, 1986). This animal model is inherited as an X-linked trait with a point mutation within the splice acceptor site of intron 6 of the canine *dystrophin* gene (Sharp *et al.* 1992). This mutation leads to deletion of exon 7 from the dystrophin mRNA and predicts a premature termination codon in exon 8. By RT–PCR technique, two in-frame dystrophin transcripts which lack either exons 3–9 or exons 5–12 were amplified from muscle, and detected a slightly truncated 390-kDa protein by Western blotting (Schatzberg *et al.* 1998). The GRMD dog leads to a severe clinicopathological phenotype similar to that of DMD (Cooper *et al.* 1988). Clinical signs are apparent at 8 weeks of age and are progressive, showing weakness, stiffness of gait and difficulty in fully opening the mouth. Serum creatine kinase (CK) levels are greatly elevated. Histopathologically, numerous necrotic and regenerating fibres together with opaque fibres, mononuclear cell infiltration, and increased fibrous tissues are observed. Tongue, diaphragm, trapezius, deltoideus, extensor carpi radialis, sartorius, and anterior tibial muscles are affected from an early stage, and fibre necrosis and regeneration are present in the tongue muscle at birth. This dog also develops a cardiomyopathy which is similar to that observed in DMD (Valentine *et al.* 1989). The GRDM model may well be the best model for assessing the effectiveness of treatment with pharmacological agents or gene therapy.

Other X-linked muscular dystrophy dogs

A dystrophin deficient dog in the Rottweiler strain has also been identified which shows similar but more severe clinical and pathological features than the GRMD dog. Recently, a new canine model of German short-haired pointer (GSHP) has also been reported (Schatzberg *et al.* 1999). This dog shows skeletal myopathy and dilated cardiomyopathy with a deletion encompassing the entire dystrophin gene.

mdx/utrn −/− mouse

Utrophin, a homologue of dystrophin, is concentrated at the neuromuscular junction which suggests a role for synaptic differentiation. In dystrophin deficient muscles, overexpression of utrophin is observed at the extra-junctional membrane which suggests a possible functional compensation. Because the *mdx* mouse shows a mild phenotype, mice deficient in both dystrophin and utrophin were generated

(Deconinck *et al.* 1997b; Grady *et al.* 1997b). This *mdx/utrn* −/− double mutant mouse exhibits a severe pathological phenotype closely resembling that seen in DMD. These mice exhibit symptoms of skeletal muscle disease including lack of mobility, abnormal breathing pattern, waddling gait, and contracted stiff limbs with a marked kyphosis. The severity progresses with age and these mice die prematurely by 20 weeks of age. These mice also exhibit a cardiomyopathic phenotype. The *mdx/utrn* −/− mouse will be a valuable model for the detailed study of the pathogenesis of human DMD and for assessing the effectiveness of any therapeutic strategies.

Models of sarcoglycanopathy

Cardiomyopathic hamster

This animal was identified by Homburger *et al.* and has been used as a disease model of cardiomyopathy and muscular dystrophy (Homburger 1979). The animal exhibits histological features of muscular dystrophy characterized by variation in muscle fibre diameter, central placed nuclei, and connective tissue proliferation. In 1995, Mizuno *et al.* Showed that the sarcoglycan complex (a subcomplex of the dystrophin and its associated protein complex) is selectively lost in the plasma membrane of muscle fibres in this BIO 14.6 hamster (Mizuno *et al.* 1995). This observation predicted that this hamster is an animal model of sarcoglycan-deficient muscular dystrophy (sarcogly-canopathy (Ozawa *et al.* 1998). Later, Nigro *et al.* and Sakamoto *et al.* independently identified a deletion in the 5′-flanking regulatory region of the δ-*sarcoglycan* gene in this animal (Nigro *et al.* 1997; Sakamoto *et al.* 1997). Interestingly, distinct sublines of hamster manifesting hypertrophic cardiomyopathy (BIO 14.6 and UMX7.1) and dilat-ed cardiomyopathy (TO-2) have been established from the original line BIO1.50. These pathological phenotypes are transmitted to descendants in each hamster line. Both hypertrophic cardiomyopathy and dilated cardiomyopathy hamster lines share a com-mon defect in the δ-sarcoglycan gene (Sakamoto *et al.* 1997). Relating to this finding in the hamster, Ben Hamida *et al.* pointed out that in human patients with sarcogly-canopathy, the clinical severity might vary, even within a single family, which is one of the important characteristics of this disease (Ben Hamida *et al.* 1983). The findings in the hamster imply that some additional factors may influence the manifestation of the phenotypes in sarcoglycanopathy. Gene transfer of the δ-sarcoglycan cDNA to the ham-ster resulted in the rescue of the cardiomyopathic and muscular dystrophic phenotype and showed that the δ-*sarcoglycan* gene was the primary gene causing both cardiomy-opathy and muscular dystrophy (Holt *et al.* 1998; Kawada *et al.* 1999; Xiao *et al.* 2000).

Sarcoglycan gene-disrupted mice

Mouse models with disruption of the genes for each sarcoglycan subunit (α-sarcoglycan: *sgca* (Duclos *et al.* 1998), β-sarcoglycan: *sgcb* (Araishi *et al.* 1999; Durbeej *et al.* 2000), γ-sarcoglycan: *sgcg* (Hack *et al.* 1998; Sasaoka *et al.* 1998), δ-sarcoglycan: *sgcd* (Coral *et al.* 1999; Hack *et al.* 2000) have been generated as in Table 1. All of the targeted models develop more severe progressive muscular dystrophy with extensive degeneration and regeneration of myofibres than in the *mdx* mouse. The loss of sarcolemmal integrity is also observed in all models resulting in increased sarcolemmal permeability and raised serum levels of muscle enzymes. Their calf and thigh muscles show pseudohypertrophic changes with fibre splitting and connective tissue proliferation. In our observation on the limb muscles of *sgcb* null mouse, the degeneration of muscle fibres including phago-cytosis and mononuclear cell infiltration is clearly found even at two weeks of age (Araishi *et al.* 1999). These degenerative changes accompanied by increase in the mass of connective tissue is pronounced at eight weeks of age. At 20 weeks of age, more than 95 per cent of myofibres contain centrally placed nuclei and variation in fibre size is prominent, however, the degenerative changes are rather reduced compared with those at eight weeks of age. After one year of age, the interstitial fat and fibrous tissue prolifer-ation is marked suggesting that the regeneration process is less active.

The *sgcb*, *sgcg* and *sgcd* null mice also develop a cardiomyopathy (Araishi *et al.* 1999; Coral *et al.* 1999; Durbeej *et al.* 2000; Hack *et al.* 1998), while the *sgca* null mouse does not (Duclos *et al.* 1998). Campbell's group reported the progressive pathologic changes in the heart of *sgcb* null and *sgcd* null mice in detail (Coral *et al.* 1999; Durbeej *et al.* 2000). The onset of degenerative changes in the myocardial tissues was relatively later than that in the skeletal muscles. After three months of age, active cellular necrosis and calcium deposits were numerously present. After five to six months, *sgc* null mice developed a severe cardiomyopathy. We also detected similar pathological changes in the heart of *sgcb* null and *sgcg* null mice at a later age. Similar cardiomyopatic changes have also been reported in *mdx/utrn* −/− mouse (Deconinck *et al.* 1997b; Grady *et al.* 1997b). Furthermore Campbell's group examined the electrophysiological function in the heart of *sgcd* null mice by ECG telemetry (Durbeej *et al.* 2000). They detected dra-matically smaller QRS amplitudes consistent with dispersion of depolarization through the ventricle in *sgcd* null mice as compared with wild and *sgca* null mice.

In relation to cardiac muscle pathological abnormalities in *sgc* null mice, Campbell's group emphasized the importance of the sarcoglycan complex in vascular smooth muscles (Coral *et al.* 1999). Two kinds of novel sarcoglycan complexes consisting of β-, γ- and δ-sarcoglycans, and β- and ε-sarcoglycans, respectively, were found in vas-cular smooth muscle and all components of them were lost in the *sgcb* null and *sgcd* null mice. They hypothesized that the loss of sarcoglycans in vascular smooth muscle must be associated with irregularities of the coronary vasculature. Both mice exhibited numerous areas of vascular constrictions associated with pre- and post-stenotic aneurysms in the vasculature of both the diaphragm and the heart. This disturbance of the vasculature preceded the onset of myocardial ischemic lesions. Interestingly approximately one-third of the *sgcd* null mice died suddenly during a treadmill exercise. Interperitoneal administration of Nicorandil, a vascular smooth muscle relaxant, was able to prevent the development of multiple myocardial ischemic lesions in *sgcd* null mice. These data suggest that the cardiomyopathic lesions in these mice are not an induced epiphenomenon caused by alterations of the cardiac muscle per se.

Models of merosin-deficient congenital muscular dystrophy

dy mouse

In 1955, a progressive fatal murine muscular dystrophy was discovered in a spontaneous mutant of the inbred strain 129 mice at the Jackson Laboratories, and designated as dystrophia musucularis (*dy*) (Michelson *et al.* 1955). The disease is inherited as an autosomal recessive trait and affected homozygous *dy/dy* mice show clinical signs of muscular dystrophy from two weeks of age, however, heterozygous *Dy/dy* and homozygous normal *Dy/Dy* are unaffected. This mouse model shows morphological similarities to the severe human muscular dystrophies. It develops muscle weakness in the hindlimbs from 3–5 weeks of age and dies of unknown cause(s) around 3–6 months of age. Histopathologically, scattered necrotic and regenerating fibres are observed from 10 days of age. Muscle fibres with centrally placed nuclei increase in number. Variation in fibre size and opaque fibres are also seen. After one month of age, the skeletal muscles are small in bulk compared with controls. Fibrous tissues are increased and hypertrophic fibres are observed. In addition to the dystrophic changes in muscle, dysmyelination in the proximal part of the sciatic nerve and the ventral and dorsal spinal roots is observed (Bradley and Jenkison 1973; Bray and Aguayo 1975; Okada *et al.* 1977; Stirling 1975; Woo *et al.* 1987). The gene responsible for *dy* has been assigned to mouse chromosome 10. In 1993, deficiency of the expression of laminin α2 chain of merosin in skeletal muscle and Schwann cells was reported and this mouse was, therefore, suggested as a model for merosin-deficient congenital muscular dystrophy (CMD) (Arahata *et al.* 1993; Sunada *et al.* 1994; Xu *et al.* 1994a). A mutation in the *laminin α2 chain* gene (*Lama2*) has not been identified yet, however, reduced amounts of mRNA and protein levels, together with linkage of both the *dy* mutation and *Lama2* to the long arm of chromosome 10 suggest that the *dy* mutation may be in the *Lama2*.

Merosin is one of the laminins containing laminin α2 chain and expressed mainly in the basal lamina of skeletal and cardiac muscles and Schwann cells of peripheral nerves. The basal lamina, which is a specialized extracellular matrix, surrounds each muscle fibre and is thought to contribute to the development of myogenic cells, regeneration after injury and muscle cell survival. In the homozygous *dy/dy* mouse, the structure of the basal lamina of the muscle fibre is severely deranged with a thin and disrupted appearance under electron microscopy (Arahata *et al.* 1993; Xu *et al.* 1994a), which is similar to human patients with merosin deficient CMD (Osari *et al.* 1996).

The brain MRI of patients with merosin-deficient CMD shows diffuse white matter changes with no notable mental involvement, which is one of the characteristic features of the disease. Some patients also show structural abnormalities of the brain. Detailed pathological features have not yet been reported, however abnormal permeability of the blood-brain barrier is suggested, because merosin is expressed around brain capillaries. Interestingly, normal brain MRI has been reported in the homozygous *dy/dy* mouse (Dubowitz *et al.* 2000).

dy²ᴶ mouse

The *dy²ᴶ* mouse was independently found to be an autosomal recessive muscular dystrophy. This mouse model is allelic to the *dy* mutant with a milder phenotype and designated *dy²ᴶ* (Meier and Southard 1970; Macpike and Meier 1976). The homozygous *dy²ᴶ/dy²ᴶ* mouse, like the homozygous *dy/dy* mouse, develops progressive muscle weakness from about three weeks of age. The earliest histological changes in the skeletal muscle appear to be more focal in the *dy²ᴶ* mouse than in the *dy* mouse. However, the changes become equally severe by eight weeks (Macpike and Meier 1976). Similar anomalies of dysmyelination of peripheral nerves in both dorsal and ventral roots have been described in the *dy²ᴶ* mouse (Weinberg *et al.* 1975). On the other hand, the *dy²ᴶ* mouse has a normal life span and does reproduce, while the *dy* mouse dies around 3–6 months of age and does not reproduce (Michelson *et al.* 1955).

The *dy²ᴶ* mouse has a splice donor site mutation (G to A replacement) in *Lama2* which results in the expression of a predominant transcript with a 171 base in-frame deletion. The translated protein has a 57 amino acid deletion (residues 34–90) and a substitution of Gln91Glu in the N-terminal domain VI. Immunoblotting study revealed a truncated N-terminal segment of laminin α2 chain, however, normal immunohistochemical staining pattern was observed. Domain VI of laminin α2 chain is presumed to be involved in self-aggregation of laminin heterotrimers (Sunada *et al.* 1995; Xu *et al.* 1994b). In fact, *in vitro* study revealed that the recombinant N-terminal fragment of laminin α2 chain with the same deletion mutation as *dy²ᴶ* disrupted polymer formation, reduced affinity to heparin, and was sensitive to proteolysis (Colognato and Yurchenco 1999).

dy³ᴷ and *dyᵂ* mice

A null mutant mice of the *Lama2* were developed and designated *dy³ᴷ* (Miyagoe *et al.* 1997) and *dyᵂ* (Kuang *et al.* 1999). These mice showed more severe dystrophic manifestations than *dy* and *dy²ᴶ* mice, with growth retardation by two to three weeks of age, waddling gait and twitching by three weeks, and death by five weeks of age. Numerous degenerating muscle fibres with phagocytosis were observed at 11 days. *In vitro* study has shown that merosin is necessary for survival of myogenic cells. Merosin promotes myotube stability by the accurate expression and membrane localization of α7β1D integrin and prevents apoptosis (Vachon *et al.* 1996; 1997). The myotubes from embryonic stem cells with homozygous disruption of the *Lama2* were unstable and showed contraction-induced degeneration along with the lack of survival, although differentiation was normal *in vitro* (Kuang *et al.* 1998). In the merosin deficient mice, involvement of apoptotic cell death was suggested by muscle fibre degeneration. Activation of caspase-3 apoptotic pathways and positive signals for TUNEL were reported in skeletal muscle fibres in *dy/dy* (Mukasa *et al.* 1999) and *dy³ᴷ/dy³ᴷ* mice (Miyagoe *et al.* 1997). In addition, abortive regeneration after muscle injury was reported in homozygous *dyᵂ/dyᵂ* mice (Kuang *et al.* 1999). These mice should be important for understanding the pathomechanisms of muscle fibre degeneration including necrosis and apoptosis together with regeneration.

The benefits of animal models

Animal studies provide a unique opportunity for investigating disease mechanisms. For example, Nonaka's group induced myofibre degeneration and regeneration by the intramuscular injection of bupivacaine in the rat which is a good model to study the pathophysiology of muscular dystrophy. (Nonaka *et al.* 1983). Matsuda *et al.* demonstrated of dystrophic muscle fibres in *mdx* mouse by vital staining with Evans Blue dye (Matsuda *et al.* 1995). This simple method of intravenous injection of the dye has been used for specific staining of degenerating myofibres and evaluating the pathological changes in mouse muscles. Coral *et al.* found vascular constrictions in the coronary artery, which may cause cardiomyopathy, by microfil perfusion in *sgc* null mice (Coral *et al.* 1999). Now animal models are being used in developing methodologies for gene therapy (for review see Allamand and Campbell; 2000). These experiments could only be done on animals. Regretfully, despite many reports of treated animal models, they are usually descriptions of the pathological changes in their muscles and are often only confirmations of those in human cases. They may be important data, which give an appraisal of the usefulness of animals as models, but their real value and benefit as experiment models will be in extending our knowledge beyond what we know in patients. The generation of induced animal models and their pathological analysis are not an end in themselves but essentially the start of research.

References

Adams, M.E., Kramarcy, N., Krall, S.P., Rossi, S.G., Rotundo, R.L., Sealock, R. *et al.* (2000). *Journal of Cellular Biology*, **150**, 1385–98.

Allamand, V. and Campbell, K.P. (2000). *Human Molecular Genetics*, **9**, 2459–67.

Arahata, K., Hayashi, Y.K., Koga, R., Goto, K., Lee, J.H., Miyagoe, Y. *et al.* (1993). *Proceedings of the Japanese Academy*, **69**, 259–64.

Araishi, K., Sasaoka, T., Imamura, M., Noguchi, S., Hama, H., Wakabayashi, E. *et al.* (1999). *Human Molecular Genetics*, **8**, 1589–98.

Araki, E., Nakamura, K., Nakao, K., Kameya, S., Kobayashi, O., Nonaka, I. *et al.* (1997). *Biochemical and Biophysical Research Communications*, **238**, 492–7.

Ben, H.M., Fardeau, M., and Attia, N. (1983). *Muscle Nerve*, **6**, 469–80.

Bittner, R.E., Anderson, L.V., Burkhardt, E., Bashir, R., Vafiadaki, E., Ivanova, S. *et al.* (1999). *Nature Genetics*, **23**, 141–2.

Bradley, W.G. and Jenkison, M. (1973). *Journal of Neurological Sciences*, **18**, 227–47.

Bray, G.M. and Aguayo, A.J. (1975). *Journal of Neuropathology and Experimental Neurology*, **34**, 517–30.

Bulfield, G., Siller, W.G., Wight, P.A., and Moore, K.J. (1984). *Proceedings of the National Academy of Sciences, USA*, **81**, 1189–92.

Chao, D.S., Silvagno, F., and Bredt, D.S. (1998). *Journal of Neurochemistry*, **71**, 784–9.

Chapman, V.M., Miller, D.R., Armstrong, D., and Caskey, C.T. (1989). *Proceedings of the National Academy of Sciences, USA*, **86**, 1292–6.

Colognato H., Y.P. (1999). *Current Biology*, **9**, 1327–30.

Cooper, B.J., Winand, N.J., Stedman, H., Valentine, B.A., Hoffman, E.P., Kunkel, L.M. *et al.* (1988). *Nature*, **334**, 154–6.

Coral, V.R., Cohn, R.D., Moore, S.A., Hill, J.A., Weiss, R.M., Davisson, R.L. *et al.* (1999). *Cell*, **98**, 465–74.

Cote, P.D., Moukhles, H., Lindenbaum, M., and Carbonetto, S. (1999). *Nature Genetics*, **23**, 338–42.

Cox, G.A., Phelps, S.F., Chapman, V.M., and Chamberlain, J.S. (1993). *Nature Genetics*, **4**, 87–93.

Crosbie, R.H., Straub, V., Yun, H.Y., Lee, J.C., Rafael, J.A., Chamberlain, J.S. *et al.* (1998). *Human Molecular Genetics*, **7**, 823–9.

Deconinck, A.E., Potter, A.C., Tinsley, J.M., Wood, S.J., Vater, R., Young, C. *et al.* (1997a). *Journal of Cellular Biology*, **136**, 883–94.

Deconinck, A.E., Rafael, J.A., Skinner, J.A., Brown, S.C., Potter, A.C., Metzinger, L. *et al.* (1997b). *Cell*, **90**, 717–27.

Dubowitz, D.J., Tyszka, J.M., Sewry, C.A., Moats, R.A., Scadeng, M., and Dubowitz, V. (2000). *Neuromuscular Disorders*, **10**, 292–8.

Duclos, F., Straub, V., Moore, S.A., Venzke, D.P., Hrstka, R.F., Crosbie, R.H. *et al.* (1998). *Journal of Cellular Biology*, **142**, 1461–71.

Durbeej, M., Cohn, R.D., Hrstka, R.F., Moore, S.A., Allamand, V. *et al.* (2000). *Molecular Cell*, **5**, 141–51.

Galbiati, F., Volonte, D., Chu, J.B., Li, M., Fine, S.W., Fu, M. *et al.* (2000). *Proceedings of the National Academy of Sciences, USA*, **97**, 9689–94.

Grady, R.M., Grange, R.W., Lau, K.S., Maimone, M.M., Nichol, M.C., Stull, J.T. *et al.* (1999). *Nature and Cellular Biology*, **1**, 215–20.

Grady, R.M., Merlie, J.P., and Sanes, J.R. (1997a). *Journal of Cellular Biology*, **136**, 871–82.

Grady, R.M., Teng, H., Nichol, M.C., Cunningham, J.C., Wilkinson, R.S., and Sanes, J.R. (1997b). *Cell*, **90**, 729–38.

Grewal, P.K., Holzfeind, P.J., Bittner, R.E., and Hewitt, J.E. (2001) *Nature Genetics*, **28**: 151–4.

Hack, A.A., Lam, M.Y., Cordier, L., Shoturma, D.I., Ly, C.T., Hadhazy, M.A. *et al.* (2000). *Journal of Cellular Science*, **113**, 2535–44.

Hack, A.A., Ly, C.T., Jiang, F., Clendenin, C.J., Sigrist, K.S., Wollmann, R.L. *et al.* (1998). *Journal of Cellular Biology*, **142**, 1279–87.

Hagiwara, Y., Sasaoka, T., Araishi, K., Imamura, M., Yorifuji, H., Nonaka, I. *et al.* (2000). *Human Molecular Genetics*, **9**, 3047–54.

Holt, K.H., Lim, L.E., Straub, V., Venzke, D.P., Duclos, F., Anderson, R.D. *et al.* (1998). *Molecular Cell*, **1**, 841–8.

Homburger, F. (1979). *Annual New York Academy of Science*, **317**, 1–17.

Huang, P.L., Dawson, T.M., Bredt, D.S., Snyder, S.H., and Fishman, M.C. (1993). *Cell*, **75**, 1273–86.

Kameya, S., Araki, E., Katsuki, M., Mizota, A., Adachi, E., Nakahara, K. *et al.* (1997). *Human Molecular Genetics*, **6**, 2195–03.

Kameya, S., Miyagoe, Y., Nonaka, I., Ikemoto, T., Endo, M., Hanaoka, K. (1999). *Journal of Biological Chemistry*, **274**, 2193–200.

Kawada, T., Nakatsuru, Y., Sakamoto, A., Koizumi, T., Shin, W.S., Okai, M.Y. *et al.* (1999). *FEBS Letters*, **458**, 405–8.

Kornegay, J.N., Tuler, S.M., Miller, D.M., and Levesque, D.C. (1988). *Muscle Nerve*, **11**, 1056–64.

Kuang, W., Xu, H., Vachon, P.H., and Engvall, E. (1998). *Experimental Cell Research*, **241**, 117–25.

Kuang, W., Xu, H., Vilquin, J.T., and Engvall, E. (1999). *Laboratory Investigations*, **79**, 1601–13.

Lebakken, C.S., Venzke, D.P., Hrstka, R.F., Consolino, C.M., Faulkner, J.A., Williamson, R.A. *et al.* (2000). *Molecular and Cellular Biology*, **20**, 1669–77.

Lefaucheur, J.P., Pastoret, C., and Sebille, A. (1995). *Anat Rec*, **242**, 70–76.

Liu, L.A. and Engvall, E. (1999). *Journal of Biology and Chemistry*, **274**, 38171–6.

Macpike, A.D. and Meier, H. (1976). *Proceedings of the Society for Experimental Biology and Medicine*, **151**, 670–2.

Mankodi, A., Logigian, E., Callahan, L., McClain, C., White, R., Henderson, D. *et al.* (2000). *Science*, **289**, 1769–73.

Matsuda, R., Nishikawa, A., and Tanaka, H. (1995). *Journal of Biochemistry (Tokyo)*, **118**, 959–64.

Mayer, U., Saher, G., Fassler, R., Bornemann, A., Echtermeyer, F., von, der, Mark, *et al.* (1997). *Nature Genetics*, **17**, 318–23.

Megeney, L.A., Kablar, B., Perry, R.L., Ying, C., May, L., and Rudnicki, M.A. (1999). *Proceedings of the National Academy of Sciences, USA*, **96**, 220–5.

Meier, H. and Southard, J.L. (1970). *Life Sciences*, **9**, 137–44.

Michelson, A.M., Russell, E.S., and Harman, P.J. (1955). *Proceedings of the National Academy of Sciences, USA*, **41**, 1079–84.

Miyagoe, Y., Hanaoka, K., Nonaka, I., Hayasaka, M., Nabeshima, Y., Arahata, K. *et al.* (1997). *FEBS Letters*, **415**, 33–9.

Mizuno, Y., Noguchi, S., Yamamoto, H., Yoshida, M., Nonaka, I., Hirai, S. *et al.* (1995). *American Journal of Pathology*, **146**, 530–6.

Mukasa, T., Momoi, T., and Momoi, M.Y. (1999). *Biochemical and Biophysical Research Communications*, **260**, 139–42.

Muntoni, F., Mateddu, A., Marchei, F., Clerk, A., and Serra, G. (1993). *Journal of Neurological Sciences*, **120**, 71–7.

Murakami, H., Takagi, A., Nanaka, S., Ishiura, S., and Sugita, H. (1980). *Jikken Dobutsu*, **29**, 475–8.

Nigro, V., Okazaki, Y., Belsito, A., Piluso, G., Matsuda, Y., Politano, L. *et al.* (1997). *Human Molecular Genetics*, **6**, 601–7.

Nonaka, I., Takagi, A., Ishiura, S., Nakase, H., and Sugita, H. (1983). *Acta Neuropathologica (Berl)*, **60**, 167–74.

Okada, E., Mizuhira, V., and Nakamura, H. (1977). *Journal of Neurological Sciences*, **33**, 243–9.

Osari, S., Kobayashi, O., Yamashita, Y., Matsuishi, T., Goto, M., Tanabe, Y. (1996). *Acta Neuropathologica*, **91**, 332–6.

Ozawa, E., Noguchi, S., Mizuno, Y., Hagiwara, Y., and Yoshida, M. (1998). *Muscle Nerve*, **21**, 421–38.

Pastoret, C. and Sebille, A. (1995). *Journal of Neurological Sciences*, **129**, 97–105.

Richard, I., Roudaut, C., Marchand, S., Baghdiguian, S., Herasse, M., Stockholm, D. *et al.* (2000). *Journal of Cellular Biology*, **151**, 1583–90.

Sakamoto, A., Ono, K., Abe, M., Jasmin, G., Eki, T., Murakami, Y. *et al.* (1997). *Proceedings of the National Academy of Sciences, USA*, **94**, 13873–8.

Sasaoka, T., Mizuno, Y., Noguchi, S., Imamura, M., Wakabayashi, E., Yoshida, M. *et al.* (1998). *American Journal of Human Genetics*, **63**, A384.

Schatzberg, S.J., Anderson, L.V., Wilton, S.D., Kornegay, J.N., Mann, C.J., Solomon, G.G. *et al.* (1998). *Muscle Nerve*, **21**, 991–8.

Schatzberg, S.J., Olby, N.J., Breen, M., Anderson, L.V., Langford, C.F., Dickens, H.F. *et al.* (1999). *Neuromuscular Disorders*, **9**, 289–95.

Sharp, N.J., Kornegay, J.N., Van, C.S., Herbstreith, M.H., Secore, S.L., Kettle, S. *et al.* (1992). *Genomics*, **13**, 115–21.

Sicinski, P., Geng, Y., Ryder, C.A., Barnard, E.A., Darlison, M.G. and Barnard, P.J. (1989). *Science*, **244**, 1578–1580.

Stedman, H.H., Sweeney, H.L., Shrager, J.B., Maguire, H.C., Panettieri, R.A., Petrof, B. *et al.* (1991). *Nature*, **352**, 536–9.

Stephens, L.E., Sutherland, A.E., Klimanskaya, I.V., Andrieux, A., Meneses, J., Pedersen, R.A. *et al.* (1995). *Genes Development*, **9**, 1883–95.

Stirling, C.A. (1975). *Journal of Anatomy*, **119**, 169–80.

Sullivan, T., Escalante, A.D., Bhatt, H., Anver, M., Bhat, N., Nagashima, K. *et al.* (1999). *Journal of Cellular Biology*, **147**, 913–20.

Sunada, Y., Bernier, S.M., Kozak, C.A., Yamada, Y., and Campbell, K.P. (1994). *Journal of Biology and Chemistry*, **269**, 13729–32.

Sunada, Y., Bernier, S.M., Utani, A., Yamada, Y., and Campbell, K.P. (1995). *Human Molecular Genetics*, **4**, 1055–61.

Sunada, Y., Ohi, H., Hase, A., Ohi, H., Hosono, T., Arata, S. *et al.* (2001). *Human Molecular Genetics*, **10**, 173–8.

Tagawa, K., Taya, C., Hayashi, Y., Nakagawa, M., Ono, Y., Fukuda, R. *et al.* (2000). *Human Molecular Genetics*, **9**, 1393–02.

Vachon, P.H., Loechel, F., Xu, H., Wewer, U.M., and Engvall, E. (1996). *Journal of Cellular Biology*, **134**, 1483–97.

Vachon, P.H., Xu, H., Liu, L., Loechel, F., Hayashi, Y., Arahata, K. *et al.* (1997). *Journal of Clinical Investigation*, **100**, 1870–81.

Valentine, B.A., Cooper, B.J., Cummings, J.F., and deLahunta, A. (1986). *Acta Neuropathologica (Berl)*, **71**, 301–10.

Valentine, B.A., Cummings, J.F., and Cooper, B.J. (1989). *American Journal of Pathology*, **135**, 671–8.

Weinberg, H.J., Spencer, P.S., and Raine, C.S. (1975). *Brain Research*, **88**, 532–7.

Williamson, R.A., Henry, M.D., Daniels, K.J., Hrstka, R.F., Lee, J.C., Sunada, Y. *et al.* (1997). *Human Molecular Genetics*, **6**, 831–41.

Woo, M., Tanabe, Y., Ishii, H., Nonaka, I., Yokoyama, M., and Esaki, K. (1987). *Journal of Neurological Sciences*, **82**, 111–22.

Xiao, X., Li, J., Tsao, Y.P., Dressman, D., Hoffman, E.P., and Watchko, J.F. (2000). *Journal of Virology*, **74**, 1436–42.

Xu, H., Christmas, P., Wu, X.-R., Wewer, U.M., and Engvall, E. (1994a). *Proceedings of the National Academy of Sciences USA*, **91**, 5572–6.

Xu, H., Wu, X.-R., Wewer, U.M., and Engvall, E. (1994b). *Nature Genetics*, **8**, 297–301.

Index

AAV, *see* adeno-associated virus
ACE polymorphism, *see* angiotensin-converting
    enzyme polymorphism
Ad, *see* adenovirus
adducted thumb, CMDs with 30–1
AD-EMD, *see* autosomal dominant EMD
adeno-associated viral vectors 267–8
adeno-associated virus (AAV) 263
adenoviral vectors 263–7
    limitations 265–7
adenovirus (Ad) 263
aminoglycosides 236
anaesthetic complications, prevention 238
ancillary examinations, cardiac disorders 205–8
angiotensin-converting enzyme (ACE)
    polymorphism, cardiac disorders 208, 257
animal models 297–309
    benefits 297, 306
    dystrophinopathy (DMD/BMD) 299–302
    FSHD 160–1
    induced 299, 300
    sarcoglycanopathies 302–4
    spontaneous 299
apoptosis, role 2
AR-EMD, *see* autosomal recessive EMD
autosomal dominant distal myopathies 179–81
autosomal dominant EMD 97, 100–2
    cardiac disorders 210
    clinical features 224
    diagnosis 104
autosomal dominant LGMD 113–14
    classification 111
autosomal recessive distal myopathies 179–81
autosomal recessive EMD 97, 100–2
    diagnosis 104
autosomal recessive LGMD 117–27
    classification 111
    sarcoglycan complex 117–21
azathioprine 234–5

basic local alignment search tool (BLAST), FSHD
    gene search 155
Becker muscular dystrophy (BMD) 72–94
    ancillary investigations 81–2, 83–4
    animal models 299–302
    cardiac disorders 209
    cardiac involvement 78, 79–80, 257
    carriers, manifesting 82–4
    clinical characteristics 78
    clinical features 74–5, 224
    cognitive impairment 80
    consensual diagnostic criteria 84–5
    contractures 79
    course of the disease 80–1

CT scanning 76–7
    diagnosis 84–6
    differential diagnosis 86
    DNA studies 73
    dystrophin analysis 74
    dystrophin studies 84
    electromyography 82
    epidemiology 73
    genetic analysis procedure 85–6
    genotype-phenotype correlation 81
    history 72–3
    manifesting carriers 82–4
    molecular genetics 73–81
    muscle histology 82, 83–4
    muscle hypertrophy 77–9
    muscle weakness 75–7
    onset 74–5
    retinal changes 80
    SCK 81–2, 83
    skeletal muscle involvement 75–9
    treatment 86–7
beta 2 agonists 236
Bethlem myopathy 113–14
*Bgl*II and *Bln*I restriction sites, FSHD 153–4
BLAST, *see* basic local alignment search tool
BMD, *see* Becker muscular dystrophy
bone marrow transplantation, cell therapy 275
brain abnormalities, CMD 10–11
breathing
    sleep disordered 248–50
    see also respiratory care

calpain 3 deficiency (LGMD2A) 121–3
cardiac disorders 202–22
    ACE polymorphism 208
    ancillary examinations 205–8
    AR-EMD 210
    BMD 209
    chest radiography 205–8
    CHF 215
    clinical evaluation 204–5
    CMD 213–14
    conduction defects 215
    cor pulmonale 214
    curative treatments 216–17
    defined 203
    detection, heart failure 204
    differential diagnosis 214
    DMD 208–9, 216, 217–18
    dystrophinopathies 208–10
    ECG 205
    echocardiography 206
    electrophysiological studies 206
    endomyocardial biopsy 207

etiologies 208
FSHD 213
future prospects 217–18
His-Purkinje system 203, 206
Holter monitoring 206
investigations 203–5, 207–8
LGMD 210–13
myotonic dystrophy 211
neuroendocrine evaluation 207
neuromuscular conditions 214
nucleopathies 210–11
pathogenesis 217–18
prophylactic measures 216
radioisotope monitoring 206–7
random association 214
recognition of muscular dystrophy 204–5
sarcoglycanopathies 212–13
SCARMD 212
therapeutic interventions 214–15
XLDCM 209–10
XLEDMD 210
cardiac involvement 4–5
BMD 78, 79–80, 257
EMD 203
MDC1A 17
cardiomyopathic hamsters 302
cardiomyopathy, prevalence and management 256–9
care, coordinated 259
carriers, manifesting
BMD 82–4
DMD 66
cataracts, CMDs and 30
caveolin 3 protein, LGMD1C 116–17
cell therapy
autologous stem cells 275–6
basic concepts 262–3
bone marrow transplantation 275
cellular sources 275
future clinical perspectives 275–6
pluripotent stem cells 274
primary myopathies 261–83
central nervous system (CNS)
abnormalities, CMD classification with 40
DMD 58–9
Fukuyama CMD 25
MDC1A 15–17
MEB 27
WWS 28
cerebellar cysts, CMDs with 29–30
cerebellar hypoplasia, CMDs with 29
chemical mismatch cleavage (CMC), BMD 85
chest infections, healthcare and treatment 255–6
chest radiography, cardiac disorders 205–8
CHF, see congestive heart failure
chromatin structure, FSHD 159–60
chromosome 1q42, MDC1A/B 20–2
clinical variability, muscular dystrophy 3
CMC, see chemical mismatch cleavage
CMD, see congenital muscular dystrophies

CNS, see central nervous system
computed tomography (CT)
BMD 76–7
TMD 175
conduction defects, cardiac disorders 215
congenital muscular dystrophies (CMD) 10–38
with adducted thumb 30–1
brain abnormalities 10–11
cardiac disorders 213–14
and cataracts 30
with cerebellar cysts 29–30
with cerebellar hypoplasia 29
classification 10–11
classification, with CNS abnormalities 40
clinical features 225
with distal join laxity 23
with epidermolysis bullosa 23
without mental retardation 11–23
with mental retardation 24–9
with normal intelligence and reduced merosin 18–22
with rigidity of spine and normal merosin 22
with unidentified gene loci 32
congestive heart failure (CHF), symptomatic treatment 215
contractures
BMD 79
DMD 228
EMD 98
coordinated care 259
cor pulmonale, cardiac disorders 214
cough in-exsufflators, chest infections 256
creatine 235
CT scanning, see computed tomography
cyclosporin 235

D4F104S1 locus, FSHD 142–8, 162
D4Z4 locus, FSHD 142–8, 151
D4Z4 repeats, FSHD 159–60, 162–3, 164, 165
DCM, see dilated cardiomyopathy
deflazacort 229–34
dehydroepiandrosterone sulphate 235
denaturing gradient gel electrophoresis (DGGE), BMD 85
desmin related disorders (MFM) 179, 180
DGC, see dystrophin-glycoprotein complex
DGGE, see denaturing gradient gel electrophoresis
dilated cardiomyopathy (DCM) 5, 65–6, 202–22
defined 203
diseases, acquired, muscle proteins and 6–8
distal joint laxity, CMDs with 23
distal muscular dystrophy, see distal myopathies
distal myopathies 173–88
classification 179–81
clinical phenotypes 173–9
differential diagnosis 181
genetics 183–5
histopathology 181–2
molecular biology 183–5
therapy and management 185

distal myopathy with pes cavus and areflexia 177, 180
distal myopathy with rimmed vacuoles (DMRV) 175–6, 182
distal myopathy with sarcoplasmic bodies 177, 180
distal myopathy with vocal cord and pharyngeal weakness (MPD2) 177, 180
distal phenotypes in other myopathies 179
distal presentation in LGMD2G 179, 180
DMD, *see* Duchenne muscular dystrophy
DMRV, *see* distal myopathy with rimmed vacuoles
DNA methylation, FSHD 160
dominant adult onset distal myopathy 177–8, 180
dominant negative mutational mechanism, FSHD 142–5
Drosophila, FSHD 161, 163
drug treatment, *see* pharmacological therapies
Duchenna de Boulogne 56
Duchenne muscular dystrophy (DMD) 1, 3, 55–71
  animal models 299–302
  cardiac disorders 208–9, 216, 217–18
  cardiac muscle 58
  carriers, female 211–12
  carriers, manifesting 66
  clinical features 55–7, 224
  CNS 58–9
  contractures 228
  diagnosis confirmation 59
  distribution, muscle weakness 56–7
  dystrophin gene 61–2
  dystrophin protein 62–4, 65
  early lower limb surgery 284–5
  electromyography 59
  female carriers 211–12
  genetics 61
  genotype-phenotype correlation 64–6
  germ-line mosaicism 67
  immunohistochemistry 66, 67
  junctional fragments 67
  management 67–8
  manifesting carriers 66
  muscle biopsy 59–60
  mutation analysis 60
  neck hyperextension 289–91
  neonatal screening 6
  NIPPV 252–4
  onset 56
  pathogenesis of weakness 62–4
  prevention 66–7
  progression 57
  SCK 56, 59, 60
  scoliosis treatment 286–9
  smooth muscle 58
  treatment 67–8, 223–39
  Western blot analysis 66, 67
Dunnigan-type familial partial lipodystrophy (OFPLD) 103
DUX4 gene, FSHD 141, 157–9, 160, 164
*dy*²ʲ mouse, MDC1A 305
*dy*³ᵏ mouse, MDC1A 305–6

dy mouse, MDC1A 304–5
dysferlin
  deficiency – LGMD2B 123–6
  MM 176
  role 128
  structural characteristics 124–5
dysferlinopathy, genetics and molecular biology 184
dysphagia 14–15, 236–8
dystrophin analysis, BMD 74
dystrophin gene-disrupted mice 300–1
dystrophin gene, DMD 61–2
dystrophin, gene transfer 264–7
dystrophin-glycoprotein complex (DGC) 125
dystrophinopathy
  autosomal recessive LGMD 119–20
  cardiac disorders 208–10
  rhabdomyolysis in 87
dystrophin protein 62
  BMD 74
  DMD 62–4, 65
dystrophin studies, BMD 84

early lower limb surgery, DMD 284–5
early onset dominant distal myopathy (MPD1) 176–7, 180
ECG, *see* electrocardiogram
echocardiography, cardiac disorders 206
*Eco*RI fragments, FSHD 142–9
EDMD, *see* Emery-Dreifuss muscular dystrophy
electrical stimulation, chronic low frequency 229
electrocardiogram (ECG) 205
electromyography, DMD 59
electrophysiological studies, cardiac disorders 206
EMD, *see* Emery-Dreifuss muscular dystrophy
emerin mutations 100–2
Emery-Dreifuss muscular dystrophy (EMD) 2, 95–108
  AD-EMD, *see* autosomal dominant EMD
  AR-EMD, *see* autosomal recessive EMD
  cardiac involvement 203
  cardiac muscle 98
  cardiomyopathy 257
  clinical features 96–7, 224
  diagnosis 104
  inheritance 98–9
  joint contractures 98
  molecular diagnosis 104
  molecular genetics 99–103
  pathology 97–8
  prevention 104
  SCK 97
  skeletal muscle 97–8
  treatment 104
  X-linking 96–7, 98–100
endomyocardial biopsy, cardiac disorders 207
epidermolysis bullosa, CMDs with 23
expiratory muscle function 248
ex vivo gene therapy 271–2

facioscapulohumeral muscular dystrophy (FSHD)
137–72
  animal models 160–1
  cardiac disorders 213
  chromatin structure 159–60
  clinical features 137–40, 224
  D4Z4 locus 142–8, 151
  D4Z4 repeats 159–60, 162–3, 164, 165
  disease mechanisms 161–3
  DNA methylation 160
  DNA rearrangements 142–6
  dominant negative mutational mechanism
    142–5
  Drosophila 161, 163
  DUX4 gene 141, 157–9, 160, 164
  enigma 165–6
  expression studies, candidate region 159
  FRG1 gene 156–7
  FRG2 gene 156–7
  gender bias 151–2
  gene, evidence for 164
  gene mapping studies 140–1
  gene, search for the 154–6, 161, 165
  gene sequences, potential 156–9
  genetic heterogeneity 141
  genetic recombination 146–8
  genotype/phenotype relationship 149–51
  histopathological changes 140
  molecular diagnosis 152–4
  monosomy, candidate region 151, 165
  monozygotic twins 151
  mouse 160–1
  PEV 162
  physical map, candidate region 141–2
  scapular fixation 291–3
  sequence homology 146–8
  somatic mosaicism 148–9, 150, 165
  subtelomeric sequence exchange 147–8, 150,
    152–3
  therapy 164–5
  'translocations' 146
  TUB4Q gene 157
  variability, clinical 139–40
feeding problems 14–15, 236–8
FER1-L3 (myoferlin) 125–6
fluorescent *in situ* hybridization (FISH)
  BMD 85
  sequence homology, FSHD 146
FRG1 gene, FSHD 156–7
FRG2 gene, FSHD 156–7
FSHD, *see* facioscapulohumeral muscular
  dystrophy
Fukuyama CMD 24–6, 39–54
  brain pathology 47
  classification 40, 41
  clinical features 24–5, 40–5
  CNS involvement 25
  eye involvement 25
  eye pathology 47–8
  genetics 48–9

  genotype-phenotype correlation 49–50
  molecular basis 49–50
  molecular genetics 26
  muscle pathology 26
  ophthalmological manifestations 44
  pathogenesis 49–50
  pathology 26, 45–8
  prenatal diagnosis 51
future clinical perspectives, gene and cell therapy
  275–6

gain-of-function mutational mechanism, FSHD
  142–5
Galveston posts, scoliosis treatment 287
gender bias, FSHD 151–2
gene correction, point mutations 270–1
gene therapy
  basic concepts 261–3
  blood born myogenic progenitors 273–4
  ex vivo therapy 271–2
  future clinical perspectives 275–6
  myoblast transplantation 271
  non-viral vectors 270
  primary myopathies 261–83
  viral vectors 263–70
genetic heterogeneity 4
genotype-phenotype correlation
  BMD 81
  DMD 64–6
  Fukuyama CMD 49–50
German short-haired pointer (GSHP) dog 301
germ-line mosaicism, DMD 67
glucocorticoids 229–34
Golden Retriever Muscular Dystrophy (GRMD)
  dog 262–3, 271, 301
GSHP, *see* German short-haired pointer dog

HDA, *see* heteroduplex analysis
heart disorders, *see* cardiac disorders
herpes simplex viral vectors 268–9
herpes simplex virus (HSV) 263
heteroduplex analysis (HDA), BMD 85
His-Purkinje system, cardiac disorders 203, 206
histology, muscle 5–6
Holter monitoring, cardiac disorders 206
HSV, *see* herpes simplex virus
hypoventilation, sleep 248–50

immunohistochemistry, DMD 66, 67
infectious diseases
  chest infections 255–6
  muscle proteins and 6–8
inspiratory muscle training 228–9, 258–9
integrin α7 deficiency 23

junctional fragments, DMD 67
juvenile-adult variable onset distal myopathy 178,
  180
juvenile onset dominant distal myopathy 178,
  180

lamins A and C mutations 100–2
  see also LMNA gene
late onset distal myopathy (LODM) 174–5, 180, 182
lentiviral vectors 263, 270
LGMD, see limb girdle muscular dystrophy
LGMD1A
  clinical and diagnostic considerations 114–15
  genetics and molecular biology 184
  molecular biology 115
LGMD1B
  cardiac disorders 210–11
  clinical and diagnostic considerations 115–16
  molecular pathology 116
  SCK 116
LGMD1C
  clinical and diagnostic considerations 116
  molecular pathology 116–17
LGMD2A – calpain 3 deficiency
  clinical and diagnostic considerations 121–2
  diagnosis 122
  molecular biology 122–3
LGMD2B – dysferlin deficiency
  clinical and diagnostic considerations 123–4
  dysferlin structural characteristics 124–5
  molecular biology 124–6
LGMD2C, cardiac disorders 212
LGMD2D
  cardiac disorders 212
  clinical features 224
LGMD2E, cardiac disorders 212–13
LGMD2F
  cardiac disorders 213
  clinical features 224
LGMD2G
  distal presentation 179
  genetics and molecular biology 185
LGMD2G – telethonin 126
LGMD2H 126–7
LGMD2I 127
limb girdle muscular dystrophy (LGMD) 1–2, 103, 109–36
  adeno-associated viral vectors 267–8
  cardiac disorders 210–13
  classification 110–13
  controversy 109–13
  diagnosis 109–13
  disease type identification 110–13
  management principles 127
  non-sarcoglycan proteins 128
  overall perspective 127–9
  subgroups 110–13
  see also autosomal dominant LGMD; autosomal recessive LGMD; LGMD**
limb surgery and orthosis 286
LMNA gene 4
  mutations 102–3
  sequence analyses 100–2
LODM, see late onset distal myopathy
Luque technique, scoliosis treatment 287

management, medical 223–46
MDC1A, see merosin-deficient congenital muscular dystrophy
mdx mouse 299–301
mdx/utrn -/- mouse 301–2
MEB, see muscle-eye-brain disease
medical management, muscular dystrophy 223–46
mental retardation
  CMDs with 24–9
  CMDs without 11–23
merosin-deficient congenital muscular dystrophy 1B (MDC1B) 20
merosin-deficient congenital muscular dystrophy (MDC1A) 12–18
  animal models 304–6
  cardiac involvement 17
  clinical features 225
  clinical findings 12–15
  CNS involvement 15–17
  feeding problems 14–15, 237
  molecular genetics 18
  muscle pathology 17–18
  peripheral nervous system involvement 17
  respiratory function 14
Meryon's disease, see Duchenne muscular dystrophy (DMD)
MFM, see myofibrillar myopathies
microcephaly-muscle hypertrophy-cerebellar hypoplasia 29
microcephaly-normal structural brain 30
microcephaly-pachygyria-peripheral neuropathy 30
MM, see Myoshi myopathy
molecular genetics
  BMD 73–81
  EMD 99–103
  Fukuyama CMD 26
  MDC1A 18
  MEB 27
  WWS 29
MPD1, see early onset dominant distal myopathy
MPD2, see distal myopathy with vocal cord and pharyngeal weakness
MPD3, see new adult onset dominant distal myopathy in a Finnish family
muscle-eye-brain disease (MEB) 26–7
  classification 40
  clinical features 26
  CNS involvement 27
  eye involvement 27
  molecular genetics 27
  muscle pathology 27
muscle histology 5–6
muscle training, inspiratory 228–9, 258–9
myoblast transplantation 271
  ex vivo therapy 271–2
myodysgenesis (myd) mouse, FSHD 160–1
myoferlin (FER1-L3) 125–6
myofibrillar myopathies (MFM) 179, 180
myogenic progenitors, blood born 273–4

Myoshi myopathy (MM) 123–4, 176, 180, 182
    genetics and molecular biology 184
myotonic dystrophy
    cardiac disorders 211
    clinical features 225

nasal intermittent positive pressure ventilation
        (NIPPV) 252–4
neck hyperextension 289–91
negative pressure ventilation 254
neonatal screening, DMD 6
neuroendocrine evaluation, cardiac disorders 207
neuromuscular conditions
    cardiac disorders 214
    ventilatory support 255
new adult onset dominant distal myopathy in a
        Finnish family (MPD3) 178, 180
NIPPV, *see* nasal intermittent positive pressure
        ventilation
nitric oxide synthase (NOS), role 2
non-viral vectors, gene therapy 270
NOS, *see* nitric oxide synthase
nucleopathies, cardiac disorders 210–11
nutritional aspects 236–8

obesity 237
oculopharyngeal muscular dystrophy 1–2
oculopharyngodistal myopathy (OPDM) 179, 180,
        189–201
    cell death 195–6
    clinical features 190–1, 225
    diagnosis 197
    dominant phenotype 191
    genetic counseling 196
    genetics 193–4
    history 189–90
    management 196–8
    molecular basis 194–6
    pathogenesis 194–6
    pathology 191–3
    prenatal diagnosis 196
    recessive phenotype 191
    SCK 191
    treatment 197
    ultrastructural features 192
OFPLD, *see* Dunnigan-type familial partial
        lipodystrophy
OPDM, *see* oculopharyngodistal myopathy
operations, post-operative respiratory
        complications 238
orthoses
    leg 227–8, 286
    spine 288–9
oxandrolone 234
oxygen therapy, chest infections 256

PAB II, *see* poly(A)-binding protein II
PABPN1 gene, *see* poly(A) binding protein nuclear
        1 gene
paediatric NIPPV 254

PCR, *see* polymerase chain reaction
peripheral nervous system involvement, MDC1A
        17
PEV, *see* position effect variegation
PFGE, *see* pulsed field gel electrophoresis
pharmacological therapies 229–38
physical therapies, muscular dystrophy 226–9
physiotherapy 226–7
pluripotent stem cells, cell transplantation 274
point mutations, gene correction 270–1
poly(A)-binding protein II (PAB II) 7
poly(A) binding protein nuclear 1 (*PABPN1*) gene
        189–90, 193–6
polymerase chain reaction (PCR), BMD 85
position effect variegation (PEV), FSHD 162
prednisolone 229–34
prednisone, *see* prednisolone
prenatal diagnosis, Fukuyama CMD 51
proteins
    disease associated 1–3
    dystrophin 62
    molecules and products, schema 62, 298
    muscle proteins, and acquired diseases 6–8
    protein defects 1–3
protein truncation test (PTT), BMD 85
pulsed field gel electrophoresis (PFGE), FSHD 143,
        148–9

quadriceps myopathy 76–7

radioisotope monitoring, cardiac disorders
        206–7
respiratory care 247–60
    chest infections 255–6
    expiratory muscle function 248
    identifying patients, respiratory complications
        250–1
    NIPPV 252–4
    respiratory function natural history 247–8
    sleep disordered breathing 248–50
    ventilatory support 251–5
respiratory complications
    identifying patients 250–1
    post-operative 238
respiratory function, natural history 247–8
respiratory muscle training 228–9, 258–9
retroviral vectors 263, 269–70
reverse transcription PCR (RT-PCR), BMD 85
rhabdomyolysis, in dystrophinopathy 87
Rideau protocol, early lower limb surgery 284
rigidity of spine, CMDs with 22
rimmed vacuoles
    OPDM 192
    see also distal myopathy with rimmed vacuoles
risks, scoliosis treatment 288–9
RT-PCR, *see* reverse transcription PCR

sarcoglycan complex
    autosomal recessive LGMD 117–21
    molecular biology 120–1

sarcoglycanopathies
  animal models 302–4
  cardiac disorders 212–13
  clinical and diagnostic considerations 118–20
  clinical features 224
  diagnosis 120
  life expectancy 119
  SCK 119
scapular fixation, FSHD 291–3
SCARMD, *see* severe childhood autosomal recessive
    muscular dystrophy
SCK, *see* serum creatine kinase
scoliosis 258
  treatment, DMD 286–9
serum creatine kinase (SCK)
  BMD 81–2
  DMD 56, 59, 60
  EMD 97
  LGMD1B 116
  OPDM 191
  sarcoglycanopathies 119
severe childhood autosomal recessive muscular
    dystrophy (SCARMD), cardiac disorders 212
sgc gene-disrupted mice 302–4
single strand confirmation polymorphism (SSCP),
    BMD 85
sleep disordered breathing 248–50
somatic mosaicism, FSHD 148–9, 150, 165
spine surgery 286–9
SSCP, *see* single strand confirmation polymorphism
stem cells, pluripotent, cell therapy 274
subtelomeric sequence exchange, FSHD 147–8,
    150, 152–3
surgical intervention, scoliosis and 258
surgical management
  early lower limb surgery 284–5
  limb surgery and orthosis 286
  muscular dystrophy 284–96
  risks 288–9
  scoliosis treatment 286–9

telethonin – LGMD2G 126
tibial muscular dystrophy (TMD) 174–5, 180,
    181–2

genetics and molecular biology 183–4
T-IPPV, *see* tracheostomy ventilation
TMD, *see* tibial muscular dystrophy
tracheostomy ventilation (T-IPPV) 254
treatment, muscular dystrophy 223–46
TUB4Q gene, FSHD 157

unidentified gene loci, CMDs 32
utrophin 301–2

variability, clinical 3
ventilatory support
  mechanisms of action 255
  respiratory care 251–5
very late onset dominant distal myopathy 178,
    180
viral vectors, gene therapy 263–70

Walker-Warburg syndrome (WWS) 27–9
  characteristics 50
  classification 40
  clinical features 27–8
  CNS involvement 28
  eye involvement 28
  molecular genetics 29
  muscle pathology 28
  ophthalmological manifestations 44
Welander distal myopathy (WDM) 173–4, 180,
    181
  genetics and molecular biology 183
Western blot analysis, DMD 66, 67
WWS, *see* Walker-Warburg syndrome

XLDCM, *see* X-linked dilated
    cardiomyopathy
XLEDMD, *see* X-linked Emery-Dreifuss muscular
    dystrophy
X-linked dilated cardiomyopathy (XLDCM),
    cardiac disorders 209–10
X-linked Emery-Dreifuss muscular dystrophy
    (XLEDMD) 95, 96–7, 98–100
  cardiac disorders 210
  clinical features 224